Alzheimer's

A Caregivers Guide and Sourcebook

THIRD EDITION

Howard Gruetzner, M.Ed.

John Wiley & Sons, Inc.

New York • Chichester • Weinheim • Brisbane • Singapore • Toronto

To Bob Herbert,
a dedicated warrior for the welfare
of the community and its people.

Published by John Wiley & Sons, Inc.
Published simultaneously in Canada

Design and production by Navta Associates, Inc.

This publication is provided to serve the reader as a supplement to professional medical guidance and treatment, and not as a substitute for professional medical care. As new medical research broadens our knowledge, changes in treatment and drug therapy are required. The author and publisher have made every effort to ensure that information regarding medical treatment is accurate and in accordance with the standards accepted at the time of publication. Readers are advised, however, to follow the product information sheet included with any drug administered and to seek professional advice before proceeding with medical treatment.

This book was sponsored by Heart of Texas Region Mental Health Mental Retardation, Waco, Texas and DePaul Center (A division of Providence Hospital, Daughters of Charity of St. Vincent DePaul), Waco, Texas

Library of Congress Cataloging-in-Publication Data

Gruetzner, Howard.
    Alzheimer's : a caregiver's guide and sourcebook / Howard Gruetzner.—3rd. ed.
      p. cm.
    Includes bibliographical references and index.
     ISBN: 978-0-471-37967-6
     1. Alzheimer's disease. I. Title.

RC523 .G78 2001   2001026232
362.1'96831—dc21

Printed in the United States of America

Contents

Preface to the Third Edition

IN THE UNITED STATES TODAY, there are five million people with Alzheimer's disease (AD), and the number is growing. The disease eventually renders the brain virtually useless, and it turns lives inside out—both the lives of the people who have Alzheimer's and the lives of those closest to them. It is a slow and irreversible disease that ultimately leads to death.

However, families confronted with Alzheimer's disease no longer must struggle through this difficult illness alone. Tremendous advances are being made in understanding the disease and devising successful care and management techniques—information that is presented in understandable terms in this book. With this information, caring for an Alzheimer's patient can be a far more positive experience than families could have thought possible.

When I began to work with people who had dementia in the early 1970s, the attitudes toward dementia were reflective of the negative social attitudes we had toward our aging citizens. There was no comprehensive, sensitive approach to evaluation and treatment. Fortunately, attitudes toward older people have changed. However, we still have much work to do to help those with Alzheimer's disease. As medications are developed that slow or delay the disease process, these people are going to be able to remain at a more functional level. They will still face many restrictions on activities such as driving. We need to be sure that we are creating opportunities for a lifestyle that is more commensurate with what they can still do and who they will always be.

This book can give both families and professionals a better understanding of the disease, the behavior of the person with the disease, and ways to cope effectively with the demands of caring for Alzheimer's patients. The first 15 chapters, based primarily on the author's 21 years of specialized work with the elderly in central Texas who suffer from Alzheimer's, depression, and other psychiatric disorders, cover symptoms and stages of Alzheimer's and provide an overview of what to expect as the illness progresses, as well as information

on the difficult transition to caregiving. There are chapters that cover depression experienced by people with Alzheimer's and family caregivers. Ways that caregivers can cope with the unique and chronic stress of caregiving are provided. A special section explores the full range of resources for Alzheimer's care available in the community—resources that can provide families with much appreciated relief from the burdens of daily care. The book also includes tips on locating diagnostic resources, home health services, and nursing home placements.

Possible causes of Alzheimer's disease are considered in Part I. Genetics has provided important clues to the cause of the disease, yet only a small percentage of cases are linked to known gene mutations. This discussion also addresses psychosocial factors that relate to AD. We can now consider risk factors for Alzheimer's, and several pathways to Alzheimer's have been identified. Other aspects of research are considered in Part II. Two chapters are designed to acquaint both caregivers and professionals with what actually happens in the brain as Alzheimer's disease progresses. Overviews of current drug treatment research, as well as other research findings that may contribute to treatment, are included. The focus of treatment has moved from finding a cure to developing drugs that slow or prevent the disease.

Care management of the dementia patient can often benefit from careful use of traditional psychiatric medications. These medications, by providing helpful ways to reduce behavioral and emotional manifestations of the disease, may also extend the period of time the affected individual can be cared for in the home appropriately. With an understanding of care management principles outlined in this book and active utilization of existing resources, caregivers will be better equipped to cope with the physical and emotional challenges confronting them.

This updated and revised edition includes four new chapters: Chapters 3, 7, 13, and 14. Chapter 3 considers depression that is associated with Alzheimer's. Depression is sometimes a response to disease-related losses. It is also associated with areas of brain damage and changes in neurotransmitters. Some depressive symptoms may be early signs of AD. Caregivers need to recognize depression so that they can seek treatment for loved ones. Depression is responsible for suffering and a greater loss of function than can be explained solely by AD. This chapter looks at treatments and approaches that caregivers can use to support loved ones who are depressed.

Our experiences with caregiving usually occur in a family setting because a family member has an acute illness or is recovering from an injury. After a fairly specific period of time, the caregiver and care recipient can resume their normal roles. Chapter 7 examines the differences between this traditional type of care and the often self-engulfing role of the Alzheimer's caregiver. When

family members are able to appreciate the changes and challenges they will face, they will be able to cope more successfully with the chronic stress of caregiving.

Caregivers are quite vulnerable to depression. Chapter 13 examines caregiver depression and factors that increase the chances of becoming clinically depressed. This chapter looks at the specific depressive disorders that caregivers are more likely to develop. It is sometimes surprising to note that the majority of caregivers who develop depression have never before experienced depressive episodes.

Chapter 14 examines chronic stress, the most significant source of caregiver depression. Initially caregivers deal with stress by making changes in the caregiving situation. However, they are also faced with problems and situations they cannot change. Other types of coping strategies are necessary. Changing the way they see the problem may be a way of reducing stress. Acceptance of situations that cannot be changed is a more successful response to an unchangeable problem than continuously trying to change it and failing. Caregivers can learn new ways of coping. Coping is one of the most valuable instruments caregivers have to deal with the stressors of caregiving. Those who are flexible and are able to employ multiple coping strategies are more successful.

I have used "person with Alzheimer's" instead of "client" or "patient" in the new chapters and updated sections of the book. I have also avoided using "Alzheimer's victim" to describe the person with Alzheimer's disease. Unfortunately, the reader will find some of these undesirable terms in other parts of the book. I hope that they will serve as reminders of the progress we are making in learning to deal with Alzheimer's and how we are learning to value those with the disease. We need to find meaningful ways to support the identity and personhood of people with AD.

I hope this guide will serve as a comprehensive reference that will make the caregiver's tasks easier, more rewarding, and more constructive. In turn, I hope it will help to make the lives of those caught in the grip of Alzheimer's disease happier, safer, and more comfortable. Finally, this book should give the reader new and meaningful ways to understand and respond to people with Alzheimer's.

Acknowledgments

I AM ESPECIALLY GRATEFUL to family, personal friends, and professional colleagues who gave their support to the first edition of this book and subsequent revisions. Observing the challenge of caring for a relative with dementia has been both revealing and rewarding. We have more information available for families caring for loved ones with Alzheimer's disease. However, it is still difficult for many family caregivers to access and use this information and resources that have been designed to help them. I hope this new edition will put valuable information into the hands of families so that they can care for themselves as they care for loved ones.

I am indebted to the staff of a local psychiatric hospital, De Paul Center, a division of Providence Hospital, Daughters of Charity of St. Vincent de Paul, and the psychiatrists associated with that hospital who provided helpful comments on the manuscript. The psychiatrists who took time to read the manuscript and comment include Stephen Mark, M.D.; Bergen Morrison, M.D.; Thomas Stidvent, M.D.; and Jack Wentworth, M.D. I also appreciate other encouraging comments from Rod Ryan, M.D., family practice physician.

Dennis Myers, Ph.D., of the Baylor University Institute of Gerontological Studies, used Part I of this book in a mental health and aging course. I appreciate Dr. Myers's comments and those of his students regarding the book's usefulness as a text. Martie Sauter of the McLennan Community College Mental Health Associates Degree Program in Waco was very generous in describing the book's usefulness for training students and caregivers.

Considerable simplification was necessary to make the chapters dealing with scientific studies on research and treatment comprehensible and meaningful. One risk of simplifying such material is that its accuracy may be compromised. I appreciate the comments made by a number of physicians including a neurosurgeon, R. H. Saxton, M.D.; a neurologist, Mark Schwartze, M.D.; a family practice physician, Edward Cooney, M.D.; a radiologist, R. L.

Zeigler, M.D. The comments of Charles Conley, M.D., a pathologist, were extremely helpful. Bill Kersh, a biologist, reviewed sections concerning the chemical changes in the brain.

Hazel Limback, deputy executive director of Heart of Texas Council of Governments, Area Agency of Aging, gave consistent support and encouragement to this project. I appreciate her concern for persons affected by Alzheimer's disease and their needs. I also appreciate the interest shown by planners from the State of Texas, Office of the Governor, and Texas Department of Aging concerning the special needs created by this disease.

Danny Fred provided tireless assistance with typing, rewriting, and editing. One of my colleagues, Samantha Anderson, provided helpful assistance with the editing and rewriting. Jeanne Levy spent extra hours typing the first draft of Part II, which no doubt seemed to have been written in a foreign language. I appreciate other typing assistance from a friend, Pam Richard, R.N., who unselfishly provided her time and support.

Katherine Gregor edited the final manuscript with professional objectivity, clarity, and sensitivity. Lynn Pearson provided tireless assistance with typing, rewriting, and editing for the entire book. She was especially helpful in keeping the manuscript simple and readable. Patty Hawk's editing of new chapters in the first revision was sensitive and supportive of the ideas I wanted to convey. Ted Scheffler, my original editor at Wiley, gave encouragement and support for the new chapters. I remain grateful to Nancy Marcus Land, with Publications Development Company of Texas, for her assistance in the production of the original book. Tom Miller, my editor at Wiley for a mass-market version and for this new revision, has been extremely supportive during a much longer completion process than either of us anticipated. My father, W. A. Gruetzner, died about the time of the first deadline.

Staff of MHMR Aging Services provided more support than they know in attending to the needs of our clients. I appreciate Vanessa Hummel, Terry Brandon, Melissa Talamantes, and Melba Ogle. My thanks go to staff who held things together during the first revision: Nata Boone, Curtis Garner, Sandra Priest, Angie Scott, Angela Antis, David Beyer, M.D., and Shamji Badhiwala, M.D. Both of these doctors continue to support our services for Alzheimer's. Nata Boone has been an important consultant to me for this edition. The following staff has been very supportive during the most recent editions: Sharon McElvany, Manuel Edquist, Jim Moore, Bob Smith, and Wesley Walker. I am very grateful to the values of this community mental health center, and the support I receive to serve people with Alzheimer's and their families. A long-time friend, Vicki Cotrell, Ph.D., was helpful in formulating some of the more difficult concepts included in earlier revisions.

Much of the research for this book and the first edition was conducted at the library of the Veteran's Administration Medical Center in Waco, Texas. I am indebted to the library staff of that facility, especially to Barbara Hobbs, for the first edition. Staff has changed, but they have been available and extremely helpful during the research for subsequent editions. I want Joann Greenwood and her staff, Sandi Cooper-Hudson, and Charmain Harbour, to know that they have accessed their outstanding resources well. I really appreciate their assistance.

When putting together ideas for this type of project, family and friends must be willing to accept the "enforced" isolation this entails. I appreciate the many gestures of support from these individuals. My wife has probably been more patient and understanding than I will ever know. I know her encouragement and love are important to me.

I want to thank my many clients and their families. They have entrusted their problems and needs to strangers, and as someone who must begin professional relationships as a stranger, I appreciate what can be learned from these other "strangers," our clients and families.

I am very pleased that Wiley has made it possible for this book to be read by more people encountering Alzheimer's. Finally, I thank my wife, Ginger, for her support of me, the writing, and the reasons I need to do it.

Special Acknowledgment

About the Poetry

MAUDE NEWTON has survived one of the most difficult experiences life can hand a person: watching her husband, Frank, move slowly, progressively toward death. Frank Newton, who had retired from a successful career in banking, real estate, and insurance in Del Rio, Texas, had Alzheimer's disease.

As Mrs. Newton went through all of the disease's stages with her husband, she began an intimate chronicle of her thoughts and feelings in verse form. "I started picking up whatever was handy—the backs of envelopes, notepaper, whatever—to write about how I was feeling at that moment," she said. "I found it was doing me a lot of good. I was verbalizing my feelings, even if just on a piece of paper." Her children insisted she save all her scribbled thoughts; later, they typed, copied, and bound the collection. Mrs. Newton's poetry introduces a number of issues in a personal, moving way, and we thank her for allowing us to reprint a few of her poems.

PART I

The Caregiver Experience

Alzheimer's disease cannot be cured. Part I focuses on what we know about this disease and what we can do to care for individuals diagnosed with Alzheimer's. A better understanding of this condition and its behavioral manifestations enables caregivers to respond more effectively to the needs of loved ones.

Our beliefs about the Alzheimer's patient and his or her behavior do not take into account the effects of brain impairment. We have no frame of reference through which brain-impaired behavior can be understood. Part I provides this perspective so that caregivers can more effectively and positively respond to the problems and needs of their loved ones.

The caregiver experience is characterized by the adaptability of the Alzheimer's patient and his or her family to this illness. Part I examines this adjustment in several ways. Stages of the illness and the family adjustment are considered. A step-by-step guide describes the experience from the time initial symptoms are noticed to the point care is planned and caregiver stress is encountered. Practical approaches to these steps are considered. Community resources are described in the last chapter of Part I since social support is such an important way for caregivers to provide for the increasing needs of their loved ones and themselves.

Twilight

It's that time again,
that time when day fades into night . . .
that time when—
if you were working late
(and I had a few minutes to wait),
I'd pick up the papers on the floor,
fluff up the pillows a bit,
and open the door to look for you.
It was good to sit on the sofa
and feel you close—
to hear about your day
and share mine with you.

It was always my favorite time of the day
when the bustle gave way
to the shared things we used to say.

Now I dread it—
I hate to sit and watch it come on—
without you.
It's just a time I must learn to endure—
to live through.

Maude S. Newton

1

What Is Alzheimer's Disease?

A Case History

Jewell Johnson had once been quite active in her neighborhood. She had also attended church regularly. These activities had not significantly changed following her husband's death three years earlier. Her friends and family had been impressed with how well she made it through the grief and kept her life going. She had always been stronger and healthier than her husband. Mrs. Johnson was now 74 and seemed to be a model for aging.

Uncharacteristic Behavior

Several months ago, her closest neighbors began to notice changes. She dropped out of church. They discovered that her feelings had been hurt. Apparently, she had made some mistakes as the treasurer of her Sunday School class, losing several hundred dollars. That was not her story, though; Mrs. Johnson insisted that someone had stolen the money. It had all been cash, and for some reason she had never deposited it in the bank.

She began to stay home more and more often. It also surprised the neighbors that she discouraged their visits. They were becoming worried about her and considered calling relatives, but her son and daughter both lived several hundred miles away and telephoned regularly. Their professional jobs made it difficult to visit very often. The pastor tried to visit, but Jewell was uncharacteristically rude to him and other church members who tried to visit her.

Household Chores and Personal Hygiene Neglected

The yard was still covered with leaves left since the fall. It was now the middle of winter. On occasion, neighbors would check on Jewell. Several times a week, her morning newspapers remained in the yard, and this gave neighbors an excuse to check on her. She always came to the door in her robe and slippers. She thanked them for the paper, making excuses that she had a cold and was resting. She refused their offers to help her. If they pursued these offers too long, she would become more restless and agitated. A few times she had shut the door abruptly.

Her closest next-door neighbor called the daughter, Joan. Joan was caught off guard because the phone conversations with her mother—while briefer and more vague—had not been that different. Her mother had always been self-reliant and independent; it was no surprise that she was so reluctant to accept help. It was strange that Jewell never told her daughter of any problems. Maybe that was why the conversations were briefer and so general. The neighbor was asked to watch after Jewell, and the daughter called her mother.

Behavior Changes Denied

The conversation was not pleasant, nor was it very long. Jewell denied any problems and told her daughter the neighbor was meddling. Jewell thought the neighbor's son was trying to get her house. The next-door neighbor had never been honest. As the paranoia became more vivid, Jewell became more upset and hung up on her daughter. Joan called the neighbor and said she would be down the following weekend.

Bills Unpaid

The next day, both the gas and electric company cut off their services to Jewell's home. In the dead of winter, they do not usually cut off the services of elderly people. The neighbor argued on Jewell's behalf but to no avail. She had not paid her bills for more than three months (about the same time she stopped attending church). Attempts to get Mrs. Johnson to the door failed. She would look out the window briefly, but that was all she would do. No one could get into the house. Neighbors called the daughter, but they could think of nothing else that would help.

Delusions Develop

Late that night, the neighbors were awakened by screaming outside Jewell's house. It was nearly freezing, and she was outside her home in a gown. She was afraid of the neighbors who tried to help calm her. She kept talking about her husband roaming around in the attic. She was afraid of him. The police were called, and when they arrived on the scene, Mrs. Johnson was frightened and still very upset. She was quite confused and could only talk about her husband in the attic. They investigated and found no sign of anyone in the attic—just as they had expected. A crisis hot line was called, and Mrs. Johnson was hospitalized since she had become a danger to herself.

Closer examination of the household was revealing. There was no food. She probably had not eaten anything to speak of for several days. The kitchen was a mess and the gas burners were still turned on, although gas service had been terminated. The police explored the rest of the household. Clothes were lying around. The toilet had not been flushed for days, and Mrs. Johnson had had some accidents in her bedroom. Newspapers lay on the living room floor rolled up and unread. Bills and other mail were heaped in piles near the newspapers.

After being stabilized in the psychiatric hospital, a thorough examination was conducted. Upon its completion, only one conclusion could explain what had happened to Mrs. Jewell Johnson over the past year. Something had obviously been wrong before her behavior changes suggested it. In fact, it was admirable that she had so successfully compensated for the difficulties she was experiencing in memory and thinking. The diagnosis was inescapable—probable Alzheimer's disease.

It was 1980, and her family and friends were bewildered. They had never heard of Alzheimer's disease (AD). They had been prepared to accept a diagnosis of "senility." Maybe depression or old age could explain her problems. In those days, older people with behavioral problems and psychiatric symptoms that now suggest dementia were hospitalized for evaluation when families could not manage them. Like the family and friends of Jewell Johnson, these individuals tried to understand what was happening and what, if anything, could be done.

Early Detection and Treatment

More people have heard of Alzheimer's disease in this new millennium and may understand that it is a condition that affects the brain. However, they may not know much more today than the family and friends of Mrs. Johnson knew in 1980. Even when Alzheimer's is suspected, too much time passes between observing symptoms and getting professional help. This is significant because treatments are now available that can slow the progression of the disease and help people with AD function better for a longer period of time.

It is important that treatment be initiated as soon as possible so that more extensive and irreversible deterioration of nerve cells in the brain can be delayed and symptoms can be managed. Then people may take part in decisions that affect them and learn to adapt to the disease. However, people still attribute symptoms of AD to other conditions and do not seek help. People who suspect that a loved one might be developing AD delay or avoid seeking a diagnosis. Since early symptoms develop slowly, they may not appear to be significant at first. Personality changes, poor judgment, and forgetfulness may be overlooked for a while. Those with early symptoms are able to compensate for them or offer other explanations that family members accept. Family members may be hesitant to seek professional help when early symptoms occur.

Alzheimer's is a disease of the brain that causes a gradual but progressive loss of abilities in memory, thinking, reasoning, judgment, orientation, and speech. It causes an inability to recognize and identify objects and carry out motor activities. People with the disease are eventually unable to perform the most basic activities of daily living such as dressing, cooking, and bathing. AD is not the result of normal aging, but it does occur more frequently in those 65 years of age or older.

More Than Simple Forgetfulness

Alzheimer's disease is far more serious than the occasional forgetfulness experienced by the elderly. In its early stages, however, the disease may be difficult to distinguish from ordinary forgetfulness. Because the disease affects the brain gradually and persons ordinarily will compensate for the early symptoms, neither the person with AD nor those around her may suspect a real problem at first. The results of Alzheimer's slow but progressive damage to the brain may not be noticed until the person experiences greater than normal life stressors, major health problems, or a situation that stretches coping abilities to the breaking point; or until major behavior problems, a driving accident, unpaid bills, or significant changes in daily functioning make denial or avoidance of what is happening impossible.

Causes of Disease—Multiple Factors

Research has made considerable progress toward understanding the disease. Ongoing research is getting closer to unlocking the secrets of the disease. AD is not a simple disease with one obvious cause. It is a complicated disease that develops as the result of a complex cascade of events that occur over a period of time and affect the brain. Alzheimer's disease results from a combination of genetic and environmental factors, as well as from other factors that are being identified. Nongenetic factors such as the free radical damage linked with oxidative stress, disease-related brain inflammation, and damage associated with brain infarcts are believed to play a role in the development of the disease. The multiple genetic and nongenetic mechanisms through which the disease develops demonstrate the difficulties researchers face in identifying a clear-cut cause that points to one definite treatment. Preventing or delaying AD involves multiple approaches.

Possible Causes

Alzheimer's (pronounced *ALTS-hi-merz*) disease was first identified in 1906 by a German neurologist, Alois Alzheimer. His subject was a 51-year-old woman who exhibited problems with memory and disorientation. Later, Alzheimer identified depression and hallucinations as additional symptoms. The woman's condition continued to deteriorate; a severe dementia was evident, and the woman eventually died at age 55 in a mental institution. An autopsy revealed that her brain had cortical atrophy and abnormalities in the cerebral cortex called neurofibrillary tangles and neuritic plaques. These changes in the brain were thought to have caused the impairment of the woman's memory, her disorientation, and her cognitive and emotional decline.

Beta-amyloid, an abnormal protein aggregating into plaques outside of neurons, is implicated as being a possible cause, or very close to the cause, of AD. The *tau* protein, aggregating into twisted tangles inside neurons, is thought by some researchers to have a causative role in the disease process. Normal *tau* protein helps bind and stabilize microtubules, which are part of the internal, skeleton-like structure of the cell. In AD, *tau* is chemically altered, which causes microtubules to fall apart. The collapse of microtubules disrupts connections over which cell communications are transported.

Genetic factors are certainly involved in the disease, but Alzheimer's is a genetically complex and heterogeneous disease. Only a small percentage of AD cases are actually caused by genetic defects. These will be considered below and in Chapter 4. Research has also identified genetic links to the disease. These genetic factors do not cause the disease, but they are associated with an increased risk of getting Alzheimer's. Scientists are identifying other factors that might confer susceptibility for developing AD, for example, high-fat diets and high cholesterol levels. More research must be conducted before these and other findings can be considered conclusive. We do know that Alzheimer's is caused by a combination of multiple causative and risk factors.

Genetic Causes and Risks

Genetic defects on three chromosomes—21, 14, and 1—are known to cause early-onset Alzheimer's in a small number of families. The disease occurs before age 60 in these individuals. Autosomal-dominant inheritance is usually involved in early-onset cases. This form of inheritance occurs in 50 percent of first-degree blood relatives, for example, siblings or children of the AD person. Since this form of the disease develops between ages 30 and 60, and occurs in families, it is frequently called early-onset familial AD. It accounts for only 5 percent of Alzheimer's disease cases. The most common form of Alzheimer's occurs in persons who are 65 and older and thus it is called late-onset.

The only gene confirmed to be involved in late-onset AD is APOE. This apolipoprotein E gene has three normally occurring forms called alleles. These alleles are designated as 2, 3, and 4. Unlike the Alzheimer's disease genes on chromosomes 21, 14, and 1 that determine the early-onset form of the disease, apoE-4 (allele 4) acts as a risk factor, but not all people with apoE-4 get AD. In contrast, having apoE-2 is a protective factor, and people with this form of apolipoprotein E are not as likely to develop AD. ApoE primarily acts as a modifier of the age at which people develop Alzheimer's.

A number of other genes may be associated with late-onset Alzheimer's. Chromosome 12, for example, may have several genes that could provide some answers about what causes AD. While all of the genetic associations found in late-onset AD may not turn out to be risk factors, they illustrate that the emerging picture of what causes late-onset Alzheimer's is very complex. Genetic factors may have a role, but they do not provide all the answers to the Alzheimer's puzzle. Large differences in age of disease onset exist for identical twins. In some cases, the disease only affects one of them. These are two compelling facts that something besides genetics is involved. Environmental factors somehow play a part. In fact, the interaction of genetic and environmental factors may account for many of the differences in when and how the disease is expressed.

Symptoms in Older People Attributed to Other Causes

Because Alzheimer's disease was originally identified in persons under 60 and other causes were considered for similar symptoms in older persons, it was thought to be rare. It wasn't until the 1970s that several investigations led to the conclusion that Alzheimer's disease was accountable for the symptoms found in older persons (Katzman, 1976). Since then, we have learned the disease is the most common type of dementia found in this population. Less than 10 percent of people with AD are under 60.

The Statistics

Five million cases of Alzheimer's disease were expected in the year 2000 (Weiner, 1996). Worldwide it is estimated that 22 million people suffer from AD. The prevalence (number of people with the disease at one time) of the disease doubles every 5 years beyond age 65. It is estimated that about 360,000 new cases (incidence) will occur each year in the United States (Brookmeyer et al., 1998). Incidence increases significantly with age. For example, from 20 to 47 percent of those over age 85 have dementia, and Alzheimer's disease accounts for over 50 percent of these cases. The U.S. population of older people will increase substantially in the near future. The aging of baby boomers will be responsible for a substantial increase in persons with the disease in the next three to four decades. By the year 2040, 14 million people in the United States are expected to have Alzheimer's (Evans, 1990).

The prevalence of Alzheimer's is not uniform among racial and ethnic groups. Some research suggests that the risk may be higher for African Americans and Hispanic Americans than for Caucasians. More research is needed to determine the basis for these differences. They may reflect different roles of environmental and genetic risks for development of AD. Non-Caucasians are living longer and will comprise an increasing percentage of the aging population in the future, especially in the older age group most vulnerable to Alzheimer's. By 2050, the non-Caucasian percentage of the aging population over age 85 will have increased from 16 percent to 34 percent.

Alzheimer's is the most common neurological disease that causes dementia, a syndrome characterized by loss of intellectual capacities and impairment of social and occupational functioning. The incidence of the disease in women is higher than in men. The disease knows no socioeconomic boundaries. Life expectancy is reduced by approximately one-third after development of AD. People with AD live an average of 8 to 10 years after diagnosis. The disease can last for up to 20 years. The rate of deterioration and severity varies.

Alzheimer's disease is the fourth leading cause of death in the United States, killing more than 100,00 people annually. But respiratory conditions, congestive heart failure, and infections, which develop in the late stages of the disease, are often given as the cause of death and make this fact less striking.

Cost of Alzheimer's Disease

Alzheimer's care is estimated to cost the United States more than $100 billion a year (Weiner, 1996). The estimated annual cost of caring for a person with mild AD is $18,408; for a person with moderate AD, the cost is $30,096. The cost for caring for a person with severe AD is $36,132.

The cost experienced by the individuals directly affected by Alzheimer's goes deeper. People with Alzheimer's lose touch with the lifestyle and relationships that have been a source of identity and self-esteem. For the sake of safety, they may be required to relinquish some responsibilities prematurely, which can result in boredom, inactivity, and a greater sense of self-loss. With the appropriate opportunities, people with AD can be more meaningfully involved in life.

Family caregivers—who provide the majority of Alzheimer's care—suffer substantial and immutable negative effects on their physical and mental health. Often they suffer a loss of self because caregiving engulfs their entire life.

Why?

I've heard it said,
"if there weren't a God
we would invent one,
for in our hour of deepest need
we must have someone—
some power on which to call."

I don't know . . .
I try hard to believe—
but we are rational creatures.
I must think,
or why was I given a mind?

I think and think
and it makes no sense.
Why would a loving Father
do this to my mate?
Why would he take from him
his mind—his pride
in being alive?

Why would he rob from him
his joy in being here?
Why leave him thus—
a poor shambling caricature
of the man he was?

Surely not for my sake—
to test my power to believe.
If so, it has defeated its purpose.
It's left me tormented and vulnerable
seeking an answer—and finding none—
and calling out—
"Oh, God—if you are my God, Why?"

Maude S. Newton

2

Symptoms and Phases of Alzheimer's Disease

Symptoms of Alzheimer's Disease

A Neurological Condition Causing Deficient Thinking and Remembering

Alzheimer's disease is a neurological condition that impairs the brain's functioning. Its exact cause is not known, but the leading theories are explored in Chapters 4 and 16. Symptoms of the illness represent deficits in many areas of how a person remembers and thinks. For instance, problems with memory may be manifested as forgetting names, dates, places, whether a bill has been paid, or something said over and over. Intellectual abilities are lost eventually. Reasoning with the affected person is no longer a successful way to understand and deal with his or her problems. Judgment about everyday situations is drastically diminished. Capacity for verbal expression gradually declines and the person with AD cannot comprehend what others say to him. As the disease progresses, he may gradually lose the ability to speak. Psychiatric symptoms such as delusions and hallucinations can occur. The person can become anxious, restless, agitated, and may even appear to be depressed. His personality will change. In fact, he may not seem to be the same person.

Alzheimer's disease has a group of symptoms characteristic of a syndrome known as *dementia*. This condition of the elderly becoming forgetful and unable to adequately care for themselves was once called senility. Terms such as senility are used less frequently to describe AD, but other terms are still used. Senile dementia, or primary degenerative dementia, may be used occasionally to describe AD. Rather than being told a family member has Alzheimer's, families frequently hear that loved ones have dementia. In some cases, neither families nor professionals clarify that diagnosis, giving the impression that loved ones have dementia but not AD.

11

There are numerous reasons why family members do not clarify that a diagnosis of dementia might actually be Alzheimer's. When a doctor makes a diagnosis, some people are not likely to question it. Families who had feared a diagnosis of Alzheimer's and then receive a diagnosis of dementia may avoid clarification. Because of denial and distress, families block diagnostic clarification, being more comfortable with any diagnosis that is not Alzheimer's. In these situations, dementia and Alzheimer's disease may be understood to be distinctly different conditions. Families are unaware that Alzheimer's is the most common type of dementia.

There are several reasons family members are not told loved ones have Alzheimer's when they probably do. The doctor may want to observe the patient longer before making the diagnosis of AD. It is difficult to get persons with AD symptoms to the doctor's office or other locations where evaluations are done. Physicians may not be able to complete their evaluation. In such cases, it may not be appropriate for them to make the diagnosis of AD. Physicians may believe the person has Alzheimer's but may not make the diagnosis. Family members who receive a general diagnosis or no diagnosis may be confused when they talk with others who are caring for people with identical symptoms diagnosed as AD.

Caregivers who do not know or understand they are taking care of a loved one with AD or another type of dementia have no reason to change how they relate to their loved one. Not being told the diagnosis is Alzheimer's disease, they will not know to seek out an Alzheimer's support group or gather information that will help them take care of their loved one. Their adaptation to the caregiving situation will be centered on psychiatric symptoms, behavioral problems, and perplexing changes in the personality of their loved one. It is important that family members clarify the diagnosis so that they have the opportunity to learn how to care for the person with AD and cope with this disease. People with Alzheimer's have the right to know about their diagnosis so that they can make important decisions about their lives and learn to cope with changes that lie ahead.

Dementia: Loss of Intellectual Abilities

Dementia, in its broader sense, indicates a loss or impairment of a person's abilities to use his or her mind. The essential feature of dementia is a loss of intellectual abilities severe enough to interfere with social or occupational functioning. An accountant with Alzheimer's disease will be unable to perform her job because of impairments in memory, reasoning, and calculation abilities. A farmer will become unable to plant and harvest crops. Buying seed and figuring out how much seed to put in planters or drills will become impossible.

Although Alzheimer's disease is the most common type of dementia, it is not the only dementing illness. Multiple strokes can cause a dementia that resembles Alzheimer's disease. Vascular dementia is the second most common type of dementia. When vascular dementia and Alzheimer's are present, stroke damage can make symptoms of AD more severe. Research focused on AD has more closely examined other conditions that cause dementia. Some are not frequently discussed; others will become more familiar and possibly diagnosed more often. The growing focus on other diseases that can cause dementia is expanding our understanding of AD. For example, a form of dementia associated with mutations of the *tau* gene has been discovered.

Although people with these mutations did not develop the plaques associated with AD, their brains were riddled with tangles. Dementia with Lewy bodies, a Lewy body variant of AD, and frontotemporal dementia appear to be more common and are difficult to differentiate from AD. Lewy bodies are abnormal lumps that develop inside of nerve cells in the brain, but their appearance varies by location. Lewy body dementia is also associated with Parkinson's disease in two areas of the brain: the substantia nigra and the locus ceruleus. Finally, the HIV-1 (human immunodeficiency virus) infection causes a severe form of dementia called HIV-1–associated dementia complex.

Depression and other psychiatric conditions can appear to be the results of dementia. In the elderly, severe depression may resemble dementia. This condition used to be called pseudodementia or "false" dementia. When severe depression is thought to cause impaired memory but memory does not improve with successful treatment of depressive symptoms, some type of dementia is probably developing.

Underlying medical conditions can cause symptoms that suggest dementia, for example, vitamin B_{12} deficiency, thyroid disturbances, and pernicious anemia. Proper treatment usually reverses the symptoms. When symptoms do not respond to medical treatments, the suspicion increases that Alzheimer's or another type of dementia is present.

Alzheimer's disease is a probable diagnosis given only after all other potential causes of dementia have been identified and treated or ruled out. Other treatable conditions can be identified in this process. An individual's functioning and quality of life may improve by treating other health problems that coexist with AD.

Some medical tests have been developed to help diagnose AD, but none are 100 percent accurate. As the accuracy of diagnosis has improved and more attention has been given to mental status and performance of activities of daily living, the process of ruling out other conditions just to make the diagnosis of AD is no longer necessary. Other possible conditions are always considered, but Alzheimer's is no longer viewed as a diagnosis of exclusion. The diagnosis can be made on the basis of history and identification of symptoms that constitute a dementia syndrome.

The diagnostic criteria for dementia of the Alzheimer's type as specified by DSM-IV (American Psychiatric Association, 1994) stipulate symptoms and how they can be recognized and measured by a person involved in the diagnostic process. Multiple cognitive deficits must have developed and be manifested by both (1) memory impairment and (2) one or more of the following cognitive disturbances: aphasia, apraxia, agnosia, and/or a disturbance in executive functioning. Executive functioning refers to cognitive abilities that involve planning, organizing, sequencing, and abstracting. (Aphasia, apraxia, and agnosia are explained later in this chapter.) Other conditions must also be met. For instance, the course of the disease must be characterized by a gradual onset and continuing cognitive decline, and not be due to other known medical or psychiatric conditions.

First Criterion for Dementia: Severe Loss of Intellectual Functioning

The first criterion for dementia is the *loss of intellectual abilities* of sufficient severity to interfere with social or occupational functioning. Not only are these abilities impaired but they are affected to the degree that the person cannot perform usual work-related activities satisfactorily. For instance, a teacher will be unable to prepare lessons and keep his presentations to the class organized and comprehensible. He may be unable to provide information that was very easy for him to grasp before the Alzheimer's process began. New academic demands may become quite stressful. In social situations he may have trouble following conversations and become confused by new points of discussion. Social demands can become more troublesome, and he may withdraw or become more anxious in social situations. His responses to other people may make less sense and may not be very well related to the topic at hand.

Routine Activities Become Increasingly Difficult

As Alzheimer's disease progresses, a person's ability to successfully carry out familiar activities of daily living will decline. The thinking abilities required to cook a meal, pay bills, clean house, bathe, dress, or even dial a telephone will diminish gradually. Because of memory problems, the person may also claim that tasks have been done, although it is quite evident they have been overlooked.

Memory Problems

Memory impairment has many manifestations during the course of Alzheimer's disease. Forgetfulness is often listed as a condition of old age, and in fact some memory loss is normal in later years. Misplacing keys or a checkbook is something all of us have experienced, regardless of our age. The memory impairment that occurs with Alzheimer's disease is much more pervasive and disabling. Problems with memory are usually the earliest and most obvious symptom of this condition. It is also a symptom that is often denied by individuals with Alzheimer's disease.

Recent memory, that is, memory for events and information experienced over the past half hour, is most affected earlier in Alzheimer's. Such memory loss obviously affects a person's daily living circumstances. Bills are not paid, the gas may be left on, appointments are missed, or keeping track of a daily routine is disturbed. Immediate recall is the ability to repeat something that has just been said. Persons with Alzheimer's disease may have good immediate recall, but little information is likely to be remembered later. New information is not easily remembered.

Recent memory problems also make it difficult for persons with an Alzheimer's-type dementia to learn new material or activities. For example, keeping up with time and place, learning new names, or remembering a shopping list, which involve recent memory abilities, become increasingly difficult as the disease progresses. Disorientation, which involves forgetting time, person, and place, can occur in Alzheimer's disease. For example, the person will reach a point when he cannot remember the day of the week, the month, or the year. Such disorientation and memory problems will contribute to the person's getting lost and will be especially evident in new situations or places.

Memories of the Past Remain Longer

Remote memory is the person's grasp of his past. For instance, this involves information about where he was born, when he was born, his parents and siblings, where he attended school, and when he graduated from school. Personal history is recorded in remote memory. Remote memory also includes facts about past presidents, wars, economic and political events. In the early stages of Alzheimer's disease, remote memory is less obviously affected but becomes more noticeably impaired over time. Direct questions or confrontations will expose gaps that exist in remote memory. Distant memories may serve as a refuge when recent memory becomes so severely affected that the individual cannot relate to what is currently happening.

Maintenance of daily routines is helpful for memory-impaired persons. Such routines can help organize a life that has become unpredictable and insecure because failing memory cannot assist the individual in controlling daily events and interactions.

The loss of intellectual functioning and impaired memory are essential ingredients in an Alzheimer's-type dementia, but several other symptoms of dementia must also be present. Some of these do not occur until later in the course of the illness and may vary considerably from one person to the next.

At least one of the following symptoms must be present for primary degenerative dementia to be diagnosed.

Faulty Judgment—Dangerous Situations

Impaired judgment and insight are symptoms manifested in the lives of persons with Alzheimer's disease. Impaired judgment occurs in many areas of the person's life and can lead to dangerous consequences. For example, the person may insist on driving the car when it is clear her ability has been seriously impaired. She may insist she can manage her finances as well as anyone, even when obviously she cannot. Cooking and lighting stoves are activities where poor judgment may become evident as well as dangerous. Of course, the dementing process is responsible for impaired judgment. However, some environments encourage rather than restrict the exercise of poor judgment. Some caregivers may be understandably anxious about confronting these kinds of behaviors, but the need to intervene usually increases with the potential risks to the Alzheimer's patients, especially when they carry with them risks to other persons. (Driving is a good example of this type of situation.)

Abilities to Discern Differences and Similarities Between Things

Impairment of abstract thinking is more difficult to recognize in everyday actions. It is more easily assessed by answers to certain types of questions. For example, proverbs such as "Haste makes waste" are difficult for persons with dementia to adequately explain. The similarities and differences between things cannot be discerned. A chair and desk are alike because both are furniture. Such associations are not likely to be made by the person with Alzheimer's disease. Defining words and concepts are other examples of tasks that require abstract thinking or reasoning.

Alzheimer's disease affects the cortex of the brain. The cortex is discussed more specifically in Chapter 16, but we should make one point here. There are several human functions controlled by the cortex, the brain's outer layer. Some of these functions involve speech and movement abilities.

Aphasia—A Problem with Speaking and Understanding Language

One disturbance of cortical functioning associated with Alzheimer's disease is *aphasia*. Aphasia is the loss of previously possessed abilities in language comprehension or production. Because of damage to the brain, an individual is unable to understand speech. Verbal expression also becomes disturbed in Alzheimer's disease. These speech deficits do not occur abruptly, as is common with a stroke. Speech abilities gradually erode. Individual variations occur during the disease process, but usually speech problems begin with some difficulty in word-finding. When talking, the person may have trouble making a point or answering a question directly. Spontaneous speech can be wordy and evasive. His comments wander around the point but never get to it. Later, word-finding problems and inability to name objects become very apparent.

Comprehension of what others say becomes impaired; thus, the person is reluctant to engage in conversation. Spoken words or combinations of words are also misused. Later, even misused words have less meaningful relationships to the words for which they are substituted. The person may even echo what is said to him. Finally, the ability to produce sounds and words is reduced because the person is having difficulty coordinating his speech apparatus. The complete inability to speak will occur in many persons during the very last stage of Alzheimer's disease.

Difficulties in Performing Purposeful Movement

Additionally, difficulties in movement can occur with Alzheimer's disease. *Apraxia* is the loss of a previously possessed ability to perform skilled and purposeful motor acts. It is not the result of weakness but rather it is brain damage that prevents a person from making an intended movement. It is sometimes hard to determine whether Alzheimer's patients have trouble dressing themselves because of memory problems and the inability to grasp the logical sequence of the task or because they are exhibiting apraxia. Later in the illness, difficulties in grasping a fork, spoon, or cup and carrying out intended movements could be due to apraxia.

Inability to Recognize Objects and People

Agnosia, an inability to recognize objects and people, is another brain disturbance in Alzheimer's disease. Agnosia is not a memory problem. Brain damage makes it impossible for information to be processed correctly. Visual information is distorted by the brain so that it is unrecognizable. The affected person may not recognize her home. At times, she may ask where her spouse is even though that spouse is sitting close by.

Number Skills Diminish and Are Lost

The ability to do mathematic calculations is also lost with Alzheimer's disease. This is not merely a problem with memory; number skills are simply lost. Addition, subtraction, and other mathematical operations cannot be done successfully. Such problems create obstacles to successful daily living, particularly in paying bills and keeping checking accounts balanced. If the person is employed in a job that requires the use of mathematics (for example, sales clerks and accountants), calculation problems may emerge before other problems are evident.

Writing Skills Progressively Erode

Writing abilities will ultimately be impaired. Initially the person may have some trouble writing paragraphs, which require him to keep up with a lot of information. Gradually the ability to write sentences will erode. Words may be used incorrectly and misspelled. Eventually the person will be unable to write his name. Reading abilities may be intact longer, although grasping the meaning of what has been read disappears sooner because of memory and intellectual problems.

Another symptom of an Alzheimer's-type dementia is difficulty in drawing and copying geometric designs. Three-dimensional figures are especially difficult to reproduce. The ability to draw or copy simpler figures will deteriorate as the disease progresses. Loss of these abilities may not seem significant, but the general loss of visual-spatial skills does impact daily living. Writing, reading, finding one's way in a neighborhood, or locating items in the home all involve visual-spatial abilities.

Personality Changes Become Noticeable Early

Personality changes occur with dementia. Usually these changes become evident after the very early stages of the illness. Some personality changes may be a reaction to unsuccessful compensations for losses in functioning; brain damage also alters the personality. With Alzheimer's disease, personality traits may become more evident and actually be accentuated. A suspicious person might become paranoid. An individual who has always reacted strongly to little troubles will react more often and more strongly to small problems. The individual's personality will change as a result of the progressive brain damage, and the person will not seem to be himself.

Delirium Must Be Ruled Out

One final condition, along with the confirmation of the previously described symptoms, must be met for a diagnosis of dementia to be possible. The individual must *show clear consciousness,* which means there is no evidence that delirium is creating the symptoms. Delirium is a clouding of one's consciousness, with a decreased awareness of the immediate environment. A person who is delirious finds it difficult to shift, focus, and sustain attention to what is occurring in his environment. His perceptions of these occurrences are disturbed. Speech may be incoherent. Disorientation and memory impairment may be present, but they are caused by the delirium, not by the dementia. Persons with Alzheimer's disease may suffer delirium at times because of underlying infections or other medical problems, which make the dementia appear to have worsened.

The symptoms we have discussed represent criteria for professionals to diagnose dementia. However, before a diagnosis can be made, the cause of the dementia must be determined. There are many conditions that can cause dementia. Alzheimer's disease may be more common, but it can be given only as a probable diagnosis when all other conditions are appropriately excluded. The history of the symptoms is extremely important, since some dementing conditions such as strokes occur abruptly. In others, like Parkinson's disease, dementia develops over a period of time comparable to Alzheimer's disease. Even if other potential causes for dementia have been ruled out, the course of the condition must be monitored. In some cases, the progression may move very rapidly or seem to stop. Such phenomena may require some cases to be reconsidered. Severe depression may mimic dementia, but with treatment the dementia-like symptoms may improve.

Dementia Can Be Caused by Treatable Conditions

Some conditions that cause dementia can be treated successfully, thus reversing the dementia. Some of the more common treatable conditions are listed. Note that these conditions do not inevitably cause dementia, and that some conditions also can cause delirium.

Reversible Causes of Dementia Symptoms and Delirium

	DELIRIUM	DEMENTIA
Depression		Yes
Congestive Heart Failure	Yes	Yes
Acute Myocardial Infarct	Yes	
Renal Failure	Yes	Yes
Hypoglycemia	Yes	Yes
Hyperglycemia	Yes	Yes
Hypothyroidism	Yes	Yes
Hyperthyroidism	Yes	Yes
Pneumonia	Yes	
Diverticulitis	Yes	
Transient Ischemia	Yes	
Stroke	Yes	Yes
Subdural Hematoma	Yes	Yes
Concussion	Yes	
Neurosyphilis	Yes	Yes
Tuberculosis	Yes	Yes
Brain Tumor	Yes	Yes
Brain Abscess	Yes	Yes
Normal Pressure Hydrocephalus (abnormal flow of spinal fluid)		Yes
Fecal Impaction	Yes	
Urinary Retention	Yes	
Sensory Deprivation States (such as blindness or deafness)	Yes	Yes

	DELIRIUM	DEMENTIA
Environmental Changes and Isolation	Yes	Yes
Electrolyte Abnormalities		Yes
Lifelong Alcoholism		Yes
Anemia	Yes	Yes
Chronic Lung Disease with Hypoxia	Yes	Yes
Deficiencies of Nutrients (such as vitamins B_{12}, folic acid, niacin)		Yes
Drug Intoxication	Yes	Yes
Bladder, Urinary Tract Infection	Yes	

This list of conditions, while incomplete, illustrates that a number of conditions can cause both dementia and delirium. It would be tragic for a diagnosis of Alzheimer's disease or another irreversible dementia to be given without the proper physical examination, as well as laboratory and other diagnostic tests. Such tests may reveal a treatable condition. The importance of the appropriate medical personnel being involved in the evaluation of dementia cannot be stressed enough.

Along with these treatable conditions, other irreversible dementias (those that cannot be treated) must be considered. Alzheimer's disease is the most common irreversible dementia, followed by vascular dementia, which is caused by multiple strokes. About 50 percent of all dementias of the elderly are caused by Alzheimer's disease, 20 to 25 percent are caused by vascular disease, and another 20 percent are caused by a combination of these two conditions. Other conditions account for less than 10 percent of the dementias. The following list represents some of the more commonly known conditions. Of course, some of these are still quite rare, for example, Creutzfeldt-Jakob disease and Pick's disease. General paresis, which is a form of central nervous system syphilis, is becoming rare with the successful treatment of syphilis.

Irreversible Dementias

Alzheimer's Disease

Pick's Disease

Vascular Dementia

Creutzfeldt-Jakob Disease

Dementia with Lewy Bodies

Kuru

General Paresis

Parkinson's Disease

Huntington's Disease

Wilson's Disease

Binswanger's Disease

Vascular Dementia Must Be Ruled Out

Vascular dementia is the second leading cause of dementia and must be ruled out when Alzheimer's disease is suspected. There is also a group of psychiatric disorders that can mimic dementia; these disorders, because they are not true dementias, are called pseudodementias. Ordinarily, depression is considered a pseudodementia when it is severe enough to create symptoms of dementia. In addition, schizophrenia can create symptoms suggestive of dementia. Without adequate personal history, it may be difficult to determine whether symptoms are caused by the thought disorder or dementia. Vascular dementia is discussed in some detail, since it is likely to be considered a potential cause of dementia in initial evaluations. (Depression, another likely candidate related to dementia, is discussed at length in Chapter 3.)

Cumulative Effects of Several Strokes Can Create Dementia

Most people are familiar with strokes, which cause varying degrees of damage to the brain. The cumulative effects of multiple strokes create dementia by damaging multiple areas of the brain. A single stroke or infarct will not usually cause dementia, even though initially this may appear to be the case. However, after the stroke, a person will usually move toward some degree of recovery. With some patients recovery may be partial, but with many recovery can be fairly complete, leaving no significant effects on everyday functioning.

Strokes Caused by Blockages in Blood Vessels or Arteries

The types and severity of strokes vary. Some strokes are caused by blockage of large- or medium-sized blood vessels. Blockage of a large artery can produce massive brain damage, impairing intellectual abilities, voluntary movements, and speech. The brain damage associated with blockage of blood vessels or small arteries may not be readily apparent. For instance, the effects of such strokes on intellectual functioning or voluntary movement are so subtle they may not be recognized. Subsequent strokes could occur, involving other small arteries. The cumulative damage of these multiple strokes likely would produce an emerging picture of dementia. When the cumulative effects of small strokes cannot be adequately observed and monitored, it is more difficult to determine whether the dementia is due to multiple small strokes or whether the deterioration of brain functioning is attributable to a primary dementia such as Alzheimer's disease.

A single stroke usually results in fairly specific symptoms that do not meet all the criteria for a diagnosis of dementia. Some of the problems caused by strokes include paralysis and restriction of voluntary movement; speech difficulties, ranging from the inability to form words clearly to problems using and comprehending words correctly (expressive and receptive aphasia); emotional instability (moods change rapidly); and impairment of memory or intellectual abilities. When symptoms are pronounced, they will also appear abruptly. If more than one stroke occurs, the deficits will appear to follow a stepwise deteriorating course. One more stroke will occur. Then the affected person will show some progress and improve. If another stroke occurs, other deficits will be evident. Some recovery will take place, but each time another stroke occurs, the overall level of abilities will deteriorate another step. The deficits will not involve all functions of the person initially, but subsequent strokes will create dementia, a vascular dementia.

One Kind of Stroke Difficult to Differentiate from Alzheimer's.

The results of one type of stroke are very difficult to differentiate from Alzheimer's disease. An *angular gyrus syndrome* involves the brain area supplied with blood and nutrients by the middle cerebral artery (Cummings and Benson, 1983). Predisposing medical factors are hypertension or cardiac disease. Aphasia, writing difficulties, calculation deficits, disorientation of right-left sides, and memory problems (actually word-finding difficulties) are some of the symptoms of this kind of stroke. The stroke patient may be apologetic about and frustrated with his language performance; however, the Alzheimer's patient will be unaware of such problems and will be more difficult to involve in conversation (Cummings and Benson, 1983).

A CAT scan (computerized axial tomography) can usually help identify larger stroke damage to the brain. However, small strokes cannot always be detected, which can be the case with the angular gyrus syndrome; often the damaged area is very small.

Vascular dementia must be ruled out before a group of symptoms can indicate an Alzheimer's-type dementia. Sometimes the professionals involved in the evaluation process may have to clearly identify differences in symptoms to make a distinction between Alzheimer's disease and vascular dementia. Laboratory tests, medical history, or even a CAT scan cannot always be helpful in making that distinction.

Even though strokes cause an abrupt appearance of symptoms, a stroke victim may not be aware of the subtle changes caused by a small stroke. Families may be unable to identify such changes in behavior, or they may attribute them to other causes. Strokes are usually painless. They may even occur while the person is sleeping. Early symptoms resulting from some strokes can include dizziness, headaches, and decreased physical and mental vigor. There may be vague physical complaints. Despite the fact that strokes can occur suddenly the onset can be gradual. Such a presentation can be easily confused with Alzheimer's disease. Many times the onset of a stroke is signaled by confusion.

Strokes can have other features that do not necessarily suggest brain damage. The affected individual may demonstrate poor judgment and insight at times. Delirium may occur, and family members may observe hallucinations. Emotional changes may be prevalent. The person who has had a stroke may not exhibit tact or sensitivity in social situations. His concern for others can diminish, and the narrowing of interests in other people and things can lead to increasing self-preoccupation. Depression is a common consequence of strokes.

Medical Conditions Create Risk for Strokes

There are many medical conditions that create risk for strokes. Hypertension, diabetes, and cardiac disease are associated with strokes and vascular dementia. Since strokes are a major cause of death, the suspicion of a stroke should never be treated lightly. If a stroke has occurred, aggressive medical treatment may prevent subsequent strokes that could lead to vascular dementia. Additionally, persons known to have Alzheimer's disease can suffer strokes. In fact, 20 to 25 percent of dementias are caused by a combination of Alzheimer's disease and vascular disease. When it is possible to prevent a stroke or subsequent strokes in an Alzheimer's patient, compounded disabilities can be avoided.

Phases of Alzheimer's Disease

Rate of progressive deterioration varies.   Many illnesses follow stages of development and recovery. With Alzheimer's, however, there is no recovery; the slow, progressive course leads to further deterioration of behavior and abilities. For some victims, particularly those under 60, the stages move rapidly, and the illness results in death within 3 to 5 years. When the onset begins at a later age, however, the disease may progress slowly for 10 years or more.

Understanding of the illness helps adjustment.   Both the person who is in the early stages of Alzheimer's and her family naturally want to know what to expect as the illness progresses. An understanding of what is to come allows the family to prepare for future stages, to ease the loved one's adjustment, and to gradually accept the disease's effect on the whole family.

Understanding stages helps both families and professionals.   The stages of the disease discussed in this chapter are essentially those developed by Dr. Barry Reisberg, associate professor of psychiatry at New York University

Medical Center. A general knowledge of these stages can help both families and professionals to do the following:

- Accurately assess and diagnose the condition
- Identify symptoms and follow their progression as the illness develops
- Determine the rate at which the illness is developing
- Have realistic expectations of the patient's capabilities
- Evaluate the adjustment of both family and patient
- Assist family with utilization of appropriate resources

Manifestations of deficits are dependent upon many factors.   Not all Alzheimer's conditions will exactly follow the gradual breakdown indicated in the following discussion of stages. There are individual variations that can be attributed to numerous factors: the person's intelligence and abilities before the illness, his personality and basic ways of coping with problems, other health problems, marital relationship, and degree of environmental support.

Stage I: Early Confusional Phase

Forgetfulness becomes a problem.   During the beginning stages of Alzheimer's, the patient may seem merely forgetful. As his memory problems worsen, however, the patient's social and occupational skills will begin to diminish noticeably. Although he will usually deny his growing memory problems and successfully compensate at times, he will not be able to catch all of his mistakes.

Confusion and slower responses affect driving.   In the early stages, it becomes harder for the person to deal with change and new things. If he travels to an unfamiliar area, he may become lost and confused. However, he probably can still travel familiar routes alone. In traffic, he will be slower to react as his powers of concentration and memory decrease.

Early problems with social conversation surface.   During this phase, the person may have trouble finding the right words to communicate his thoughts. Problems in recalling the names of new people and recent conversations may be increasingly apparent. Similarly, he may retain little information from books, magazines, or television shows.

Personality changes appear.   The person will begin to lose his spontaneity and sparkle. Socially speaking, he will be slower and less discriminating in what he says and does. His lessened initiative, energy, and drive will be noticeable. He will become more easily upset, anxious, and angry as a result of the uncertainties created by his memory problems. This anxiety, most evident when the person is in demanding social or work-related situations, may cause him to completely avoid unfamiliar or difficult situations.

Denial conceals recognition of early problems.   Despite a person's degree of impairment during this early stage, his family may be aware of only a few specific problems. The individual will be using his remaining strengths to cover for his deficits. This denial often leads family members to discount the severity of the person's problems. A person going through the first stages of Alzheimer's disease seems distressed, but the reasons are often a mystery to those closest to him.

Early emotional symptoms are brought to the attention of mental health professionals.   At this point, because the symptoms seem to be emotional rather than physical, psychiatrists and other mental health professionals are most likely to be called upon for diagnosis and treatment. Medications might be considered to manage the emotional symptoms. It is important to note that not all persons who exhibit characteristics of the first stage of Alzheimer's disease actually have Alzheimer's. However, if the symptoms of Alzheimer's are present, a diagnosis should be sought, even though it may be distressing to face the full implications of the person's behavior. A person with Alzheimer's will change gradually but dramatically, and it is both unfair and unrealistic to go on treating the person exactly as in the past.

The disease process results in changes in abilities and actions.   It is critical to understand that AD problems are not caused by mere laziness, carelessness, or momentary irrational behavior. The disease is the culprit, and the caregiver must begin to prepare himself for the worsening of problems as his loved one slowly declines.

Stage II: Late Confusional Phase

Memory problems more evident.   As Alzheimer's disease progresses, problems with memory become more evident and somewhat more pervasive. For example, the person's retention of current events declines. She will easily lose the thread of a story and have noticeable difficulties in following conversations. Her responses will fail to correspond to the situation. Likewise, her memory of personal history may become foggy.

Decision making and financial management deteriorate.   Making plans or decisions becomes extremely difficult for the person and equally as frustrating for the family. Family members may feel the need to help their relative with her finances and other important responsibilities as it becomes obvious that she is not handling them well.

Denial of the problem makes the family's job more difficult.   The affected relative may not welcome assistance. She still may be denying her problems and may see any assistance as interference. The caregiver may see the loved one's refusal to admit both her problems and her need for help as impaired judgment. These differences in perception can begin to generate even more conflict within the family. In addition, the person with AD may choose to avoid social situations altogether as they become too difficult to handle.

Driving becomes riskier.   The person's driving also becomes a source of concern. At this stage, the Alzheimer's patient probably can travel familiar routes with reasonable safety. However, she is vulnerable to mistakes and improper responses to unforeseen situations. She may overreact or not react at all to potentially dangerous traffic conditions. The family should seriously consider curtailing or eliminating driving opportunities.

Orientation in time and place affected.   Some aspects of the person's memory—her orientation to time, place, and person—may still be intact at this stage. However, difficulties in concentrating may make it tough to recall these things or to recall the events of the past few minutes or the past week. In contrast, memories of the distant past can be surprisingly clear and accurate. She may speak more often about past events and avoid conversations about current events.

Supervision means supportive assistance.   The AD person will need some supervision and daily support during this stage. Although she is not disabled in all aspects of life, she will need help in more complex areas such as handling finances and paying bills. The mixture of stress and detailed organization necessary to file income tax reports, balance a checkbook, and pay bills may be more than she can handle.

The person with AD becomes self-absorbed and depressed.   As the person sees her capabilities slipping away, she is likely to become increasingly self-absorbed and insensitive to the feelings of others. Often, the person sinks into depression, making her situation even worse. The caregiver, trying to assist a loved one with problems she denies having, can easily feel rejected and unappreciated.

Stage III: Early Dementia

Dependency increases the caregiver's load.   By this time, the person with Alzheimer's has become quite dependent on others for her care. That dependency increases the caregiver's sense of responsibility for meeting all of the person's needs and keeping her safe from harm. It is difficult for someone who is not involved in the actual care to understand how much must be done daily.

In fact, other family members may fail to support the primary caregiver because they cannot envision how strenuous the mental and physical demands of daily caregiving are. A person in the early dementia phase requires:

- Help in initiating most activities
- Someone to help her "think"
- Hands-on care as her dependencies increase
- Help in expressing her needs

The victim should not drive.   A person who is exhibiting symptoms of early dementia is a hazardous driver. For example, she may increase her speed or drive through stop signs unknowingly. Likewise, stressful situations encountered while driving can dramatically affect her judgment. Family members therefore must take it upon themselves to ensure that the patient does not drive.

Memory gaps trigger insecurity and defensive behavior.   Even though her problems are obvious to everyone around, the patient may continue to deny and shield her mistakes. In conversations she may fabricate information that seems irrelevant or absurd. Actually, she is valiantly trying to fill in information gaps created by memory loss. The patient is trying to pull together pieces of her own reality in order to maintain a meaningful life.

As her memory deteriorates, a heightened sense of insecurity can develop into suspicion and paranoia. Judgment and reasoning deteriorate further. Suspiciousness may be accompanied by anger, even when a family member tries to prove the accusations or suspicions are unfounded. Agitated behavior may develop.

Emotional reactions become more prominent.   The patient's emotional instability comes from a mixture of psychological, social, and neurological sources. During this stage, the Alzheimer's patient may have periodic crying spells and abrupt mood changes, with or without obvious causes. Such instability can be frightening and aggravating to families. Soothing, calming approaches that convey support and understanding are good responses on the caregiver's part.

Memory deficits fluctuate.   Fluctuations in memory on an almost moment-to-moment basis are not uncommon in Stage III. Caregivers should realize that such fluctuations are a normal part of the disease, making the best of those days when their relative seems better, and avoiding despondency when she seems worse.

Logical, sequential reasoning and actions diminish.   The person's ability to recall the correct sequences of behavior and tasks becomes seriously impaired. This inability may show up in areas such as dressing or grooming, where she may complete only part of the task.

Independence encouraged.   Usually, she can continue to perform part of her daily routine with help. It is easy, however, to increase her dependency unnecessarily by assuming certain things are too intricate for her to complete. For example, by Stage III she will need help in selecting properly matched and appropriate clothing, but this does not mean she cannot still dress herself. Some persons with Alzheimer's will want to wear the same clothes every day, without changing or washing them. Although this kind of behavior will tempt caregivers to take over the entire task, the patient should be encouraged to care for herself as long as possible.

Simple decisions become overwhelming.   During early dementia, a person will have difficulty making even simple decisions concerning eating or dressing. But the caregiver still can offer simple alternatives that require a yes or no response. It may be helpful to suggest a choice of two necessary alternatives, such as bathing or picking up the dirty clothes. This increases the chance that the patient will undertake at least one desirable course of action.

Social withdrawal accompanied by impaired thinking capacity.   The affected person can be expected to withdraw from both social and task-oriented activities. Her decreasing thinking and reasoning abilities will make her less flexible and less able to adjust to stressful situations. If she is pushed, she will become both overly anxious and angry; if she is pushed too often, she will refuse to do even necessary stressful activities. Nonetheless, she may still enjoy some social situations. For example, going to church or the movies may still be fairly undemanding, while visiting with longtime friends may be overwhelming.

Caregivers require support.   At this point, caregivers need considerable emotional support and relief from their full-time responsibilities. Family members, friends, and neighbors can provide both the support and the relief the primary caregiver needs, whether it is by sitting with the relative, doing chores, or visiting. Caregivers should carefully monitor their own ability to handle the demands placed upon them, and they should not hesitate to ask for help as needed.

Stage IV: Middle Dementia

The person with AD reacts more severely to loss of abilities.   Major changes occur as the disease progresses from early to middle dementia, and the involvement of caregivers increases considerably. Throughout the illness, the patient may have been fairly successful in using denial to protect herself from the realization that her mind is slipping away. However, denial is becoming a less effective protector. Withdrawal is being replaced by tendencies toward agitation, paranoia, and delusions. The need for security cannot be satisfied by the person's mind. At this point, the environment can meet this need through structure, routine, and caring.

Delusions.   Delusions often reflect fears of loss and imagined threats in the external world. Spouses may be accused of being unfaithful. Neighbors and friends may be blamed for unbelievable things.

Sleep disturbances and hallucinations.   During this phase, the patient's sleep is more often disrupted and erratic. She may be awakened by hallucinations or delusional fears that make it almost impossible to sleep, and she may begin to wander at night.

Repetitive behavior.   A number of emotional changes appear during the middle dementia stage. They may include compulsive symptoms such as pulling clothes out of drawers and replacing them over and over. The person may not be able to hold onto her thoughts long enough to complete a course of action. Obsessive thoughts or repetitive ideas and concerns may be more evident in some persons.

Movement and coordination difficulties.   Problems with movement and coordination may become more obvious now and interfere markedly with performance. The person will develop difficulties with walking and with the purposeful, coordinated movements required for dressing, eating, brushing her teeth, and so forth. Eating difficulties may contribute to weight loss; alternatively, excessive eating may become a problem.

Help with daily activities is essential.   At this point, the AD person requires assistance with most activities of daily living. The caregiver must carefully and sensitively adjust social and behavioral expectations of the patient downward. The individual must not be placed in situations that could lead to emotional overload; she could overreact in violent and frightening ways.

Sources of violent behavior.   Much of the violent behavior of persons with Alzheimer's disease is triggered by excessive environmental demands. The person is unable to comprehend what behavior is expected of her and may respond inappropriately. Pressure to respond to situations promptly further accentuates inappropriate responses. Too many choices or options can precipitate more anxiety and agitation or may lead to further withdrawal.

Bathing problems emerge.   The middle dementia stage brings a real fear of bathing. This fear is often misinterpreted by caregivers as simple stubbornness and uncooperativeness. But actually, the person's fear of bathing is related to reasonable concerns. The patient forgets how to adjust water temperature and how to use the soap and washcloth. Her impaired coordination creates difficulties in getting in and out of the tub, and she may fear falling. In addition, the patient has lost her sense of the social importance of personal hygiene. To reduce conflict over bathing, the caregiver may substitute towel washing for a tub bath or reduce the frequency of bathing. Sometimes the patient may accept a hot bath as a way to relieve tensions, especially when it is combined with a soothing body massage.

Loss of touch with events and experiences.   Persons in middle dementia are generally unaware of their surroundings, the time of year, the year itself, and other indications of time and place. Memory abilities deteriorate to a fragmentary knowledge of home address and whereabouts. Getting lost becomes almost inevitable and is a real worry for caregivers. The patient may be able to distinguish strangers from familiar persons, but often she cannot identify the person on whom she is most dependent, her spouse. She will usually know her own name and have some sketchy recall of her past, but she is largely unaware of all recent events and experiences. She may give pieces of information which have no clear meaning. For the victim of Alzheimer's, the world has become frightening and largely unmanageable. The loss of cognitive, memory, and perceptual abilities prevents her from organizing the pieces of her life into a meaningful whole.

Caregiving becomes lonelier and more isolating.   At this stage, caregiving takes up most of the day and night, yet the caregiver receives little or no recognition from the patient. Kindness is rarely seen, unless it is read into some small action or gesture. This is extremely difficult for many caregivers to accept, since they naturally seek gratitude and approval from their relative.

If the caregiver assumes solitary care for the person with AD, he is likely to become severely isolated, both physically and socially. Friends no longer visit, and community activities are restricted. The greatest isolation is created by the inability of the patient to relate to the caregiver. All decisions fall on his shoulders. There are no rewards and appreciation for the caregiving, unless the caregiver finds ways to affirm himself and compensate for the emotional isolation and separation.

Caregiver must hire help or place the person in an institution.   By this stage, the emotional burdens of caregiving force those involved to make difficult decisions about whether to hire in-home help or possibly place the person in an institution. In Stage IV, hiring full-time assistance is the ideal situation for caregivers. However, it is costly to hire experienced full-time help; thus, part-time help may be the best alternative. But the primary caregiver must have some relief from the consuming tasks of direct care and supervision. In addition, the patient may need some form of psychiatric or other professional mental health assistance.

Caregivers need support groups.   Even with help, the caregiver's role may become so demanding as to totally overwhelm his life. The patient's sleeping problems are likely to disrupt the caregiver's sleep; her agitation makes management more perplexing and tiring; her delusional beliefs are painful and frightening. A family support group can help. The caregiver may also feel a need for individual counseling and assistance in securing other supportive resources.

The caregiver should call upon the whole family for help and support as needed. Major decisions regarding other arrangements for the patient's final weeks, months, or years are forthcoming, and few caregivers should be making such decisions without some degree of family input and support.

When family members do not support the most appropriate course of action, the primary caregiver must be reassured by others that he is making the correct decisions. Conflicts may develop because relatives do not understand the implications of the illness and the daily strains of caregiving.

Stage V: Late Dementia

Such phrases as "a long good-bye" or an "unending death" have been used to describe the disease's final stage. Caregivers must give so much for so small a response that often all the questions of life seem to be best summed up in one word—"WHY?"

Recognize limitations of caregiving.   Decisions now must be made without the loved one's nod of approval. Notions of what is best or what she would have wanted compete with the fact that one must decide alone. As narrow as the person's life has become, it is still valuable to the family, and it is hard to say good-bye. Nonetheless, one hopes to see the suffering end. Although the caregiver may want to keep his loved one at home, an institution may be the only realistic alternative when he can no longer provide full-time care.

Denial may continue to protect the person with AD from the emotional impact of the illness. She may still be able to smile, to laugh, and to appear to enjoy life at times.

Less of everything.   The emotional experience of life can go on even though the words have been lost. Behaviorally, the person is as likely to be amenable as she is to be difficult. The need for tranquilizers lessens because her behavior has become more easily managed.

Her motor abilities will continue to deteriorate and eventually her ability to walk, sit, and smile will be lost, as well as her control of bladder and colon functions. The loss may be uneven: a person who is still walking may be found on the floor or caught as she falls because she suddenly has forgotten how to walk. Such cases may require medical attention to ensure that a stroke or transient ischemic attack (condition in which blood supply to the brain is temporarily interrupted) has not occurred.

Addressing movement problems.   It is important to help the person with Alzheimer's to walk as long as she is able. She will not be able to use a walker, since she has lost her coordination, but guardrails and other supports can help. In addition, rearranging furniture to provide support and eliminating barriers (such as loose rugs) will help. The use of geriatric chairs and other confining devices should be avoided as much as possible; such confinement increases agitation and restlessness.

Eating difficulties.   During this final stage, the patient will eventually lose the ability to chew and swallow food. The caregiver may have to cut the food into, small pieces or prepare an almost totally soft diet. If the patient refuses to eat, other methods of feeding must be considered.

Need more structured, highly supervised care.   As brain activity becomes severely disturbed, the patient is increasingly vulnerable to seizures as well as aspiration, pneumonia, infection, and other illnesses. She will need assistance in eating, since choking, blockage, or other problems in breathing and swallowing can occur. Respiratory problems can worsen through decreased activity, particularly when the person becomes bedridden.

The final reconciliation.   Stupor occurs in this terminal stage and leads finally to coma and death. Throughout the illness, the caregiver has had to meet one challenge after another in caring for his loved one. Human contact has made a real difference to the AD person. Such contact is still important, even if the person is seemingly unable to respond. Patience and kindness, though they require great strength, are necessary. A touch, a loving voice, and the presence of a loved one help keep a person physically and emotionally alive, even when she can no longer reach out to anyone.

3

Depression and the Person with Alzheimer's Disease

Persons with Alzheimer's disease can develop other health problems that can further restrict their capacity to function in social situations and ordinary activities of daily living. While pronounced changes in behavior and psychiatric symptoms may be associated with Alzheimer's disease, these symptoms can result from other health problems as well, when they appear abruptly. There is, however, another health problem that is commonly seen with Alzheimer's disease. It is essential that caregivers be able to recognize it and respond to it appropriately. This problem is depression, and it has significant impact on the person with AD and his or her caregivers. When suffering from depression, people with Alzheimer's disease are known to be more distressed and agitated and to have greater problems with functioning and performing activities of daily living. Family members experience more stress and burden because of the increased dysfunction and mood-related disturbances experienced by their loved ones. This is not the occasional experience of being down in the dumps. It is more serious, yet depression is very difficult to diagnose with AD.

Identifying depression with AD is more difficult because depressive symptoms are often transitory, or less severe and pervasive, than those seen in major depressive disorders. Depression and Alzheimer's share symptoms, and some symptoms of depression may actually represent early signs of AD. Depression may not always occur when we would most expect it, so we need to reconsider our assumptions on when and why people with AD get depressed. For example, people who are aware of dementia symptoms and understand what it means to have Alzheimer's might have a greater risk of becoming depressed at an early stage of dementia. This psychological reaction

33

to loss does not, however, explain the fact that depression occurs in people who not only have little awareness of dementia symptoms but who have more severely advanced dementia (Devanand, 1999). Nevertheless, people with AD who have less severe cognitive impairment or more severe functional impairment have a higher risk of becoming depressed (Payne, 1998).

Recent research has determined that depressive symptoms may develop as long as 3 years before some people are diagnosed with Alzheimer's disease (Visser, 2000). While some depression is mild and has transitory symptoms, depressive disorders found with Alzheimer's disease can be severe. We can conclude several things about depression with Alzheimer's disease: it is common, has multiple causes, and occurs at different points in the disease process. The severity of symptoms varies and the presentation of symptoms may depend on the stage during which depression develops. We may find that differences in onset and symptom presentation may actually characterize different types of depression. We still have more to learn about depression and Alzheimer's.

Some problems attributed to dementia may be caused by depression. Depressed people with Alzheimer's are more likely to be agitated and have behavioral problems that are more difficult to manage. They are more likely to suffer delusions. They are prone to exhibit greater impairment in dressing, grooming, eating, bathing, and other activities of daily living. Persons with depression and AD may exhibit more cognitive impairment. Depression may be difficult to identify with Alzheimer's, but unlike Alzheimer's disease, it can be treated.

Recognizing and treating depression creates significant benefits for persons with AD and their caregivers. It reduces their distress and suffering. It improves their mood and outlook. It increases their energy and improves their ability to function in activities of daily living. Communication and relationships improve and cooperativeness is more likely. Treatment of depression also reduces the distress of caregivers and substantially decreases their burden of care. In some instances, depression may herald the arrival of Alzheimer's. Depressive symptoms may be seen when cognitive impairment is not yet severe enough to meet the criteria for dementia. Depressive symptoms may represent a prodromal stage of AD—that is, signs that appear before the symptoms of the disease can be recognized. Early recognition and treatment of AD and depression are important.

This chapter discusses the ways caregivers can recognize and manage depression. Symptoms shared by depression and Alzheimer's are discussed. Risk factors for depression and the types of depression more frequently experienced by persons with AD are presented. The unique association that appears to exist between some types of depression and AD are considered. Causes of AD-related depression are examined and different treatments are discussed. Approaches that can be effectively utilized by caregivers are included.

Risk Factors for Depression

Depression or depressive symptoms are common in Alzheimer's disease. But the difficulties of making the diagnosis of depression are suggested by the wide variation in rates of prevalence. From 0 to 86 percent of people with Alzheimer's suffer depression or manifest some of its symptoms (Migliorelli et al., 1995). Depressive symptoms rather than the actual clinical depression may account for such widely varying estimates.

Depression and Alzheimer's share some symptoms, which can be an obstacle in identifying AD with coexisting depression. Poor concentration may create problems with memory that resemble the impairment characteristic of Alzheimer's; the apathy of Alzheimer's resembles the loss of interest or desire common with depression. Nevertheless, major depression affects from 30 to 50 percent of the individuals who develop Alzheimer's (Backman et al., 1996). Persons with Alzheimer's are also known to develop another depressive disorder called dysthymic disorder.

Major depression is a serious, acute form of depression with symptoms that must be present for at least 2 weeks. It is caused by biochemical changes in levels of neurotransmitters in the brain. In Alzheimer's disease some of the anatomical changes in some parts of the brain may play a role. Dysthymic disorder is a chronic type of depression. Its symptoms must be present for at least 2 years. This disorder is affected more by such factors as personality, personal losses, and environmental stressors.

Some persons with Alzheimer's have a higher risk for depression. A personal or family history of depression increases the risk of developing depression with Alzheimer's. Women with AD have a greater risk for depression. The presence of delusions and early-onset dementia increase the risk for depression.

Early-onset Alzheimer's occurs in persons who may be in their early 40s to late 50s. This is an important psychosocial period of adult development. Children are getting older. Some are still dependent on parents; others are likely to be in school or beginning careers and families. Individuals affected by AD may be at the peak of achievement. They may be looking at other activities or roles to occupy them as they enter their 60s. It may be a time for relationships to be strengthened and for couples to do things that had been postponed so that they could accommodate the needs of children and careers. Alzheimer's disease interferes.

Persons with dementia, particularly early onset, can experience a great sense of loss of themselves and the life they had envisioned. The activities that had supported their sense of self as spouse, parent, and employee are threatened. The time they had expected to have is getting short. These circumstances can precipitate depression as the person developing Alzheimer's is sensitive to the impact the disease process will have on his future. Alzheimer's-related depression may be related to psychosocial changes; it can also be related to changes in brain chemistry created by brain damage.

Depression, as we understand it, is more frequently observed during the early to middle stages of AD, but it can develop in the later stages. People are thought to have more awareness of the disease and its effects on their lives before the disease process advances. This awareness is more likely to precipitate psychological reactions to losses. An individual's awareness, insight, and capacity to cope determine the risk for some forms of depressive disorders. The risk for people who cope well and who have good social support is not as great. When it occurs early in the disease process, AD depression looks much like non-AD depression. But not all depression associated with Alzheimer's results from poor coping skills or deficiencies in social support. Some depression may have less to do with the risk factors just noted.

There may be several types of depression affecting people with AD. Some precede signs of dementia. Others develop after symptoms of dementia have been identified. Depression is considered during the diagnostic work-up for dementia. It is one condition to rule out, since it has an effect on cognition, memory, and behavior. But after the diagnosis, health professionals may not be as aware of depressive symptoms, since Alzheimer's and depression share some symptoms. After the diagnosis, caregivers are in the best position to recognize signs and symptoms of depression.

Signs and Symptoms of Depression

Passive Symptoms and Agitation

Some depressive symptoms resemble symptoms of Alzheimer's disease more than others do. These are called passive symptoms. They include apathy, social withdrawal, and lower level of activity. Loss of interest and spontaneity, slowed gait and motor responses, limited emotional expressions, and a decrease in talking are examples of other passive symptoms shared by depression and dementia.

Passive symptoms due to dementia tend to increase as the severity of the disease progresses. They indicate that more significant functional impairment has occurred. However, when the disease progression has not advanced into the later stages and passive symptoms are pervasive, the possibility that depression is their source must be considered.

Let's consider this example. John was recently diagnosed with Alzheimer's disease. He initiates very little speech. He shows little interest in activities that he used to enjoy and is apathetic about matters that were once quite important to him. John is quite withdrawn and inactive. His memory is mildly impaired and it is difficult for him to think and solve problems. If John did not also have symptoms of AD, his symptoms might suggest depression. If he had difficulty sleeping, didn't care to eat, appeared sad, and became tearful when questioned about how he was feeling, the chance of his being depressed would be even greater. Evidence of feeling worthless, hopeless, and helpless would leave no doubt that he was suffering from serious depression.

When Alzheimer's is more advanced and passive symptoms are predominant, recognizing depression is even more difficult. Since passive symptoms are also seen in dementia, they are not reliable as indicators of depression associated with AD. We need to look for other symptoms to make the distinction between dementia and depression. For example, if John expressed feelings of being worthless and feeling helpless, his chance of being depressed would be much greater. Expressions of not wanting to live, other thoughts about death, and suicidal ideation would be important indications of depression.

People with Alzheimer's are less able to describe what they are feeling. It may be more difficult to recognize low self-esteem, hopelessness, and thoughts about death. Caregivers still need to explore how loved ones are feeling. We can help loved ones find ways to communicate their thoughts and feelings. Depressed persons are more comfortable opening up when they are approached in the spirit of patience and empathy. Sometimes by softly questioning the experience of the person with AD, we discover that a physical problem is responsible for a lack of activity and withdrawal to the bedroom. Or if the complaints are vague, they might suggest depression.

Passive Symptoms May Represent Coping

Passive symptoms of Alzheimer's disease might represent an attempt to cope with situations that are uncomfortable or overwhelming. There are other psychological defenses that people with AD use. The most common is denial, which is used to avoid confrontations that focus on the reality of impairment. People with AD may be coping by withdrawing from stressful situations. They may be trying to maintain some degree of control over the demands their environment is exerting on them. They may, for example, refuse to respond to requests they don't know how to handle. Their silent withdrawal from demands needs to be viewed differently, since such behavior may represent efforts to save face. Passive symptoms could represent psychological defenses that assist the individual in preserving mental and emotional equilibrium that prevents painful exposure of impairment.

Passive behaviors resulting from Alzheimer's are not very responsive to interventions. Passive symptoms due to depression are more responsive to treatment than those resulting from AD. These are examined in the discussion of specific symptoms of depression.

Agitation and Depression

Agitation and agitated behavior describe a wide range of disruptive and disturbing behavior in people with Alzheimer's. Agitated behaviors include restlessness, irritability, pacing, and wandering. Resistance to help, and verbal and physical aggression, are other agitated behaviors. These behaviors are often difficult for caregivers to manage when helping loved ones with activities of daily living such as dressing and bathing, or preventing them from entering an unsafe situation. Agitated behavior is a common occurrence at some point in the AD process. Caregivers may provoke this behavior when they are making stressful demands or may create an upsetting situation for the care recipient because they are so agitated themselves. However, some agitated behavior in people with AD may occur because of underlying depression.

Depression, Alzheimer's, and Memory Impairment

Memory problems in the elderly used to be attributed to old age; the label "senile" was sometimes used. Hardening of the arteries, poor circulation, or lack of oxygen were thought to be responsible. Efforts to ameliorate this situation with oxygen failed. Eventually, the connection of symptoms seen in older persons was made with those Dr. Alzheimer identified in a middle-aged woman. Alzheimer's disease, not old age or eccentricities of old age, was responsible for problems with memory, loss of function, and other behavioral and psychiatric symptoms.

Memory impairment can be caused by conditions other than Alzheimer's. Some medications can cause mental confusion and depression. Memory impairment can result from other psychiatric conditions when psychosis and poor concentration are present. Depression is another potential source of memory problems. Treating possible depression is an important approach to diagnosing suspected cases of dementia so that other sources of memory deficits can be ruled out. However, dementia and not depression is usually responsible for the underlying memory problems that often accompany depression. Memory impairment can occur with major depression, but memory functions improve when there are concomitant improvements in mood and other depressive symptoms. When other depressive symptoms are treated successfully and memory impairment persists, Alzheimer's disease or a similar type of dementia may be present.

Depression and Alzheimer's may be linked in some other ways. Some researchers believe severe depression may cause damage that makes the brain more vulnerable to a disease process such as Alzheimer's. Others believe that damage associated with Alzheimer's makes the brain more susceptible to depression. Some depressive signs such as loss of interest in daily activities and apathy have been identified as early indications of AD. These do not occur as psychological reactions to cognitive impairment because the cognitive impairment is not yet very evident. They are the result of behavioral and affective changes associated with changing chemical and physical properties of the brain.

Alzheimer's with depression has many different faces. Some depressive episodes that occur for the first time in later life are suspected of being precursors of Alzheimer's. It is possible that certain presentations of depression seen with Alzheimer's may represent a subtype of Alzheimer's. Depressive symptoms may appear before symptoms of dementia because of specific areas of structural damage to the brain and neurochemical changes that have been activated by the disease process. Signs and symptoms of dementia become evident later in the disease progression.

To summarize, memory problems that do not respond to successful treatment of other depressive symptoms are probably not caused by depression. Memory impairment in such cases is probably related to a medical condition. Some illnesses may be treatable, but in older persons this situation raises major concerns that a type of dementia is developing. Indeed, follow-up of these late-onset cases usually confirms a dementia of the Alzheimer's type. Having the first episode of depression late in life may be an early sign of AD, especially when significant cognitive impairment characterizes the depression. Depression can be treated successfully when it coexists with Alzheimer's. Memory problems related to depression abate with improvement in depressive symptoms.

Depressive Symptoms and Disorders

Depression is not just a matter of feeling blue for a few days about something that happened to you. Depression is a group of symptoms that an individual must have had for a specific period of time. Persons with dementia can develop major depressive or dysthymic disorders. Major depressive disorder may be called major depression. This type of depression is more severe than dysthymic disorder. Major depression can cause symptoms that suggest dementia and must be ruled out as a cause of cognitive impairment and loss of functioning. Dysthymic disorder is a chronic presentation of depression. Fewer symptoms are required than for a major depressive episode; these must have been present for at least two years. In a major depressive episode, either a depressed mood, or loss of interest or pleasure in nearly all activities, must have been present for at least two weeks.

Major depressive episodes and dysthymic disorders can be difficult to differentiate on the basis of symptoms alone. Since it is more important for caregivers to recognize signs and symptoms of depression than determine which disorder is present, there is no need to discuss diagnostic criteria further. Caregivers need to seek professional help when they observe symptoms that suggest depression. Medical professionals will find their observations quite helpful.

Symptoms of these disorders can include the following:

- Diminished ability to concentrate or think, or to make decisions.
- Depressed mood suggested by reports of feeling empty, sad, down in the dumps, tearful or crying excessively.
- Difficulties with sleep, especially awaking in the middle of the night or early morning and unable to get back to sleep. Getting to sleep may also be a problem. Sleeping too much is seen less frequently.
- Fatigue or loss of energy.
- Feelings of worthlessness; excessive or inappropriate guilt that may have delusional content.
- Loss of self-esteem.
- Feelings of hopelessness.
- Significant changes in appetite and weight.
- Recurrent thoughts of death, recurrent suicidal ideation without a plan, or specific plan for committing suicide.

These symptoms cause significant distress in social, occupational, or other important areas of the depressed individual's life. Now let's examine symptoms of depression and presentations of similar symptoms that occur in AD.

Depressive Symptoms and Cognitive Functions

Depression has a significant impact on cognitive functions. Abrupt cognitive decline is more likely to be a sign of depression; slowly declining cognitive function is more common in Alzheimer's disease. Attention and concentration are necessary for information to be received clearly so that it can be stored in our short-term memory. Since these activities and cognitive processes such as problem solving and learning are susceptible to depression, memory impairment sometimes appears to be a symptom of depression. While memory impairment is observed with depression, particularly in older people, it is a result rather than a symptom of depression. It is a problem that results from poor concentration and attention—problems that make it very difficult for information to be stored in more permanent memory. Information stored in longterm memory is extremely difficult for seriously depressed individuals to retrieve.

Depressed persons often have difficulties concentrating, remembering, and thinking. They are unable to make simple decisions. Persons with Alzheimer's deny or minimize their memory problems. They might try to put the blame on something or someone else. They will acknowledge they have memory problems if offered that option in a nonconfrontive, compassionate manner. The diminished ability to think, concentrate, or be able to make decisions represents an important cluster of depressive symptoms that are sometimes viewed primarily as problems with memory.

Depressed Mood

Other core symptom clusters of depression point to a sad mood and thoughts and feelings that go along with being blue. Whereas dementia is distinguished by the impairment of memory and the capacity to think and reason, depression is characterized as a mood disorder. This depressed or dysphoric mood is a primary symptom in most cases of depression. It can be expressed as a feeling of general dissatisfaction, discomfort, or unpleasantness. Comments of depressed people suggest feelings of vast emptiness or deep sadness. Feelings of hopelessness are frequently expressed. Crying or tearfulness frequently accompanies a depressed mood. And yet some depressed persons feel nothing at all and appear emotionally flat. Others look the part: moving slowly and with great effort, looking sad and tired, and responding slowly and ponderously to questions.

Signs of a depressed mood can be helpful in determining how much cognitive impairment is due to AD. People who are depressed often have a sadder mood in the morning and may be more confused. Their mood and performance tend to improve later in the day. People with AD tend to be at their best earlier in the day. Their cognitive ability fades later in the day and they are less able to cope with the demands of daily living. Sometimes they show more confusion and agitation later in the day and into the evening. These are signs of sundowning.

Sundowning appears to be more common in the moderate to severe stages of AD. It may be present when the person with AD becomes more agitated, restless, anxious, active, confused, or combative in the late afternoon or evening. When caregivers first observe these behaviors, they need to be certain that they are not a reaction to distressing stimuli such as unrealistic demands, aggravating activities, noise, pain, or other types of physical discomfort.

Sundowning may be caused by buildup of physical and mental fatigue that peaks later in the day. Disorientation due to reduced daylight and increased shadows may contribute to it. There is evidence that Alzheimer's disease causes damage to a specific part of the brain that controls the body's internal clock or circadian rhythms. This causes a major disruption in an individual's normal sleep-wake cycle.

Several approaches to sundowning problems maybe helpful to caregivers. First, be sure that some stimulation is not creating the problems, for example, too much caffeine. Restrict caffeine intake to the morning. The use of bright, even lighting has produced positive results; glare should be eliminated. Caregivers should be flexible with expectations and respond calmly with reassurance to loved ones. Consult with a physician to make sure that anxiety, restlessness, and agitation are not related to medical conditions or medication. Professional help should be sought if these approaches fail. Major tranquilizers may be necessary to manage behavior problems related to sundowning.

Sleep Difficulties

Having trouble sleeping or sleeping too much are symptoms of depression. Both of these disturbances are also seen in Alzheimer's disease. Trouble getting to sleep can be caused by agitation associated with activities initiated before bedtime, such as bathing. Another time might be more suitable for some of these activities. Worries and fears can prevent or delay sleep. Hallucinations or delusional beliefs can cause sleep problems. A person might be afraid to go to sleep. Because of her confusion, she may believe she must do something like go home or go to work.

Medications, especially those given for agitation or sleep, can be sedating and cause daytime dozing. So can antihistamines and anticonvulsants. Changes in medications, times they are given, or dosage might help solve these problems. Sleep/wake cycles can be reversed when persons frequently sleep during the day and lay wakeful much of the night. This may contribute to more disorientation and confusion. To resume a more natural sleep/wake cycle, caregivers should pay more attention to getting the person up on time in the morning than putting her to bed at a specific time at night.

Although allowing care recipients to sleep during the day may decrease the caregivers demands during this time, it will likely increase demands on them at night when they need sleep themselves. Boredom during the day is another common reason for sleep problems. A lack of meaningful and stimulating activity during the day may foster dozing or napping. Exercise and movement during the day can be a good sleep aid. Sleep during the day may be a way to avoid dealing with a demanding or confusing environment.

Some people sleep excessively during the day because they have not been able to sleep well during the night. They are catching up on needed rest, which may be beneficial if it does not interfere with sleep at night. Persons who are tired become more agitated and disagreeable. Problems managing behavior can lead to problems with nighttime sleeping. Sometimes sundowning can be ushered in with increasing agitation in the middle to late afternoon. More rest may help reduce the agitation and fatigue.

Sleep disturbances are a frequent complaint of depressed people. They involve getting to sleep and awaking in the middle of the night or early in the morning. Sleeping too much can also occur. Ruminative thoughts, regrets, and worries are common. Anxiety is often present. Some people just lay awake and do not get sleepy.

Awaking in the middle of the night can be quite disruptive. Sometimes it is due to nightmares. In other cases, persons who are depressed become aware of bothersome thoughts regarding past or future situations after they wake up. They become more alert due to their struggle to get the unwanted thoughts off of their mind so that they can get back to sleep. Depressed individuals may also awake very early in the morning and may not be able to get back to sleep for some of the same reasons already noted.

Problems with sleep are often an important treatment focus of either Alzheimer's care or depression. In either case, caregivers need to address this problem so that they do not face the prospect of losing sleep themselves.

Fatigue or Loss of Energy

Sleep problems contribute to another cluster of depressive symptoms: fatigue or loss of energy. People with depression frequently complain about being tired and not having the energy to do anything. Often fatigue or a lack of energy is given as explanations for not getting dressed, not getting out of bed, or not performing other daily activities. People may resist doing things because of their mental state, yet depression has considerable impact on physical functioning and the perception of physical symptoms.

Depression and Physical Complaints

Depressed people commonly report physical complaints such as fatigue, headaches, indigestion, constipation, dizzy spells, chest tightness or pain, urinary disturbances, and loss of sexual drive. When these physical concerns are repeatedly expressed and other symptoms of depression are observed, depression is likely present. But since physical symptoms could suggest other medical problems, consultation with a physician should be considered.

Some people express more physical than emotional symptoms when they are depressed. Their reports of physical symptoms mask the emotional aspects of their depression. Sometimes depressed persons may be more guarded about expressing their emotional concerns because these represent a weakness they are unwilling to expose to others.

Feelings of Worthlessness and Guilt

Feelings of worthlessness and excessive or inappropriate guilt represent another cluster of depressive symptoms. Delusions or false beliefs may reflect these perceptions. The guilt is not merely that of self-reproach or guilt about being sick. Excessive guilt can, however, arise from what a person believes has caused Alzheimer's disease. Sins of omission or commission—the things a person has failed to do or should not have done—are believed to be the cause of the disease. This kind of guilt is usually present when there is a great deal of other unfinished business in relationships with another family member. The guilt is irrational, yet the person cannot be dissuaded from her beliefs. Some people refuse help because they believe they are worthless and deserve to be punished. Depressed persons have low self-esteem with feelings of hopelessness.

It is difficult for caregivers to respond to these symptoms. Considering the situation in which they occur, they are demoralizing. Caregivers may not believe they can offer loved ones hope because of Alzheimer's poor prognosis. However, depression exacerbates difficulties that may have been attributed solely to Alzheimer's. For example, a depressed mood paints a very dismal future. Caregivers exposed to this type of mental/emotional landscape may find it harder to keep a healthy perspective about caregiving situations and offer the support a loved one needs. There can be realistic hope found in the successful treatment of depression and improvement in function and outlook. Symptoms of being worthless and hopeless, getting upset, and giving up decrease with an improvement in mood.

Changes in Appetite and Weight

Depression involves changes in appetite and weight. Persons with Alzheimer's sometimes do not eat because they forget to eat or are unable to feed themselves. Weight loss and what appears to be a problem with appetite can occur with Alzheimer's disease. Problems with weight and appetite occur as important symptoms of depression for other reasons.

Depression is responsible for either significant weight loss or weight gain. These symptoms can be related to major ongoing changes in appetite and eating habits. There are several explanations. Food may not taste good. Often people just don't have the desire to eat anything. They are not hungry. Others overeat to ward off anxiety or fill up their emptiness. Some people with excessive guilt or feelings of worthlessness starve themselves as punishment. They have a desire to die. Weight loss can occur even when depressed persons are eating. This is also a basis for concern, since weight loss occurs with other health problems.

Eating difficulties associated with the dementia syndrome of Alzheimer's disease are somewhat different. People who report they are eating lose weight because they are not eating at all or are eating less than they remember. This is most likely to occur when these people are alone or unsupervised much of the time. It is common for them to report they are eating as they always have. They have no memory or evidence of what they prepared. They will also decline food because they believe they have already eaten. Some have eating binges and crave sweets. These possibilities must be ruled out as the source of weight changes before depression is implicated as the cause.

Thoughts of Death and Suicide

Recurrent thoughts of death, suicide, or plans to commit suicide are very serious symptoms of depression. It does not seem possible that individuals with Alzheimer's disease would be capable of taking purposeful action toward a goal such as suicide. They can and they do. National news has carried stories about Alzheimer's-related suicides. Assisted suicide also occurs. Many of these suicides have been driven by depression. There are also cases where spouses have killed the person with Alzheimer's and then killed themselves.

Factors other than depression may be involved in suicidal behavior and completed suicide. Depressed persons with Alzheimer's can feel so badly about themselves and their future that death is viewed as the only way to escape their pain. They may have concerns about financial matters and becoming a burden to their family. Alcohol may exacerbate suicidal ideation and risk. The diminishing quality of life may be another factor. Some persons with Alzheimer's who are affected by these factors but are not depressed may also choose to end their life.

Loss of Interest and Pleasure

Apathy, boredom, and withdrawal represent another important cluster of depressive symptoms: a significant loss of interest or pleasure in most, if not all, activities. This loss is pervasive. No interest or pleasure can be derived from activities that had been enjoyable before. In Alzheimer's, apathy and boredom occur because people may not be able to initiate or maintain involvement in activities. They might want to do something but may not understand how to plan or start an activity. Structure, routine, and encouragement are usually needed. Step-by step instructions aid as well. Providing assistance or alternate activities may be helpful.

When depression is also present, other factors need to be considered. The person needs to be offered activities that have been pleasant in the past. Whenever possible, encourage her to make a choice. Too many choices may be overwhelming, so make the decision for your loved one.

Barriers to participation must be identified and corrected. For example, caregivers need to see how a lack of energy or being overly challenged makes activities less attractive. Noise, poor lighting, and too many distractions sabotage the best of intentions. Patiently encouraging and rewarding an individual's gradual efforts to become involved can be helpful.

It also helps to remind persons of the ways they will benefit from doing things. For example, before you go walking, invite them to remember how often they have felt more relaxed and had more energy. Have them remember pretty sights and pleasant sounds. Some activities are more enjoyable because of the other people who are involved or the places you might go. Other factors such as weather, time of day, time required to get to an activity, and noise or crowds must be considered. This may be an opportunity for caregivers to be involved in something they can also enjoy.

Mental anguish and physical suffering characterize a depressive disorder. Even minor depression in people with Alzheimer's can lead to disability, behavioral disturbances, decreased self-care, and sudden decreases in functioning and psychological well-being. Angry outbursts, increased apathy, and the reappearance of aggression need to be evaluated because these behaviors can be atypical presentations of depression. The causes of depression in Alzheimer's disease are complicated; it is likely that it has multiple causes.

Causes of Depression with Alzheimer's Disease

The depression seen with Alzheimer's is caused by the interaction of psychological and physiological factors. Some people who develop Alzheimer's may be more genetically vulnerable to depression. Some have had previous episodes of depression or have continued to suffer chronic depression. Some cases of Alzheimer's actually appear to begin as depression. It is only later that symptoms of a dementia are recognized.

AD causes brain damage that results in a loss of neurons and neurotransmitters. These physical and chemical changes contribute to problems with mood, behavior, and cognition. A greater loss of neurons in some parts of the brain predisposes some individuals with AD to depression. Neurotransmitters such as norepinephrine and serotonin are depleted in AD. Both are implicated in mood disorders. It may be that the loss of the neurotransmitter acetylcholine can influence mood as well as behavior. Depression caused primarily by underlying biological factors can be influenced by psychological factors, but these are not necessary for its development. A good example is the biological type of depression that occurs during the individual's relative unawareness of AD or its symptoms. Depression is also observed in more advanced AD.

Psychological factors predispose people with AD to depression. Certain coping and personality styles, lack of social support, major concurrent illnesses, and complications created by losses increase vulnerability to depression. People who cannot live up to their expectations in the face of AD may be more inclined to suffer guilt and loss of self-esteem. Depression may develop when an overwhelming sense of failure prevails despite their best efforts. People who have depended too much upon others may be more fearful of becoming a burden and being abandoned, and are more likely to become anxious and depressed. People who have suffered previous bouts of depression are more vulnerable to subsequent episodes of depression.

Psychological defenses such as denial may be used to cope with loss and trauma. The degree of awareness a person has of deficits that result from AD may foster depression, which is suggested by studies indicating that nondepressed Alzheimer's patients show more denial than those who are depressed (Migliorelli et al., 1995). But is the denial an indication of lack of awareness or a true psychological defense? Are we assuming denial occurs when a lack of awareness negates the recognition of a problem?

Awareness and insight may be factors involved in the development of depression. We may believe that the more we are aware of negative events, the more they will hurt us. Our reaction is influenced by our perception of what happens and what the event means to us. Is it a threat or is there no reason for concern? People with awareness of the problem may be more vulnerable to a reactive depression than those who are relatively unaware of the disease and its effects on them. They can be overcome by recognition of what is happening, which is why we believe depression occurs more frequently in the earlier stages of the disease. But people with awareness may have a greater need for defenses such as denial to protect them from the implications of what they perceive to be happening to them. They have more cognitive abilities remaining to cope with Alzheimer's disease. Awareness doesn't automatically cause depression. Nor does lack of awareness exclude people with Alzheimer's from developing depression.

Actual losses trigger depression. So can threatened or symbolic losses. People whose identity and well-being are solely defined by activities and interests that cannot be continued or replaced experience a significant threat to personal identity and self-esteem. They may feel they have less worth and are not valued as competent people like they were before Alzheimer's developed. When loved ones restrict their participation in activities and roles, it hurts them—even if they cannot understand the reasons for such behavior.

Caregivers must, of course, take steps to ensure the safety of the person with dementia. These measures sometimes introduce conflict because the person with Alzheimer's perceives them to be unfair. They set off a series of losses that have considerable impact on self-esteem, personal control, and life satisfaction. Restrictions on driving, managing finances, and cooking represent losses that are not easy to understand or accept. Some people feel these safety measures take away everything that is important.

Memory loss whittles away at the identity, competence, and self-esteem of a person with Alzheimer's. The caregiving situation can be quite negative because it strikes at the same characteristics of an individual's personality. These daily assaults on the person's view of himself represent a potential source of depression. Gradually, the person's view of self is severely threatened, and to the extent that it depends on performance, it may be very hard to accept. Self-esteem is severely challenged by losses of function.

People with Alzheimer's receive lots of negative messages about what they cannot do. They need positive messages about themselves and their value to loved ones. Cooperating with or helping the caregiver is an important adaptation to limitations caused by the disease. It might help to hear that the family caregiver appreciates this behavior.

People with AD often receive negative messages because caregivers need to justify the assistance they offer. Let's look at what happens when the caregiver takes over paying bills. The person with AD is no longer able to pay bills but denies she has a problem despite the fact that she cannot determine what bills need to be paid and is unable to fill out a check correctly. Nevertheless, she objects to her husband's assistance. He tells her she doesn't know what she is doing and shouldn't be trusted with money. There are better ways to explain this problem. It is one of many personal affronts to her competence and integrity. For persons who have based their identity and self-esteem on accomplishments and high standards of personal competence, these encounters may be quite painful.

The relationship caregivers have had with loved ones and the quality of their interactions can play an important role in the development of depression. Caregivers may be the only ones who can give positive and meaningful feedback. Since they know what is important to the person with AD, they are in the best position to reward behavior. Caregivers must be aware of their own vulnerability to stress and depression. Depression can be contagious. Caring for a depressed person who has Alzheimer's increases this risk. It is possible for caregivers to develop depression before the care recipient. Depressed caregivers will have more difficulties relating to loved ones. There are several reasons for them to seek treatment for depression. One is to be able to be more positively involved with a loved one's care.

Treatment for Depression

Caregivers are in a unique position to see signs of depression in loved ones and then get help for them. Medical or mental health professionals will then determine if depression is present and suggest treatments. Medical problems or medications may be responsible for some depressive symptoms. During the evaluation, caregivers can be of help to the professionals providing treatment. History of the person thought to be depressed is essential, and the family caregivers may be a valuable source of information. They can also help loved ones deal with the treatment situation.

Caregivers can make an important contribution to the recovery of the depressed person. Their relationship with the depressed person enables them to validate the identity and self-esteem of this person. They can bring up experiences and memories from the past that portray the person in meaningful ways. Professionals are at a disadvantage without a family caregiver's observations and feedback about treatment-related changes. Depressed persons and their caregivers can benefit from supportive relationships with these professional helpers.

There are several approaches to treating depression. Pharmacological treatment is often recommended. Therapy can benefit the depressed person and it can also involve the caregivers. Often a combination of medication and therapy increases the chances for successful treatment. Supportive education regarding AD, depression, and caregiving is essential. In addition to educational resources, caregivers may need more social and emotional support.

Pharmacological Treatments

Depression with Alzheimer's is usually responsive to antidepressant medication. Newer antidepressant medications are good alternatives to the older class of antidepressants called tricyclics (see table of antidepressants in Chapter 18). Tricyclic antidepressants have a higher potential for side effects, especially those that increase confusion and memory loss. People with dementia are at greater risk of developing delirium when taking tricyclic antidepressants such as amitriptyline or doxepin, which are more likely to increase cognitive impairment. When a tricyclic antidepressant is needed, desipramine or nortriptyline would be more useful.

Newer antidepressants are called new-generation antidepressants and include several different classifications. The most familiar class is known as selective serotonin reuptake inhibitors, or SSRIs. Zoloft, Prozac, Paxil, Celexa, and Luvox are the trade names of current SSRIs. (The reader may refer to Chapter 18 to match trade names with generic names.) They work by selectively preventing nerve cells from eliminating the neurotransmitter serotonin. Other new-generation antidepressants include Effexor, Wellbutrin, Remeron, and Serzone. These antidepressants act on chemical changes in neurotransmitters thought to be involved in depression.

New-generation antidepressants act more specifically on chemical imbalances involved in depression. Although side effects such as dry mouth, nausea, anxiety, agitation, gastrointestinal complaints, and insomnia might occur, they usually abate after adjustment to the medication.

The same antidepressant is not appropriate for everyone. Some work more effectively for certain depressive symptoms than others. Slight differences in the therapeutic action of these medications and their side effects are important for physicians to consider so that they can maximize positive outcomes and minimize negative effects. Serzone and Remeron, for instance, might aid sleep at night but might also increase drowsiness during the day. Effexor might cause headache, nausea, and elevated blood pressure. Since it does not interact with other medications, it might be the safer choice for people taking multiple medications.

In older people taking antidepressants there is the risk of postural hypotension, which increases the risk of falling when arising from a chair or the bed. If the person appears dizzy as she is getting up, she should be encouraged to get up slowly. If this doesn't help and the risk of falling remains, medication changes need to be made.

New medications such as Aricept are being developed. Exelon was approved for release in April 2000. Several others will probably be available this year. It is necessary to monitor how antidepressants and other medications work together. Recently, a possible interaction between Aricept and Paxil was reported. Paxil may slow the metabolism of Aricept, and higher levels of Aricept cause side effects. Insomnia, confusion, irritability, and severe diarrhea are examples. Some side effects could be serious. A physician or pharmacist should be consulted about possible side effects all medications.

Each individual is different. The antidepressant effective for one person may not work as well for another. Several may need to be tried to find the appropriate medication for a specific individual. If side effects are going to occur, they usually appear within the first few weeks. Individualizing medication regimens—that is, finding the most effective dosage and time of day to take the medication—is one approach to reducing side effects. Within two weeks to a month it is usually possible to determine if a particular medication will be effective. Some symptom relief may be evident sooner.

Anxiety and agitation frequently occur with depression. If these symptoms develop after taking an SSRI, they may be side effects of the medication. These symptoms are usually temporary and subside as the body adjusts to the medication. If there are problems with sleep, another antidepressant, Desyrel, may be added. This antidepressant is also helpful in treating agitated depression.

Some antidepressants are proving to be useful in treating other behavior symptoms seen with dementia. Paxil has been effective in treating verbal agitation. Trazodone is used to treat agitation and is helpful in addressing insomnia. Citalopram, a relatively new antidepressant, has been found to be useful in treating fear, panic, irritability, and restlessness, as well as depressed mood. In addition to its effectiveness with depressed mood, Luvox has shown some promise in treating anxiety, irritability, fear, panic, restlessness, and confusion. Results are mixed, but the use of antidepressants in treating behavioral symptoms seen with Alzheimer's disease is encouraging.

Mood and behavioral disturbances are common features of depression and AD. Other psychiatric symptoms can develop with depression that are disturbing and create an even greater load of stress for caregivers. These symptoms include delusions, hallucinations, and agitation. Frequently, behavior management is more difficult because severe sleep disturbances, greater resistance to help, and attempts to leave the household accompany the symptoms. When other approaches are not successful, another pharmacological approach needs to be considered.

Newer forms of major tranquilizers, called atypical antipsychotics, like new antidepressants, are more selective in action and have a better side effect profile than older medications. They are helpful in managing delusions, hallucinations, agitation, aggressiveness resulting form psychosis, and severe sleep disturbances associated with these symptoms.

Nonpharmacological Treatments

Other approaches that do not include antidepressant medications can also be helpful. In many cases, these should be considered before medications if the depression and associated symptoms are mild. Depressed individuals with Alzheimer's disease can benefit from therapy, supportive interactions with caregivers and other family members, exercise, and structured daily activities. Caregiver education about depression and Alzheimer's is important, since the reaction of the caregiver directly affects a love one's adaptation to supportive care for AD and recovery from depression. The following suggestions are supportive actions for needs associated with depression or AD:

- Respond to loved ones with empathy, patience, and unconditional positive regard.

- Show and reassure loved ones that you are there to help and support them.

- Give the impression the two of you can learn to deal with what happens, and when you can't, it's okay, and it may be a good idea to get some help.

- Provide ideas about a few things that might be helpful to think or do. Whenever you see something positive and helpful, let it be known, for example, "I appreciate the way you went on and got dressed early today."

- Reinforce the intrinsic value of the person and avoid being carried away with the negatives of the moment. Things can change if you let them.

- Suggest a positive response to replace a loved one's self-effacing remarks, for example, "I may not be able to do this now, but I'm still a good person," or "I can't do it now, but maybe I will later," instead of "I'm just not worth anything anymore," or "I can't do anything right."

- Identify and increase the number of activities that have been enjoyable, for example, walking, listening to music, doing crafts, visiting friends, or going to a place that is associated with pleasant memories.

- Plan outings with friends who the person enjoys being with to give yourself a break from doing things that have become too tiresome and annoying.

- Choose to do things with a loved one that are more likely to be enjoyable and meaningful to both of you; if an activity is going to be beneficial to you and will have no negative effect on a loved one, do it.

- Help loved ones get started on specific tasks or activities instead of communicating an expectation that is too vague to them. Verbal assistance, physical assistance, and helping the person get started serve as cues for a desired behavior.

- Once the person is involved in the task, encourage and reinforce desirable behavior intermittently to maintain attention and the current level of participation and cooperation.

- Be positive and give meaningful praise and appreciation for attention, effort and completion of tasks and activities. Use a step-wise approach to shape the behaviors that you believe are possible so that you can reward the person each step of the way. These steps also provide helpful cues to move the person onto the next level.

- Have realistic expectations so that the person has a chance for success (increase the positives and decrease the negatives). Depression heightens awareness of negatives, which lead to greater frustration and demoralization. Again, break complex tasks down into simple steps and provide verbal, physical, and visual cues to help a loved one complete a behavior more independently and successfully.

- Having more realistic expectations of loved ones also reduces your own frustration; thus, you feel better about what they are able to do.

- Look at your beliefs about how loved ones (or you for that matter) are doing things. Do you still hold onto expectations that communicate negative messages to them when they cannot succeed at a previous level of functioning?

- Loosen up. So many things that used to be so important, for example, bathing daily, are probably not matters of life and death.

- The individual may be incompetent in terms of skills but is still a person of value. Remind your loved one of his human value and help him understand that one or more diseases are causing the problems and no one blames him.

- Take every opportunity to reward the specific successes loved ones enjoy. Getting a shirt on or finding something may be important to them. Also, let loved ones know you appreciate who they are to you. For example, point out enduring and unique personality traits you notice. Recognition of these characteristics supports their personhood.

- Neither Alzheimer's nor depression is responsible for all problems. Look at what you believe about this. Caregivers—because of how they interpret and respond to needs—may be the source of some problems. We cannot overlook the influence of other health conditions or the effects of the environment as sources of problems.

- Remember that some problems can be corrected and other you must learn to accept.

- Avoid negative and degrading comments, for example, it is more supportive to say, "It will help if you will do this with me now" than "You can't do anything right anymore."

- Create an environment that is familiar, warm, and comfortable and reduces demands and anxieties. Loud noise can be irritating; dark rooms are depressing.

- Provide positive stimulation to offset boredom, loss of interest, and initiative.

- Physical exercise such as walking or performing simple movements regularly is an excellent way to deal with depression and stress (physical exercise is now thought to be a protective factor for Alzheimer's as it has been for other major diseases).

- Build in opportunities for relaxation and rest to offset fatigue and confusion that increase late in the day.

- Engage in topics of conversation that the person can enjoy and relate to. Pictures, music, style of clothes, old cars, jobs, and a train ride long ago can all be useful in triggering memories filled with recognition and meaning (don't make the mistake of overcorrecting or being too picky about accuracy).

- Use a similar approach to trigger memories about the relationship that you share.

- Look for opportunities to find humor in what is happening and lighten things up.
- Laugh *with* or *about,* but not *at.*
- Avoid disturbing relationship and interpersonal situations. Relational factors contribute to depression. The face you wear will be the face loved ones see. They will respond in kind.
- Evaluate your own emotional state and then put more effort into taking care of yourself.

People with Alzheimer's can benefit from therapy. Caregivers can also benefit from therapy and more formalized problem solving. They can learn to think and respond differently to problems when habitual responses are no longer effective. Professional helpers can assist with identifying community resources. They can find new ways to view, interpret, and respond to the situations that are persistent and troublesome.

Therapy is a source of support for both caregivers and the family member identified as "patient" or "client." There may be longstanding problems in the relationship that cannot be handled in the present situation. Dealing with the losses may be especially difficult. Some coping strategies may not only be ineffective but may be a source of problems for caregivers and care recipients. For example, if you have habitually used avoidance to manage problems by keeping them at a distance, you have a greater risk of depression. Nothing is ever solved and problems eventually pile up.

Depression is common with Alzheimer's disease. Treatment reduces distress. Greater disability associated with depression can be reversed and the individual's functioning in daily life can be enhanced. The chance of restoring more positive aspects of the caregiver's relationship is greater as treatment reduces the impact of depression. These factors translate into a better quality of life for persons with AD and the loved ones caring for them.

Grief and Coping

Grief and coping provide hope for suffering and help people adjust to loss and stress. The grieving process may involve some depressive symptoms. It may actually lead to depression because of complications with the mourning process. But grief is a normal process of healing. Grief is a response to loss. People with AD and loved ones face multiple losses. Other losses are not apparent when impaired memory is the focal point. Losses threaten the dignity and sense of worth of persons with Alzheimer's. It is ironic that restrictions to protect them from harm diminish self-esteem and whittle away at their sense of self. We need to understand how they feel about their losses and appreciate their efforts to hold on to self-defining activities and important roles. We need to grasp the differences between coping with issues related to Alzheimer's and being overwhelmed by demands we make of people with AD. Then we can support their adaptation rather than hinder it; affirm their sense of self and personal identity instead of undermine it; lift up their value in our lives rather than negate it.

People with Alzheimer's make efforts to cope with changes that affect them. We may be able to recognize some manifestations of grief that represent coping responses. Some behavioral and emotional responses may be disturbing, yet they represent a person's reaction to losses and threats to self—for example, anger, resentment, shame, and hopeless resignation to change. Too often we view these behaviors as problems we must manage or fix without appreciating their function. They may be windows to an individual's subjective experience. These expressions of self-protection or protest may reveal a great deal more to us about how loved ones are coping—where they are in the process of adapting to the impact the disease has had and will have on what they can do and who they are. What does humiliation and frustration mean to them when they cannot remember how to do something? What is it like to have another person speak for them?

Their sense of identity, or view of self, may be gradually eroded by impaired memory and the losses of meaningful roles, relationships, and activities. Their efforts to cope may help protect sense of self, autonomy, security, comfort, territory, independence, self-worth, competence, or rights. Some of their reactions may represent attempts to prevent subsequent losses. These are more difficult to accept because the reasons for the changes that create the losses cannot be understood.

Sometimes these losses are collectively portrayed as a "loss of self," and it is tempting to view people with advanced dementia as beings who have very little left to suggest who they once were. But there are parts of self that transcend that sense of self saved in memory. The parts of self that extend beyond memory have been called personhood and include feelings, emotions, and reactions of the persons with dementia (Kitwood, 1993). When caregivers place restrictions on activities such as cooking or driving, the agitated response of people with Alzheimer's may be a defense of their identity.

Some of the behavior we label as uncooperative or resistant may be a form of protest. It might represent an attempt to preserve self. We may be able to understand it as a manifestation of grief or another form of adaptation. Then we have the chance to understand what the emotional experience of people with AD means and how it relates to their sense of loss and preservation of personhood. This perspective may be important in addressing depressive symptoms more appropriately.

We examine some views of the grief process. Then we look at how people with Alzheimer's view and adapt to what is happening to them. One view of the grief process addresses how people adapt to loss of self (Cohen, 1991). I don't believe that complete self-loss occurs. Many images that were saved in memory are faded or erased, but there is still much of the person present in emotional responses and moments of clarity and awareness. We need to understand and appreciate the experience of people with Alzheimer's and support their adaptive attempts and coping efforts as they go through the following stages:

Recognition and concern: awareness that something is wrong.

Denial: the belief that "this could not be happening to me."

Anger/guilt/sadness: reaction to "Why is it happening to me?"

Coping: efforts to adapt to what cannot be changed, for example, "If I am to go on with my life, I must . . ."

Maturation: living each day as fully as possible.

Separation from self: sense of self is lost, but needs for attachment continue, and needs for security and comfort increase.

As they struggle to adapt, people with Alzheimer's try to hold on to what makes them unique and vital. We are challenged to treat them as individuals who are still fully vested with all rights of personhood even though they may no longer be able to exercise them. Perhaps by being more aware of how loved ones are trying to cope and how they are trying to accept losses, we can respond to needs of personhood that rise above our concerns about how well they can remember or perform. When we experience a loss of such magnitude, it becomes important to know we are not alone. We feel more secure with the reassurance that our sense of loss is important to another person, especially those who love and respect us. And the person who is closest to us will comfort us. So it is for people with Alzheimer's—in spite of the eventual decay of the memories they have of themselves, these needs remain and may even be greater, as cognitive impairment makes it more difficult for people with this disease to cope with greater unpredictability in a world that is defined by immediacy.

Another view of grief involves the sequence of denial, anger, depression, acceptance, and reconstruction. There are parallels to this in AD. Grief is a dynamic process of healing that takes work, not just time. It does not follow the nice, orderly sequence suggested by stages. The experience may be difficult for people with dementia to complete before the continuity of their experience is fragmented into momentary glimpses of recognition of themselves and a quickly fading view of what was lost.

The disease process itself compromises the abilities that enable us to make some sense of loss and work through it. Impairment of memory, reasoning, and other skills necessary for coping with grief are affected by AD and make successful resolution of losses more difficult. The diagnosis of Alzheimer's may not mean a loss of self. It does, however, create another enigma.

This enigma is born in the changing sense of self. The changes in self-defining activities and roles weaken and fragment the sense of "who one is." So do the impairments intrinsic to the disease. One study of the self in dementia notes that the sense of "who one is" is often in a state of flux (Harris and Sterin et al., 1999). And being ourselves becomes more difficult when others view us as becoming someone different because of things we do that really are not like us.

Losses occur on multiple levels and are another source of this changing sense of self. Imagine how we would be affected by a loss of meaningful roles in our life, loss of independence, loss of competency, loss of respect and self-worth, and loss of memory. Then imagine how we are defined by our relationships with other people. Alzheimer's is the source of these losses. We need to listen to these themes of loss because they are a threat to the personal identity of people with Alzheimer's.

The emotional reactions of people with Alzheimer's can be linked to efforts to maintain their sense of self (Harris and Sterin et al., 1999). They commonly express frustration, embarrassment, humiliation, anger, despondency, fear, disempowerment and uselessness. Sometimes they have these feelings about their losses but direct them toward loved ones or themselves.

People with Alzheimer's use multiple coping strategies to maintain their sense of self and to have a sense of control. Harris and Sterin found that maintaining a daily routine, making lists and keeping a calendar, receiving support from family members, attending support groups, having a sense of humor, and calling on their faith were effective coping strategies. People with other skills and experiences developed coping skills unique to them, which is something that caregivers can examine. There may be coping approaches that loved ones used before the illness that can be employed with a little encouragement and assistance.

Harris and Sterin identified different patterns of dealing with the challenges of the disease and its threat to self. These reactions provide a picture of adaptation based on coping statements that often gave greater direction and purpose to the person's life.

I'll live until I die. People with this belief were fighters who were actively involved in living with the disease. This is a stance in which people with AD take control of the disease and their life the best they can. People with this belief looked for ways to keep control and engaged in activities that defined them.

I accept what I have. These people were surprised with their diagnosis but accepted it and adjusted their new life to it. They did not harm their sense of self by fitting their personal identity into new roles.

There is nothing wrong with me. People with this belief denied their situation and could not accept the diagnosis. The diagnosis was too devastating and they expressed denial as anger toward the people caring for them. They denied symptoms of the disease. Denial was necessary for these people to maintain their sense of self.

I'm just struggling to get through the day. Persons with this perspective were not having much success battling AD. Living with it was overwhelming and they tried to hide the disease from others close to them. They were trying to cope with the impact of having Alzheimer's and understand its effect on self-identity.

I'm giving up. People with this belief were strong but could no longer cope with the disease and remain themselves. Perhaps this means they chose to accept the fate of Alzheimer's. Maybe this belief gave them more freedom. Maybe they gave up and let go of important aspects of themselves.

These statements offer clues that help us understand the basis for some of the behaviors of persons with AD. They are still more than people we used to know. They can be characterized in many ways. We need to find descriptions befitting their personhood. We will be more supportive partners if we have a clearer picture of how loved ones are trying to deal with the disease.

All of the people involved in this study have shared something personal about what it is like to live with progressive memory loss. Self-identity, self-esteem, and self-concept are all at stake. Three values were found to be extremely important for defining a sense of self congruent with whom they had always been. Caregivers should attend to these values in every reasonable way. Persons with Alzheimer's value meaningful productivity, autonomy, and comfort and security. If their identity is to be maintained and these values are to be honored, it will largely be up to others to provide for them. This affirmation of the person will certainly be another way to ease losses and decrease the impact of depression.

4

Possible Causes of Alzheimer's Disease

Many clues to Alzheimer's disease have been identified but have yet to converge on a single causal explanation. There is growing evidence that Alzheimer's is a complex disease caused by multiple factors, and these factors must act in some sequence or combination for the disease to be expressed. The abnormal protein, beta-amyloid, provides a good example. It is associated with at least one genetic cause of the disease and is implicated in causing the death of neurons. Some believe it has a very central and precipitating role in the development of the disease. Despite evidence of its many associations with different aspects of the disease, the role of beta-amyloid remains a topic of intense scientific investigation.

Of the causes being considered, genetic factors are the only ones that definitely cause the disease in a small percentage of cases. Genetic factors and theories concerning slow viruses, the immune system, and brain inflammation are discussed in this chapter. Excess aluminum intake is also discussed.

It also appears highly likely that certain psychosocial factors can influence the development of Alzheimer's disease and the severity of its symptoms. We therefore look at environment, psychiatric history, social and sensory deprivation, and one's sense of support and control.

What Does Not Cause Alzheimer's

A word also seems in order about what does *not* cause Alzheimer's disease. It is not caused by simple old age, hardening of the arteries, or stroke. Most importantly, it is not caused by the person's character or behavior. "Bad" or "lazy" people do not develop Alzheimer's disease any more often than "good"

59

people. No one has ever "deserved" to get Alzheimer's disease. Although caregivers and others struggling to understand the inexplicable may be tempted to create such explanations, perhaps subconsciously, it can only make a difficult situation unnecessarily harder to imagine that the victim or anyone else is to blame for the disease. The seemingly "crazy" behavior of an Alzheimer's victim is brought about by very real physical and chemical changes in the brain (see Chapter 16) over which the person has no control. Let us hope the true causes of these changes and of the disease itself can be identified soon.

The Genetic Theory

Genes and Genetic Factors Linked to Alzheimer's Disease

Genes and genetic factors have significant roles in Alzheimer's disease. Evidence links genes on five chromosomes—1, 12, 14, 19, and 21—to the disease today. In the early 1990s, chromosome 21 held much of the interest of those conducting genetic research. Researchers found evidence of other genes for late-onset Alzheimer's on chromosome 12 (Stephenson, 1997). Although replications have not supported this finding, there are other suspect genes in this area. These will eventually add more to our understanding of AD.

Genetic factors were already known to have a part in the development of other brain diseases. Huntington's chorea and Down's syndrome are two examples. Alzheimer's disease and Down's syndrome have several features in common. The amyloid plaques and neurofibrillary tangles that occur in Alzheimer's disease are found in the brain tissue of individuals with Down's syndrome. Individuals with Down's syndrome invariably develop Alzheimer's disease if they live past age 40. There are extra copies of chromosome 21 in people with Down's syndrome. This association of Alzheimer's with chromosome 21 has brought new energy to genetic inquiry.

Familial Alzheimer's Linked to Chromosome 21

Subsequent research has shown that a genetic defect on chromosome 21 accounts for a pattern of genetic transmission known as autosomal-dominant inheritance in a very small number of families with early-onset Alzheimer's disease (St. George-Hyslop et al., 1987). This research indicates that 50 percent of first degree relatives (parents, brothers or sisters, and children) will develop the disease. The defect on chromosome 21 also includes gene mutations involved in the formation of the abnormal amyloid protein.

APP Gene

The amyloid precursor protein (APP) gene is on the long arm of chromosome 21. It is involved in the daily maintenance of nerve cells and regulates the common brain protein for which it is named, amyloid precursor protein. APP is the parent protein of the amyloid that is found in the plaques and walls of small blood vessels in cases of Alzheimer's disease (DeKosky, 1996). The APP molecule, as it interacts with the nerve cell membrane, gets cut into fragments by two enzymes: beta-secretase and gamma-secretase. One of those fragments results in the abnormal protein, beta-amyloid.

Less than twenty families worldwide have the amyloid precursor protein gene mutations (Roses, 1996).

Members of these families represent less than 10 percent of all early-onset familial Alzheimer's disease—that is, families in which there are multiple cases of Alzheimer's, the onset commonly occurring before age 65. The autosomal-dominant transmission due to genetic defects on chromosome 21 is an example of this type of AD. Early-onset familial Alzheimer's disease is uncommon in the general population and probably comprises less than 5 percent of all Alzheimer's disease cases. Families with the mutation in the amyloid precursor protein gene on chromosome 21 have typical presentations of Alzheimer's except that the age onset is usually in the 40s or 50s. Occasionally, age of onset is in the 60s. The younger age of onset may be associated with the APOE e4 allele.

Familial and Sporadic Cases

Chromosomal links have been sought to explain other family pedigrees in which the disease seemed to be following some pattern of inheritance. A small number of families with some type of inheritance pattern affecting several generations have been identified around the world. In addition to chromosome 21, autosomal-dominant patterns of inheritance have been linked to chromosomes 1 and 14. The familial form of Alzheimer's disease is caused by inheritance of gene mutations linked to these chromosomes. Another gene, apolipoprotein E (apoE), figures in the age of onset primarily in the sporadic form of AD. These cases are of late onset and occur at 60 years or more of age. This gene is on chromosome 19 and is a susceptibility gene, since it influences the age of onset and to a degree a person's risk of having Alzheimer's.

Chromosome 14 has gene mutations in the presenilin 1 gene. Presenilin 1 (PS-1) accounts for the majority of familial AD cases. These represent less than 5 percent of all disease cases; the remaining 95 percent are sporadic with seemingly random occurrence (Roses, 1996). The age of onset for persons with PS-1 is usually in the 40s or early 50s. Onset in the 30s and early 60s has been reported, but onset after age 65 is quite rare. Age of onset is not influenced by apoE. Disease progression is relatively rapid, occurring over a period of 6 to 7 years. These cases are associated with seizures, involuntary muscle contraction (myoclonus), and language deficits.

Less than 1 percent of AD cases are caused by mutations in the presenilin 2 (PS-2) gene on chromosome 1. Most of the families affected are of Volga German ancestry living in the United States, Italian kindred, and one of Spanish descent. The age of onset is much wider and extends from 40 to 75 years. ApoE is not associated with age of onset. The duration of the disease in these cases is 11 years.

Most familial cases are early onset, but findings connected with a gene mutation on chromosome 19 identified both an increased risk for the common late-onset Alzheimer's disease (Corder et al., 1993), and a protein (apolipoprotein E) that binds to beta-amyloid. Thus, three chromosomes (1, 14, and 21) are associated with an autosomal mode of inheritance; another, chromosome 19, is associated with a complex mode that indicates risk or susceptibility to Alzheimer's. The gene on chromosome 12 is also thought to increase susceptibility.

ApoE Genes

The most common type of Alzheimer's disease, late onset (age 65 and older), is primarily a sporadic form of AD. From 50 to 75 percent of late-onset cases are associated with the inheritance of various forms of the apolipoprotein E (apoE) gene, found on chromosome 19 and already well known as a carrier of cholesterol in the blood (Roses, 1996). In addition to being a risk factor for Alzheimer's, apoE is known to have an important role in blood vessel changes and is a risk factor for stroke. In animal studies the apolipoprotein E has been linked to deposits of amyloid in blood vessels of the brain. In humans these deposits develop into a condition called cerebral amyloid angiopathy, which is the cause of about one-third of bleeding strokes. One form of apoE, E4, has been established as a risk factor for AD. Apparently it is a risk factor for cerebral hemorrhage as well because the E4 form is more likely to lead to blood vessel damage in the brain. ApoE may be responsible for this kind of amyloid buildup, which may explain why vascular dementia frequently coexists with Alzheimer's.

There are three forms, or alleles, of the apolipoprotein E gene: apoE2, apoE3, and apoE4. ApoE3 is the most common form in the general population; more than 50 percent of the population has a matched pair of the apoE3 allele. ApoE4 increases the risk of developing Alzheimer's. People who inherit two apoE4 genes—one from the father and one from the mother—are at least eight times more likely to develop the disease than those who have two of the more common apoE3 alleles. Having one or two of the E4 alleles also seems to influence the age at which symptoms develop. The least common allele, apoE2, may actually lower the risk for developing Alzheimer's disease.

ApoE4 and Amyloid

Interest in apoE4 is high for another reason. It binds rapidly and tightly to beta-amyloid; apoE3 does not. The apoE4 protein causes the normally soluble beta-amyloid to become insoluble. This might increase the deposition of beta-amyloid in the brain. ApoE4 is thought to have a role in regulating the very protein from which beta-amyloid is formed—amyloid precursor protein.

Genetic screening

ApoE4 is a risk factor for developing Alzheimer's disease. The general use of tests to identify persons at risk of developing Alzheimer's on the basis of their apoE status is of interest. Predictive testing is available for the autosomal-dominant genes. However, apoE status cannot tell whether someone will get Alzheimer's disease. Some people with the gene do not develop Alzheimer's; others without it do. Having an E4 allele does not definitely predict AD until symptoms are present.

Genetic factors provide the basis for understanding some of the ways Alzheimer's disease develops. Even these, however, do not account for that many cases. Alzheimer's is caused by the interaction among multiple factors. Findings associated with genetics continue to connect more of the numbers in the Alzheimer's puzzle. Other genes, as yet unidentified, are likely to help us make more connections in our understanding of the causes of the disease. Other undetermined factors involving the environment must act as triggers for the development of the disease and interact with genetic factors.

The Viral Theory

An Extremely Slow and Infectious Virus May Be the Cause

Another theory holds that Alzheimer's disease is caused by an extremely slow, infectious virus that may take several decades to incubate. Other neurological disorders have been found to be caused by such viruses; these include kuru, Creutzfeldt-Jakob disease, and Gerstmann-Straussler syndrome (Prusiner, 1984). These viruses are similar to a viral agent that causes the neurological disorder, scrapie, in sheep and goats. This infectious agent, a prion, is much smaller than conventional viruses.

It Has Never Been Shown That Alzheimer's Can Be Transmitted

To prove that such a virus for Alzheimer's disease exists, clinical studies would have to show that the disease can be transmitted. So far, laboratory tests attempting to transmit the disease from brain tissue to animals have failed. It may be, however, that the animals simply were not susceptible to the disease or that the incubation period for the disease is longer than the duration of the studies (Prusiner, 1984). (Kuru and Creutzfeldt-Jakob disease, for example, are known to incubate for 20 to 30 years.) Such a long incubation period would seem consistent with the late age of onset usually found in Alzheimer's.

Some studies have explored the theory that Alzheimer's is caused by a combination of viral and familial/genetic factors. Others have suggested a relationship between amyloid plaques and viral-like agents. Since no hard evidence exists to either confirm or deny the idea that Alzheimer's is caused by a virus, this theory must remain an active area for further research.

The Immune System Theory

Age Is the Strongest Risk Factor

Increasing chronological age is the strongest risk factor for Alzheimer's disease. The elderly tend to get more autoimmune diseases such as cancer, late-onset diabetes, and rheumatoid arthritis (Nandy et al., 1983). Other neurological diseases, including multiple sclerosis and Huntington's chorea, are known to involve immune system alterations; several studies report abnormalities of brain immune function may contribute to the progression of Alzheimer's disease (Peskind, 1996). Loss of neurons and the appearance of plaques and tangles may be partly mediated by mechanisms of the immune system (Rogers et al., 1992).

A chronic inflammatory state affects the AD brain. This is not the inflammation we associate with a wound—the redness, pain, heat, and swelling. It refers to the primary reactions characteristic of the brain's immune response. The possibility exists that an immune system attack might be responsible for much of the neuronal destruction in Alzheimer's disease (McGreer and McGreer, 1996). The inflammatory response of the brain may be associated with the production of beta-amyloid. Inflammation may be a reaction to neurotoxic effects on nerve cells before the serious degeneration. The finding that nonsteriodal anti-inflammatory drugs might decrease the risk of developing Alzheimer's (Breitner and Gau, 1994) lends additional support to the suggestion that altered brain immune function is somehow involved. Even with evidence that the basic processes of immune response and inflammation can be observed in the Alzheimer's brain, one important question remains. Do immune mechanisms in this disease merely reflect natural processes that help the damaged brain heal, or might these mechanisms be a source of the damage (Rogers et al., 1992)?

The Aluminum Theory

High Levels of Aluminum in the Brain May Cause Alzheimer's

Some researchers have theorized that neurofibrillary tangles in Alzheimer's disease and other dementias could be caused by an excess of aluminum in the brain. The concentration of aluminum in the human brain is known to increase with age (Yates, 1979; Jenike, 1985). Abnormally high levels of aluminum have been found in the brains of persons suffering from other dementias (Thienhaus, 1985), though these may well be unrelated to the disease. Together these indications suggest that high levels of aluminum may possibly be related to Alzheimer's disease, though there is certainly no conclusive proof.

Chelation Therapy Not Proven Helpful

Some health practitioners advertise chelation therapy and imply that this therapy will reduce aluminum levels and thus improve the impairments that characterize Alzheimer's disease. Chelation is a chemotherapeutic treatment for metal poisoning. There is simply no scientific support for using chelation for Alzheimer's treatment. Often these clinics fail to properly diagnose Alzheimer's disease, assuming that the patient's problems are caused by treatable "vascular dementia." Since chelation therapy is expensive, can produce serious side effects, and has never been proved to help Alzheimer's patients, such treatment should be discouraged. Too often it simply drains the pocketbooks of families desperate for a cure.

Concern about aluminum has led many families to worry about the risks of using aluminum cookware and aluminum-rich antacids and other medications. Though there is no evidence that prolonged use of these products affects Alzheimer's in any way, some researchers suggest that people may wish to request medications with less aluminum from their doctors (Shore and Wyatt, 1983) if their medications are extremely high in this element.

Psychosocial Factors and Dementia

Negative Psychosocial Factors Create Obstacles

Psychosocial factors can have powerful effects, both positive and negative, on everyone. On the positive side, such things as an adequate income, consistent family support, and a comfortable home environment make caring for a person with dementia much less burdensome. On the negative side, serious health problems, excessive family conflicts, and the absence of daily routines can create obstacles in the care of and adjustment to Alzheimer's disease. Viewed in this context, psychosocial factors can have a definite relationship to how a person with Alzheimer's disease will fare in the long run.

In addition, feelings about the causes of the disease can influence both the caregivers' attitudes and those of the family toward Alzheimer's patients. Family members sometimes wonder whether there is anything in their relative's history that could have caused or contributed to his or her condition. Family members sometimes blame severe, recent illnesses for precipitating symptoms of dementia. However, if their relative's condition meets criteria for Alzheimer's disease, these other medical problems will have already been ruled out as the cause of the dementia.

Medical Trauma Can Precipitate Symptoms

We have seen a few cases in which the aftermath of traumatic medical conditions or reactions to severe losses or psychosocial stressors seem to contribute to the progression of Alzheimer's disease. Sometimes, a person traumatized by serious medical conditions will begin to exhibit symptoms of dementia. Usually, these symptoms preceded the illness in a very subtle form, but become more pronounced afterward. Additionally, unlike the hospital-type delirium that occurs with older persons, these symptoms do not disappear. In fact, the person's intellectual and memory abilities not only fail to return but continue to deteriorate. These medical conditions do not cause Alzheimer's disease; they simply precipitate a worsening of the process.

Reactions to the Loss of a Spouse Can Hide Symptoms of Dementia

In the case of reactions to losses or other stressors, the most common situation is the loss of a spouse. Prior to the spouse's death, the surviving spouse will often seem to be handling things relatively well, considering the demands of care and the emotional adjustment. Any subtle symptoms of dementia can be explained as normal reactions to the circumstances. We have also seen cases where the medically ill spouse was the "cognitive" manager of the care situation. He or she kept household activities, bills, and medications under control. These persons, even though physically ill, were caregivers in a sense for the spouse who was later found to have an Alzheimer's-type dementia. When this significant other dies or goes to a nursing home, the spouse left at home may experience substantial loss of organization, routine, and support. Grief and/or depression may be observed.

The grief or depression may not immediately appear, but it may emerge later as reactions to coping with dramatic life changes. It may be difficult initially to determine whether the impairments of memory and intellectual abilities are the symptoms of dementia or reactions to what has happened. Pseudodementia may be present in the form of depression, which can coexist with Alzheimer's disease.

Medical problems and significant psychosocial losses can enhance the symptoms of Alzheimer's disease. Again, these events do not cause the disease; they accentuate symptoms that were already developing insidiously.

No Connection Between Past Events and Alzheimer's Disease

Families sometimes try to blame psychosocial stressors or other past events in a person's life for Alzheimer's disease, even though there is no connection. Relative's beliefs at times center on things that should or should not have been done (e.g., he should have worked harder, or he worked too hard). Family members may point to some specific event in the past that brought about changes in their relative's behavior. For example, they may say their relative never was the same after his parents died or after he lost a job 15 years ago or after he had a knock-down drag-out fight with his brother. They may try to resurrect these problems as explanations for Alzheimer's disease. Behavioral changes, indeed, may have occurred in their relative after these kinds of events, yet there is no reason to believe these events caused the degenerative brain disease.

When a person affected by Alzheimer's disease has had a troubled life long before the illness began, there may be considerable hard feelings and conflicts within his family. Family members may be both bitter and resentful of things they believe their affected relative did to them or others. In this case, what the family says is the cause for Alzheimer's disease, they really think of as deserved punishment. Hostility and anger can erupt, and caregiving may be difficult for such family members to provide. This situation increases the risk for abuse. However, the affected relative's "sin" of commission or omission did not cause the Alzheimer's-type condition.

The family adjustment process can sometimes bring up beliefs about why the loved one has developed Alzheimer's disease. These beliefs, unlike those just described, usually represent family members' attempts to come to terms with this illness.

A History of Psychiatric Problems Does Not Increase Risk

People who have had psychiatric problems are not necessarily more susceptible to Alzheimer's disease. However, some families may believe that psychiatric illnesses, such as chronic depression, are responsible for later brain disorders. There is virtually no evidence for this contention. One research report suggests that persons with Alzheimer's disease do seem to have a higher incidence of psychiatric episodes, especially depression, which occur much earlier than the onset of the disease's symptoms (Agbayewa, 1986).

Psychiatric Episodes Often Precursors to More Obvious Symptoms of Dementia

The author of this research suggests that the psychiatric episodes could conceivably represent prodromal stages of the illness. In addition to depression, paranoid disorders were strongly implicated as potential forerunners of the

Alzheimer's type dementia (Agbayewa, 1986). This area of research should be continued; however, the reported findings should be viewed cautiously. Currently, only depressive symptoms like loss of interest and lack of initiative have been identified as possible prodromal signs of AD.

Psychiatric symptoms can be manifested during the course of Alzheimer's disease. Delusions, hallucinations, agitation, anxiety, depression, and catastrophic reactions can all occur. Psychiatric manifestations, their intensity and duration, can vary from one individual to another. The environment, which includes the family, has some influence.

Sensory Impairments Contribute to Hallucinations and Delusions

Sensory impairments such as existing visual and hearing problems contribute to individual variations. For instance, persons with significant hearing impairment can be more susceptible to auditory hallucinations, even when they do not have Alzheimer's disease. Limitations in reasoning and interpretation of sounds in Alzheimer's create a greater chance of hallucinations, and delusions sometimes develop out of these hallucinations.

Hallucinations represent an abnormality in perception. These misperceptions occur without any external evidence of what is reported to have been experienced through the senses: hearing, vision, touch, smell, and taste. While the external reality validating the hallucination does not exist, the sensory evidence of the hallucination is very real to people having this experience. Sometimes it is a relief for these people to know that while the experience is real to them, it is not really happening: Their hearing or vision is distorted for some reason. It's comforting for them to know that they are safe and you will not let anyone or anything hurt them. Hallucinations should be distinguished from illusions. Illusions involve a misperception of an external stimulus. Illusions, like hallucinations, are more common in the advanced stages of Alzheimer's.

Delusions represent an abnormality in thought. These false beliefs cannot be explained by either established facts or the person's cultural background and beliefs. Delusional beliefs can be so fixed that no factual evidence contradicting the belief will be accepted. Frequently, people with strong and fixed delusional beliefs become angry and vehement when these beliefs are challenged because they feel they are being attacked personally. Individuals with Alzheimer's disease develop delusions. Disease-related impairments of memory, cognition, and the loss of the capacity to reason and logically solve problems contribute to this condition. Delusions are more common in the middle to late stages of the disease.

Several delusions are common. People with AD accuse family and friends of stealing their personal possessions when they are unable to locate them. When the false belief that someone is stealing from them becomes entrenched, people with Alzheimer's sometimes put more effort into hiding things in illogical places, thus reinforcing the belief that things are being stolen because even caregivers cannot find them. Blaming others for stealing things is an attempt to account for the AD person's inability to understand memory deficits.

Another delusion seen in persons with AD is particularly painful to spouses who have made caring for loved ones the center of their shrinking world. A person with AD may accuse her spouse of having an affair, often with a friend or neighbor or other person who has not been forgotten. This belief may be a response to the insecurity and social disconnection that result from memory loss and other impairments of brain function. Sometimes these impairments dismantle the familiarity and intimacy that have been a basis for trust. Agnosia is one such impairment. It disturbs the ability to recognize familiar persons, places, and things. Delusional beliefs may develop because of it. Family members may be accused of being imposters. The person with AD demands to know what you (her spouse) have done with her spouse. The face or voice of a person to whom she has been married for 50 years becomes unrecognizable.

Personality factors enter into psychiatric symptoms accompanying Alzheimer's disease. By the time an individual develops this condition, his personality traits are well defined. Enduring characteristics of the person, how he behaves socially, and how he typically responds to situations are indicators of his personality. Suspicious and paranoid types may become more agitated and distrustful when they have Alzheimer's disease. A person who has always been dependent will become more dependent and insecure.

A Familiar, Well-Organized, Comfortable Environment Minimizes Coping Problems

Environmental factors, including physical arrangement and social and psychological overtones, exert considerable influences on how individuals cope with Alzheimer's disease. The caregiving environment will also determine to a degree the effectiveness and endurance of the caregiver. A familiar, well-organized, and comfortable environment can be supportive of Alzheimer's care. Good lighting during the day and enough lighting at night to help the patient find the bathroom can be helpful. Later, signs can be used to indicate the bathroom door. A poster with important reminders, names, and phone numbers can increase the security of some Alzheimer's patients when the caregiver must be gone for a short while. The house can be secured at night to prevent the patient's wandering outside the home. Additionally, the household can be run in a calm, relaxed manner to reduce unnecessary noise and unsettling distractions.

Social Contact Important for Both Patient and Caregiver

Complete social isolation is harmful for both the caregiver and the patient. Outside social contact need not be lengthy for the Alzheimer's patient, but some degree of consistency from friends and other family helps maintain a sense of a social bond. For example, the length of visits can be preset and arranged to include both the patient and the caregiver. When the patient begins to tire and withdraw somewhat from the conversation, the visitor can spend some focused time with the caregiver, satisfying both persons' need for social interaction. At times, those who have Alzheimer's disease are self-conscious about their limitations and may leave the room even when visitors are still there. Both visitors and caregiver should accept the departure without protest; the patient should not be forced to stay. Additionally, caregivers need to reassure the affected relatives that they are loved and accepted in spite of the disease.

Psychological Environment

The psychological environment should be encouraging and supportive. A calm atmosphere has a more relaxing effect on both the patient and the caregiver. Of course, some stimulation and activity must be preserved according to the capabilities of the person receiving the care. Too many demands may create more restlessness and agitation. The affected relative should no longer be held accountable for many of his mistakes and errors in judgment. The caregiver's insistent correction can result in more reactive responses from the patient. Any opportunity to support the self-esteem of the Alzheimer's patient must be acted upon. Meaningful rewards are important, even for helping with the smallest of tasks.

In this book, a great deal of emphasis is placed on the beliefs of family members concerning the changed behavior of their affected relative. When families can understand more of their relative's behavior from the perspective of brain impairment, they can relate more successfully to that behavior. Their responses can be more sensitive without as much anger and frustration. Uninformed and overburdened caregivers have attributed intricate intellectual plans to loved ones, believing that the brain-impaired person consciously followed these plans to get what he wanted or to repay the caregiver for some supposed insult. It is questionable whether an Alzheimer's patient can respond in such a premeditated manner. It is more likely he is reacting to something in the environment or to his own misinterpretations.

Isolation Has a Profound Effect on Elderly Persons

From our community work in geriatric mental health, we have seen the profound effects that isolation can have on the elderly. They are referred to us for treatment when they seem to be a danger to themselves or seem unable to provide for their most basic needs. Most often family or neighbors notice unusual or frightening behavior and call us for help. When we go to the home to check out these reports, we often find the house in disarray, cans of open food in the cabinets, decomposing items in the refrigerator, and unopened take-out lunches from the senior center on the counter. Sometimes we find the person just lying on the floor in a heap. In some instances, these people may be defensive when they see us, but often they try to be cordial and friendly. They are bewildered by troubles they cannot seem to handle on their own, but they are frightened to allow strangers to help them (a reasonable response even if the strangers are part of a geriatric mental health team).

In these cases, symptoms of dementia are often present. Many of these persons will eventually be diagnosed as having Alzheimer's disease. Occasionally, reversible medical conditions or pseudodementia are found to be responsible for the functional impairments.

Hearing and Visual Impairments Contribute to Isolation

Hearing and visual impairments often contribute to isolation in the elderly. Sensory and social deprivations are known to have a significant impact on a person's functioning, and in the elderly individual with dementia, they may play a role in precipitating delusions and hallucinations. Interestingly, the hallucinations and delusions in this context may be attempts at creating stimulation in a world that has shrunk to the parameters of a couple of rooms. The isolated person with dementia is stuck between the insecurity of memory problems and the fear of other people taking over his life.

Reaction to Nursing Home Placement Influenced by Benefits Perceived in the Move

Eventually the Alzheimer's patient may have to be placed in a nursing home or other 24-hour facility. Placing a family member in a nursing home is a difficult decision. Relocation effects on the patient are influenced by the person's perception of loss of control along with other aspects of the move.

Thus, it is *how* the living situation changes, not the change itself, that is important. If the relocation improves the person's living situation, its effects will not be detrimental. For example, persons make a better adjustment to a nursing home relocation if they perceive the care as better, have easier accessibility to their physician, have meaningful things to do, and have the opportunity to make friends.

These factors increase security and, consequently, the person's sense of control, because there is more positively defined predictability in his life. However, of the factors that indicate quality, one is more significant than all the others: the extent of social support the person perceives himself to receive. It is the emotional response induced by the change, not the change itself, that is vital (Henry, 1986).

More advanced Alzheimer's patients do not have the intellectual capacity necessary to adjust to a new environment without considerable assistance. However, they may relate most often—at a basic emotional level—to what is happening to and around them, as their ability to reason and make intellectual judgments fades.

These observations have applications to caregiving even when there is no relocation in the immediate future. A strong sense of social support is critical to persons with Alzheimer's disease whether they are living in nursing homes or in their own homes. Deprived environments can precipitate excessive disability and learned helplessness, while supportive and stimulating environments encourage individuals to maintain more control of their life and be a little more involved in the world outside of themselves.

Uncertainty and Risk

Not knowing what causes Alzheimer's is a psychosocial factor of the disease that often has negative effects on dementia patients and their caregivers. Family history has been a known risk factor; persons who have a first-degree relative with Alzheimer's may have a fourfold increase in risk for getting the disease (Weiner and Gray, 1996). Women have a higher risk than men do. Aging is the best-established risk factor. The older we get, the greater our chances of developing the disease.

Other risk factors have been identified: head injury associated with hospitalization or loss of consciousness, history of severe depression, history of Parkinson's disease in a first-degree relative, and possibly advanced maternal age (Katzman, 1996). Lower educational level may increase the risk; more years of formal education may delay or decrease the chance of developing Alzheimer's later in life. Anti-inflammatories and estrogen have been implicated as having a role in reducing risk.

Culture and environment may carry risk factors. For example, a recent study has drawn the tentative conclusion that Japanese American men who have moved from Japan to Hawaii are more susceptible to developing Alzheimer's disease (White et al., 1996). Another example of the role of environment is seen in twin studies. Identical twins are genetically the same, but AD develops in only about half of identical twin pairs. When identical twins develop Alzheimer's, their age at time of diagnosis may differ by as much as 15 years. Environmental factors appear to influence genetic predisposition. Some research suggests that African Americans and Hispanics have a higher risk for developing AD. The apoE4 allele may be a source of some of the increased risk. It is not clear how culture or environment accounts for these differences.

Most negative and positive risk factors are beyond our control. There is one notable exception: educational level. It appears that there is some degree of truth to the old idea that we will lose our mental capacity if we fail to use it. Learning at any age is generative or regenerative from a neurobiological perspective.

Community Resources

For this long moment in time, while we wait for a cure or treatment, we must use what we know to make the lives of individuals with Alzheimer's disease as well as the family caregivers safer and more meaningful. Other approaches to long-term care must be developed. Many communities are still lacking the resources to support Alzheimer's services, such as day and respite care. Families often feel less helpless in dealing with this illness if they are involved in support groups. Political action has already paid off for Alzheimer's research, but more research and care options are needed. Families can work with their own legislators or city officials to gather more support for funding vital services. Area agencies on aging can help develop options.

Families Must Not Be Afraid to Seek Available Help

Just doing something about the situation often counteracts feelings of helplessness and hopelessness. Families must be willing to seek help when they need it, particularly when help is available. Certainly Alzheimer's disease can be described in tragic terms, but there are other tragedies that can often be prevented. One example is the suffering that families experience when they are unwilling to seek help that is available. Another example is the suffering added to the lives of persons experiencing or dealing with Alzheimer's disease by insensitive professionals who project their own hopelessness onto those they are charged with helping. Such needless pain can and must be prevented.

5

Six Common Myths
About Alzheimer's

Many misconceptions exist about the nature of Alzheimer's disease. Lacking adequate information about the disease, families commonly hold mistaken notions about the disease itself, old age, and their own role in caring for the person with Alzheimer's. In addition, they may harbor unnecessary fears about the likelihood that they will inherit the disease from their relative.

Because our beliefs are the basis for our actions, it is important that families have an accurate understanding of Alzheimer's and its significance. The following are some of the most common myths about Alzheimer's, followed by a correct assessment of the pertinent issues.

Myth 1: Alzheimer's Symptoms Are a Normal Sign of Old Age

Some of the early symptoms of Alzheimer's, such as forgetfulness, do correspond to our common notions of aging; but Alzheimer's is a disease and should not be confused with the aging process. This becomes clear as the disease progresses and the person's deterioration becomes more dramatic.

In terms of memory loss, for example, it is true that a degree of increased forgetfulness commonly accompanies aging. Older persons may find it more difficult to recall the details of past events. However, the memory loss caused by Alzheimer's is far more severe and progressive in nature. Eventually the disease destroys not just the memory of details but all memory of the event itself. The person in time will forget not only the events of the past but what she did that morning, who her spouse is, where she lives, even her own name. These are not the normal consequences of aging.

Myth 2: Senility Is the Usual Cause of Problems in Old Age

Senility is a blanket term that has long been used to cover a wide-ranging variety of symptoms. In this sense, it is a damaging notion and a term to be avoided. An assumed diagnosis of senility obscures the real problem at hand and increases the difficulty of getting correct treatment for the older person's condition or impairment. The older person may assume her condition is irreversible, when treatment may in fact be readily available. In addition, the myth of senility reinforces the negative and mistaken belief that all persons must become helpless and useless with age.

Common Hearing and Visual Problems Produce Misleading Views

If an older person has difficulty relating to others or conducting her affairs, many problems other than senility or Alzheimer's disease may be the source. For example, the person may suffer from impaired hearing or vision. Her failure to clearly follow a conversation or respond to something in the environment may make it seem that her thought processes are impaired, when actually she has simply not seen or heard what happened. Additionally, the impaired person may begin to avoid situations where her problem is most apparent or troublesome. A person who is hard of hearing may avoid crowds, while a person with poor sight may become confused in social situations because everyone's face looks the same. Often older persons are unwilling to admit these impairments, which can add to confusion about the source of their problems.

Medical Problems Produce Emotional and Behavioral Changes Labeled as Senility

Medical conditions also may be at the root of the older person's problems. Congestive heart failure may cause weakness, fatigue, mental confusion, forgetfulness, and other symptoms mistaken for senility. Hyperthyroidism may cause apathy, depression, lethargy, impaired memory, and slow responses in the elderly. Hypothyroidism has similar symptoms in the elderly, with weakness and fatigue a little more prominent. Both of these illnesses have a slow, progressive onset similar to that of Alzheimer's disease. Persons suffering from these problems should receive a full medical evaluation, and family members should not just assume that the problem is old age.

Other conditions that may be confused with Alzheimer's include B_{12} deficiencies, pernicious anemia, electrolyte imbalances, normal pressure hydrocephalus, hypoglycemia, and a range of infections. Infections of the urinary system, for example, may cause confusion, apathy, and inattentiveness before other symptoms are apparent. It is therefore essential that experienced medical personnel rule out all other possible causes for the older person's problems before arriving at a diagnosis of Alzheimer's.

Medications

Often medication prescribed for a medical condition can cause side effects similar to Alzheimer's symptoms, such as confusion, forgetfulness, tremors, and slower responses. This can be a particular problem when the older person is taking several medications at one time to treat different conditions. If problems are apparent, they should be brought promptly to the attention of the doctor or doctors involved. When a number of doctors and pharmacies are involved with different medications, there is a greater chance that medication-related problems will develop. It is therefore extremely important to provide all professionals involved with an up-to-date regimen of medications.

Depression

Psychological problems such as depression often are passed off as senility as well. It is common for older persons to experience some depression as they face the loss of health, friends, spouse, home, as well as their own death. Such major life changes late in life may lead to mental conditions requiring a psychiatrist's care, such as severe depression, anxiety, or paranoia. The person may not seem "crazy," but fear and insecurity in the face of real losses or perceived threats may be interfering with her ability to effectively cope with life.

Depression can in turn lead to complaints about memory problems. The person may see even minor memory lapses as evidence that she is becoming senile. In fact, however, she may simply be suffering from lapses in attention and concentration caused by the depression. One difference between the symptoms of depression and those of Alzheimer's is that, while the depressed person may not recognize her depression, she will rarely deny the resulting problems. Alzheimer's victims, in contrast, tend to deny all evidence of the disease.

A Belief in Senility Stops People from Seeking Help

The myth of senility and the lack of dignity associated with it often prevent older persons from seeking treatment for conditions that are in fact reversible. Family members should encourage older persons to seek medical treatment for the problems they encounter and should not let them assume that senility is a necessary consequence of old age.

Myth 3: Nothing Can Be Done for the Person with Alzheimer's

Proper Care Important in the Management of the Illness

It is true that at present we have no cure for Alzheimer's disease. The disease is progressive and leads ultimately to death. However, there is much that can be done to make the victim's last months or years more meaningful, pleasant, and comfortable.

Medical Care

Alzheimer's patients benefit from both proper medical care and informed behavior management. Thus, the family should involve health professionals in their loved one's care as early as possible, and they should continue to seek professional opinions throughout the disease.

Psychiatric Care

Psychiatrists and other mental health professionals can successfully treat the depression or other psychological symptoms that frequently develop. Doctors and nutritionists can provide help with meal preparation, special diets, and nutritional supplements as the person's appetite and eating abilities deteriorate. Careful attention to the use of medications will prevent unnecessary and prolonged side effects.

Other Medical Problems

Treatment of coexisting medical problems is also very important. It should not be assumed that all of the person's physical and mental symptoms are caused by the disease. Persons with Alzheimer's are especially vulnerable to the common viruses, colds, and infections that affect us all, including pneumonia, and these conditions should receive prompt medical attention.

Myth 4: Alzheimer's Is Strictly a Mental Illness

Psychiatric Symptoms

Many of the changes initially observed in the Alzheimer's patient seem to be personality disorders or other psychological problems. Furthermore, because Alzheimer's disease primarily affects the brain, it is in a sense a "mental" illness. However, Alzheimer's disease is a degenerative medical condition and not a psychiatric disorder.

Psychiatric symptoms are a significant part of the illness. As the brain gradually loses its capacity to perform normal functions we take for granted, the individual becomes increasingly insecure and unable to relate to her daily world. In time her personality is completely altered.

Psychiatric or Medical Condition?

Society's recognition of the medical nature of Alzheimer's is fairly recent, yet confusion about whether it is a mental or medical illness still occurs. This is frequently seen in the errors that occur in insurance billings. Insurance payments can vary significantly depending on whether Alzheimer's is coded as a psychiatric or medical condition. Fortunately, the diagnosis and treatment of behavioral problems, psychiatric problems, family counseling, and psychological counseling are usually covered. Again, problems with coverage are more likely to be related to how services are coded, who provides the service, and who is listed as the provider of the service. There are Medicare and Medicaid restrictions on what is allowable service when the person with Alzheimer's is not expected to benefit from the service—for example, Medicare will not cover psychotherapy because the person with AD would not benefit because he or she is cognitively impaired. Many coverage issues have not yet been resolved, and they reflect the insurance companies' strictly medical view of needs. Insurance claim staff should be able to answer questions about coverage when caregivers are setting up an appointment with a professional service provider. The Alzheimer's Association has a good Web site discussion of "Insurance Coverage and Reimbursement" and related topics at **http://www.alz.org/hc/insurance.htm**. They also have a Medicare Advocacy Project listed.

Misleading Diagnostic Findings of Good Health

The impression that Alzheimer's is a mental illness may be supported when a diagnosis of general "good health" is coupled with a diagnosis of Alzheimer's disease. What medical professionals mean by such a diagnosis, however, is that no other medical problems have been found, or other conditions are so successfully controlled that the individual is in otherwise satisfactory health.

Myth 5: Only the Family Should Care for the Person with Alzheimer's

Family Care Is Supportive and Necessary

In most cases, it is certainly best if the affected person can stay at home with her spouse or family as long as possible. The love and regular interaction a family can provide usually helps the person retain her abilities longer and helps ease her difficult adjustment to the disease.

Other Resources

However, not all spouses or children have the resources to care properly for their loved one. Even those who do have the resources eventually may have to call upon outside care when the disease reaches its later stages and caregiving becomes an utterly exhausting experience.

Caregivers Should Be Careful About Overinvolvement

Overinvolvement, or the feeling that the caregiver must do everything herself, is a common reaction to the disease. Often it represents a stage in the family member's adjustment to the disease (see Chapter 9). The caregiver imagines that she can hold back the disease by doing everything herself, and her grief leads her to become extremely protective of the person with Alzheimer's. She may also feel reluctant to seek outside help because of shame and the stigmas associated with mental conditions.

Primary Caregivers Must Accept Help

However, the family, and in particular the primary caregiver, must learn to accept help. The burden of caring for an Alzheimer's patient can otherwise cause serious problems for the caregiver and alienate her from friends and family who want to share the caregiving role. The caregiver should not hesitate to call upon community resources as well, such as those discussed in detail in Chapter 15. Without these resources, the burden of care can become overwhelming.

Myth 6: All Relatives of People with Alzheimer's Are Likely to Inherit the Disease

Facts of Genetic Risk

It is common for relatives of people with Alzheimer's to be concerned that they may have a genetic predisposition toward the disease. When the first edition of this book was published in 1988, a few families in which early-onset Alzheimer's (before age 65, usually starting in the 40s or 50s) was documented were known to have a pattern of autosomal-dominant inheritance. If one parent had a defective gene, each child had a 50 percent chance of inheriting the gene. These persons would not necessarily develop the disease at an early age, or ever develop it. For the individuals at risk in this family, waiting determined whether they developed AD.

Familial Alzheimer's Disease

The families knew, however, that some members would eventually develop familial Alzheimer's because members of other generations were known to have had it. From one generation to the next, the disease continued to appear in yet another family member. Early-onset Alzheimer's cases are likely to represent this form of the disease. It may develop in some persons when they are in their early 30s.

Early-Onset Alzheimer's

These early-onset forms of familial Alzheimer's disease with autosomal-dominant inheritance are rare. They are associated with mutations of genes on three different chromosomes: 1 (presenilin 2 gene), 14 (presenilin 1 gene), and 21 (amyloid precursor protein gene). Members of these families may have a basis for concern. Family history of known or suspected Alzheimer's must be documented. It may not be easy or even possible in some family histories to track and document instances of Alzheimer's disease. Genetic mutations are not identified in all early-onset cases. It is likely there are still other genes to be identified for this form of the disease. Since other early-onset cases appear to be more sporadic; interaction between both genetic and nongenetic factors may be present.

Late-Onset Alzheimer's

For late-onset (age 65 and older) Alzheimer's disease it has been more difficult to establish the role of genetic inheritance. Experts estimate that roughly 98 percent of patients develop late-onset Alzheimer's (Stephenson, 1997). Some late-onset familial and sporadic forms of the disease have been linked to the apoE gene on chromosome 19. There are three forms, or alleles, of this gene: E2, E3, and E4. ApoE4 accounts for about 50 percent of late-onset Alzheimer's disease and is the form of apoE that increases a person's susceptibility to the disease. Persons with familial and sporadic forms of AD have this gene, and whether a person has one or two E4 genes influences the degree of the risk, as well as at what age Alzheimer's disease develops.

Late-Onset Alzheimer's Is Genetically Complex

Late-onset Alzheimer's is beginning to look like a more genetically complex disease. While the apoE4 allele influences when susceptible complex persons might develop AD, in persons who survive to very old age (about age 84 and older), it has no bearing on whether they will develop the disease (Meyer et al., 1998). Late-set Alzheimer's may involve other genetic influences. There is very good reason to continue the search for other genetic evidence linked to the most common form of the disease. Some of these genetic factors may be on chromosome 12. One of several possibilities involves a protein called alpha 2-macroglobulin produced by a protease inhibitor gene in a region of chromosome 12 (Blacker et al., 1998). This genetic finding suggests another potential factor that carries susceptibility for late-onset AD. Genetic research has given us a better view of what is involved in Alzheimer's, and there are likely other genes that confer risk.

Genetic Tests

The identification of the apoE gene and its association with Alzheimer's has created interest in the use of a genetic screening test that might identify or predict AD risk. ApoE is not a consistent biological marker for the disease; screening for it would miss some persons with Alzheimer's and falsely identify others. For this reason, a public policy statement concerning genetic testing was issued at a conference sponsored by the National Institute on Aging and Alzheimer's Association in October 1995. ApoE testing is appropriate for use in research settings that incorporate much broader protocols for diagnostic purposes and consider apoE testing only when persons are concerned about symptoms suggesting AD. Genetic counseling is recommended for research volunteers and their families so that they can learn about the genetics of the disease, the tests being used, and the meaning of results.

For families facing the possibility or the very real fact of an inherited form of Alzheimer's, involvement with research centers provides the chance for information, care, and support. They can see that, although the numbers may be small, other families are also dealing with the ongoing plague that AD unleashes on them. Family members who collaborate with researchers in a meaningful way and feel they are making a contribution may gain a greater sense of mastery over this part of their life.

6

Coping: A Step-by-Step Guide to the Caregiver's Experience

A Hypothetical Case History

Eleanor is becoming increasingly concerned about her husband Bill. He has made some errors in his checkbook, which are uncharacteristic, and twice recently he has gotten lost driving in unfamiliar parts of town. Yet when she brings her concerns up, he becomes angry and denies everything. At first, she associated these problems with getting old. Bill does have early cataracts and does not see well. But now he is becoming suspicious of her and the neighbors. Recently she was shocked when he confronted a neighbor about stealing tools out of the garage. He had never done anything like that before.

During the last few years, Eleanor has heard a great deal about Alzheimer's disease. She is afraid that something like that might be happening to Bill. Her husband is slowly changing, and she feels a growing pressure to do something. But what? Should she talk to the family doctor or a psychiatrist? It has always been difficult to get Bill to see a doctor, and Bill keeps insisting that he has no problems. Bill's behavior is becoming embarrassing to Eleanor, which makes her reluctant to do things with her friends. She does not know how to tell the children about her fears, and since they both live out of state, they have not seen for themselves what is happening to their father. Whenever Eleanor thinks about the changes in Bill, she feels alone and afraid.

Responding to Alzheimer's Symptoms Is Difficult

Eleanor's predicament is typical of the difficult situation in which relatives of persons in the early stages of Alzheimer's often find themselves. They feel certain that something is very wrong, but they do not know what they should do to help. Never having experienced anything like this before and afraid that the problem may be more serious than they can bear, they feel at a loss to identify the first step.

Knowing What Lies Ahead Helps

This chapter seeks to alleviate the confusion and anxiety that caregivers experience by offering a step-by-step guide to the process of coping with Alzheimer's disease. It outlines the steps that caregivers will need to take and offers helpful, practical advice for what to do at each stage. By clearly identifying the disease process and the challenges that lie ahead for the caregiver, the information in this chapter aims to relieve the anxiety caregivers feel in facing an unknown threat. The following are the steps discussed in depth in this chapter:

1. Noticing initial symptoms
2. Confirming suspicions
3. Seeking information
4. Taking action
5. Weighing findings
6. Identifying resources
7. Planning care
8. Managing caregiver stress

1. Noticing Initial Symptoms

All illnesses have symptoms. If the problem is a physical one, the symptoms are likely to be familiar physical complaints such as fever, headache, nausea, fatigue, and specific areas of pain. The signs of mental illness can be more difficult to identify, yet symptoms are still present. Persons suffering from depression, for example, may not recognize that they are depressed, yet they often report symptoms. Similarly, persons with Alzheimer's may experience symptoms but fail to attribute them to a brain condition.

Early Symptoms

With Alzheimer's, symptoms observed early in the illness are likely to be behavioral or emotional, and the person's distress is usually psychological. He probably will not associate his initial problems with an intellectual function such as memory or suspect that a serious illness is the cause. Though a spouse or other relative may observe slight changes in the person's normal behavior, it is difficult to take these changes seriously at first.

Denial of Symptoms

The affected person may feel that acknowledging his difficulties would create unnecessary worries for his family or place his job in jeopardy. He may feel that he can overcome these problems if he tries harder.

Often, when he discovers that he can do little about his memory problems, he will become noticeably anxious, frustrated, and irritable, with the possibility of depression developing. It is common for the affected person to point out memory lapses of other family members to distract attention from his own growing difficulties.

Symptoms Become Harder to Ignore

However, the person's memory problems, as well as his emotional and behavioral reactions, will begin eventually to create genuine concern among family members. They will begin to wonder if perhaps the changes and deficiencies they are noticing might be symptoms of something larger.

2. Confirming Suspicions

Families Must Seek Professional Help

Families usually discuss early concerns with other family and friends first. As initial doubts become more persistent, they generally feel a need to share their concerns with a health professional who can positively confirm or deny their suspicions.

It is important to consult a health professional as soon as possible, since a preliminary medical consultation will:

- Clarify the seriousness of the problems
- Verify the need for action
- Ensure prompt treatment even if the condition is not in fact Alzheimer's

Often, it is difficult to get the person to agree to see a doctor, and many families are reluctant to take a relative to a health professional without consent. When this problem arises, the family may wish to consult a doctor or a mental health professional on their own. Contact with a professional can accomplish the following:

- Give initial feedback on whether the symptoms described sound like those associated with Alzheimer's.
- Suggest where to go for a comprehensive evaluation of the relative's condition, and explain the costs and time involved.
- Address the fears, doubts, and confusion of family members about what needs to be done. (This area alone justifies contact with a professional familiar with Alzheimer's disease.)

If the family can provide the professional with a list of problems and examples of symptoms observed, this will help the professional make a determination of their loved one's condition.

Use of Behavior Profile

Included in Appendix A is a Behavior Profile which is a comprehensive listing of difficulties ranging from orientation to behavior problems. This scale is helpful for families in documenting problems and their frequency. The profile also provides the caregiver with an opportunity to determine how stressful he finds a particular behavior. It will be useful later in the illness to determine the amount of assistance a person requires and specific behaviors that require more intervention and supportive counseling.

Families Should Establish a Clear History of Symptoms

The history of symptoms and problems is extremely important in making an accurate diagnosis. Families should note how long they have observed various symptoms in their relative. A number of illnesses such as depression and strokes without motor impairment have symptoms that are very similar to those characteristic of Alzheimer's disease. A good history of such symptoms will reflect whether they developed suddenly or over an extended period. Such information becomes significant in the evaluation of this illness.

3. Seeking Information

In addition to consulting a family doctor, neurologist, psychiatrist, or other mental health professional, the family may wish to seek information on Alzheimer's disease from an Alzheimer's family support group or an Alzheimer's resource center. Family support meetings can put a family in touch with vital local resources as well as with professionals who are experienced in diagnosing Alzheimer's disease.

4. Taking Action

A Full Evaluation Involves Several Health Professionals

An appointment with the family physician may be the starting point for the evaluative process, with basic tests ordered. Often the physician may refer his patient to another professional for evaluation, such as a neurologist, a psychiatrist, or a mental health center.

Since the family has decided to act, they want results and some answers. What will help? What can be done to manage the situation even though no cure exists? The family probably expects a medication to manage symptoms.

The family's need for information accelerates after the implications of the diagnosis are recognized.

A Second Opinion May Be Necessary

If a physician gives the diagnosis of Alzheimer's after minimal testing, the family may experience a letdown that can create distrust, lack of confidence in the physician, and real dissatisfaction. A similar situation exists when an incorrect diagnosis of senility or hardening of the arteries is given to informed family members who are keenly aware of their loved one's extreme degree of impairment. Not all doctors are experts in diagnosing and managing the disease, and families should not hesitate to seek a second opinion if they feel skeptical with the first diagnosis. If Alzheimer's is suspected, a doctor with a particular expertise in the disease should be consulted—even if this means traveling to another city.

5. Weighing Findings

After initial diagnostic evaluations have been completed, family members are faced with several tasks including:

a. Questioning the diagnosis and considering the need for a second opinion

b. Understanding the implications of this diagnosis, particularly when confusing, conflicting, or inaccurate information and advice from both professional and nonprofessional sources must be reconciled

c. Reaching a family consensus about what needs to be done now and in the future, and by whom

d. Deciding whether others should be told about the Alzheimer's condition.

6. Identifying Resources

Alzheimer's as yet cannot be cured. However, some of the related problems can be managed and even treated with medication and proper behavioral management.

Before embarking upon a plan of management for the disease and care for the person affected, family members need to realistically assess their personal resources in both emotional and financial terms and examine those offered in the community. Resources are determined by the following factors:

a. The physical health of the most likely primary caregiver

b. The availability of community support and resources

c. The caregiver's living situation and the proximity of other involved family members

d. The family's financial resources and the AD person's eligibility for publicly funded services

e. The strength of the caregiver's marital relationship (Can it withstand the stresses of continuous caregiving?)

f The availability of transportation

g. The availability of family, friends, or paid help to take over care of the patient for several hours at least twice a week

h. The availability of persons who fill the role of confidant

Compensating for Changes Personal/Social Supports

Caregivers must realize that the support system of friends and family that has helped them in previous times of trouble may not be enough to get them through the stresses of caring for their loved one. Alzheimer's caregiving can last a long time. The family caregiver must assess the potential support available during the caregiving process as realistically as possible.

The caregiver can use the Personal/Social Support Resources form in Appendix A to assess the degree of support that is currently available. Caregivers must realize that they need support for themselves, too. If the affected family member has been the primary source of support, new resources must be actively sought out.

7. Planning Care

Planning the care of a person with Alzheimer's can seem to be a confusing and perhaps even unnecessary task (especially when the patient is not exhibiting serious management problems). However, as time moves on and the disease progresses, it will become obvious that a plan is necessary.

In-Home Care List

To begin the care planning process, a Family In-Home Behavior Care List is included in Appendix A. The items on the list will help a family identify areas in which their relative needs assistance and how much assistance is needed. Caregivers must begin to prioritize needs, and they must decide who best can deliver the needed help. They must realize that their lives are changed by the disease, and they must change their approaches accordingly.

Problem Behavior Needs Careful Consideration

Other approaches to problem solving should be considered in family care planning.

a. When do problem behaviors occur, and what else is happening when these problems surface? (For example, is the person more difficult and irritable when the television is playing loudly?)

b. What occurs before or after the undesired behavior? Are these events or conditions producing and rewarding the undesired behavior?

c. How frequently does the problem occur? Is it really that big a problem?

d. How severe or dangerous is the problem?

e. Can advance planning reduce opportunities for the problem behavior to occur?

Case Example of Problem Solving

Emma started calling for her' husband at night after she had gone to bed. He usually helped her to bed about 10 P.M. and then stayed up a while alone. She usually awoke in a panic calling for her husband, somewhat confused. Her husband always turned the bedroom light off before going into the den for his quiet time. Because she was so afraid, her husband always ran to her rescue, most often holding her and falling asleep with her. Night after night, she became frightened when she awoke in the dark. As a consequence, her husband had very little time to himself.

Emma's husband realized he was reinforcing her behavior—the calls at night increased. He also realized that waking in the dark might be frightening to Emma. To deal with the problem he did several things:

- He spent more intimate time with his wife before she went to sleep.

- He left a lamp on in the bedroom while she was asleep.

- When she called for him, he called back to her, reassuring her he was just down the hall in the den. Most of the time Emma went back to sleep, and her husband could continue relaxing alone.

8. Managing Caregiver Stress

Stress from Caregiving Not Necessarily a Result of the Alzheimer's Condition

Too often the stress of caregiving is attributed solely to the condition of the relative with Alzheimer's. As his condition worsens, the stress experienced by the family caregiver increases. This point of view fails to appreciate other aspects of the caregiving situation, which in turn can make it more difficult for the caregiver to cope effectively with the needs of his relative. More contact from friends and relatives provides for social and emotional support needs, which have increased during the caregiver's physical isolation due to the solitary care situation. Utilization of available resources can allow the caregiver to participate more in the community.

Other Factors

The age of the caregiver may influence the degree of stress he experiences. Younger caregivers may have other career and family responsibilities that conflict with full assumption of the caregiving role. The type of role change created by caregiving also influences the degree of stress. For example, female caregivers may resent a return to the caregiver role after raising children and finding a satisfying career. Some men, in contrast, may view the change associated with a new "provider" role more satisfying. Nurturing his ill spouse offers the male a way to repay his wife for her earlier role in family nurturing.

Caregivers Need to Help Themselves

The stresses of caregiving are not simply the result of the continued deterioration of the relative affected. The well-being of the family caregiver is essential. One of the purposes for an Alzheimer's family support group is to help family members cope successfully with the illness. Counseling also can be sought. Caregivers may prevent some stress by utilizing their personal/social support resources.

Caregivers can do much to help themselves. They should explore community services, and they must recognize their limitations, especially during a long period of intense care. Without outside support, caregivers can develop stress-induced illnesses such as depression and anxiety (see Chapters 3, 13, and 14). Men who are depressed have a greater risk of heart conditions. Medical problems such as hypertension, diabetes, and heart conditions may worsen because of prolonged stress and negligent self-care.

A Stress Test

The Care Management Stress form included in Appendix A can help families identify specific stress areas. The areas include stress created by family expectations, isolation, problem behaviors, an uncertain future, and the inherent burden of day-to-day care. In responding to the items, the caregiver should note the frequency of each response and his emotional response to each statement, and should make care decisions accordingly.

A Stress Scale for Institutional Caregivers

Staff of nursing homes and other institutionals also can experience stress as they see the consequences of the illness daily. A Staff Stress Measure is included in Appendix A. Training and other educational opportunities can help staff understand Alzheimer's, deal with behavior effectively and compassionately, and manage the stress associated with such care.

Both the Care Management Stress form and the Staff Stress Measure can be scored. The higher the score, the higher is the potential for stress. More importantly, caregivers can identify particularly stressful areas and give them more attention.

Managing Stress

Managing stress is an ongoing activity. Different features of the patient's progressive condition precipitate new problems and stressors. For example, the first time the Alzheimer's patient fails to recognize his spouse may be so shocking that the caregiver's adjustment is set back considerably.

Stress Is Likely to Grow

As the patient's condition worsens, the stress felt by the caregiver is likely to grow. He should therefore be willing to continuously reassess the possibility of seeking outside help in some form. These resources range from day or respite care to psychiatric hospitalization or nursing home admission. Outpatient mental health services also should be considered as the burdens placed on the caregiver mount.

Look for Positive Experiences in Caregiving

There are many ways to change the negatives of this illness into some unexpected positives. Opportunities actually surface from the most unexpected situations, which may lead to new experiences or back to old experiences and activities that seemed to have been lost.

Some Examples of the Positive Aspects of Caregiving

Thomas became the caregiver for his wife about six months ago. He had been doing the cooking and washing. Then his wife required help with bathing and dressing as well. His "hands-on" care began to increase.

After years of working hard while his wife Janet reared their six children (and some would say their seven grandchildren), Thomas saw that he had the chance to give back to Janet all the love and care she had so willingly given to her entire family.

Joanne was almost devastated when she first learned that her husband Ted had Alzheimer's disease. Months later, she became involved in a local Alzheimer's family support group. Over the next few months, she came to know a number of other people in situations like hers. They became close friends and confidantes—something she never thought she would have. For two years she benefitted from their support and concern, and they from hers. When Ted died, these friends stood by her along with her family.

Feelings

I've had my wounds
and I'm not sure
anyone knows how to heal them.

The doctors and my friends,
family and others
tell me—

"You've lost so much,
you've nursed your loved one
through a baffling disease—

"You've been ignored
drawn taut—
suffered and cried.

"Now that he
is in a nursing home
and you have help
in caring for him,
you are now free
to live your own life.

"Get out and go—
join clubs—be with people—
develop some hobbies—
travel a bit."

I'm trying—I'm trying—
I know they love me—
in many ways, they're right—

But there are times
when I feel like
crawling into a corner
like a sick cat
and just licking my wounds—

Maybe, maybe—for just a time
There's not much wrong with that.

Maude S. Newton

7

From Family Care to Alzheimer's Care: Preparing for Caregiving

When family members learn that Alzheimer's disease accounts for changes they have observed in a loved one's memory and other abilities, they must absorb this news and consider its meaning. What impact will it have on the present and the future? Who will be the caregiver? They will have questions about caregiving. What does Alzheimer's caregiving involve? How is it different from the things family members ordinarily do for each other when someone is ill? If they cannot provide the care, what will they do? These are the kind of choices that families face when they prepare for the transition from family caregiving to Alzheimer's caregiving.

The Roots of Caregiving

Our orientation to caregiving is grounded in our experiences with traditional family care. Caregiving was a part of the parenting role, or a response to another family member who was ill. Children grow up. Many illnesses are temporary, and the family member usually functions independently again. Unlike the Alzheimer's situation, there was probably no reason for caregivers to do anything differently to take care of themselves. These intervals of caregiving are a normal part of family life. Alzheimer's care draws from these caregiving experiences, but the differences between the two situations are significant.

In this chapter we examine these differences and identify ways that caregivers might handle problems. Alzheimer's disease is a degenerative condition. Alzheimer's care has many of the problems commonly observed by caregivers involved with chronic health problems.

We are frequently concerned about caregivers, partly because they provide exhaustive care for an average of eight years. However, we rarely look at their reasons for helping. Motivation is an aspect of caregiving that is seldom discussed. It has an important association with coping. It affects adaptability to the caregiver role and resiliency.

Business and Safety Issues

There are some very basic issues that caregivers should address early. They need to be acquainted with family finances and how they will be managed to provide for needs of the patient and the caregiver. Legal matters such as wills, durable power of attorney, and directives (e.g., a living will) should be in order. Caregivers should be familiar with insurance policies. Alzheimer's care requires caregivers to learn how to make many adjustments so that they will be in a better position to manage what lies ahead.

Household changes are necessary to ensure safety. This "childproofing" helps prevent accidents and other problems. Prescriptions and poisons must be placed in safe, secure locations. Weapons and sharp objects should not be accessible to persons with Alzheimer's. Fire and smoke alarms should be installed. Stoves and microwaves should be adapted so that they are safe when the person with AD attempts to use them. Water heaters should be adjusted to prevent injury. Unplugging appliances not in use or having them out of sight might be necessary. Gates should be locked and yards kept safe. Tools and equipment should be safely secured. A safety or double lock may be installed in doors.

People with Alzheimer's may not be able to pay bills, but they can agree to items and services sold over the phone, through the mail, or on television. Aggressive salespersons do not screen out people with dementia. Address these potential problems before you are unpleasantly surprised. Remember that loved ones may agree not to do things, but these agreements are lost to their forgetfulness.

Driving is a very difficult issue to address. People with moderate dementia should not be driving. The use of a driving test, however, can backfire. People with early to moderate dementia have passed both the written and driving part of tests to get their licenses renewed. Caregivers may enlist the help of professionals, but most likely they must handle this issue alone.

New Views of Behavior

Alzheimer's disease is not like other diseases caregivers might have encountered. Psychological and behavioral changes are associated with symptoms of impaired memory and cognition. Caregivers need to learn how to interpret and positively respond to these symptoms and the needs they create. This requires a different view of what causes behavior and who is responsible for it. We have learned to hold each other responsible for our behavior, but this perspective cannot be fairly and reliably applied to persons with a dementia such as Alzheimer's disease. We have used logic, reasoning, and insight as our primary means of identifying, discussing, and solving problems. These traits become less and less available to people with Alzheimer's.

Caregivers must learn to solve problems differently. Reasoning leads to arguments that lead to bigger problems. Rather than explain why something must be done, use imagination and creative approaches to get loved ones to be agreeable to things that need to be done. Here are some examples. When dealing with the driving issue, it is easier to disable the car, or make it disappear to the repair shop indefinitely, than to convince the driver he cannot drive it because he has Alzheimer's. If visits to a doctor are a problem, go out and do something that is fun a few hours before the appointment. As you start to head home, say that you almost forgot that you had an appointment. Since you are close by, you will keep it. Doing things that might be resisted usually work out well when placed within the context of pleasant activities.

Developing another frame of reference to view and understand behavior is critical. Disease-related impairments contribute to behavioral problems. Attributing all changes to impairment, however, creates a situation in which treatable causes of problems can be overlooked. Behavior can be influenced by multiple factors. Caregiver attitudes and demands, and environmental features such as noise and unfamiliarity, contribute to behavioral problems and psychiatric symptoms. Unidentified medical conditions are possible sources of problems, especially in more advanced stages when bladder and kidney infections can cause significant changes in behavior and mental status. Learning how to understand and respond to behavior is an important goal for the transition into Alzheimer's care. It should be at the top of a list of things for caregivers to learn. Trying to change the behavior of loved ones can sometimes create more problems. Caregivers need to look at how their own behavior affects the behavior of care recipients.

Caregivers need to be aware of how their behavior is perceived for other reasons. They may behave like a caregiver yet may be expected to act like they have always acted as a husband, wife, or child. When a spouse or adult child responds to problems as a caregiver, the person with Alzheimer's may not be able to understand the basis for the change in behavior. Why is the wife who never stood up to her husband telling him he cannot drive his car anymore? When a caregiver changes a longstanding behavioral pattern, the person with Alzheimer's will not understand the reason. He may interpret the reason as having something to do with him. He may wonder why this nice person he has lived with for 40 years is suddenly getting so mean. An explanation will usually make matters worse. The person with AD cannot appreciate or accept the reason things have changed.

How Loved Ones Perceive You

Even if you respond appropriately to behavioral changes, doing what is best does not mean that your efforts will be well received. Limiting and controlling the activities of people with Alzheimer's will trigger unacceptable and childish responses. You may witness a tantrum. The person's self-pitying behavior might even make you feel guilty.

People with AD will not be able to cope well with the changes you must initiate as caregiver. They may respond in less adaptive, more immature ways. Because they are not getting to do what they want to do, your behavior will seem unfair to them. They will become angry and argue. This is reminiscent of a child's response to parental authority. Caregivers are empowered to be soft and nurturing, but they must also recognize they have responsibilities that cannot be exercised without empowering themselves to take charge. They can not gauge their performance as caregiver by the popularity of their decisions.

It is difficult to take a stand against the will of someone who used to have a different role in your relationship. It is much easier to be a caregiver if taking care of someone means granting the person's wishes and being rewarded for it. We usually characterize caregiving in terms of the nurturing aspects of the role because it reminds us of how our original parental caregivers responded when we were hurt or frightened. When they responded to us with warmth and comfort, and gave us what we desired, we perceived them as good parents. But nurturing is only one dimension of parental caregiving.

We saw the other dimension of a parental caregiver as strict, controlling, and having authority and power. We had to toe the line when the parent with authority was around. This person corrected and disciplined us. But this was also the same parental caregiver who protected us and stood up for us in tough circumstances. In different circumstances and different cultures, nurture and authority are associated with different parents. Both are needed to care for loved ones.

Caregivers need to exercise nurture and authority. Sometimes setting limits and taking charge will be extremely important; in other situations loved ones will need nurture from their caregivers. Some caregivers may find it more natural to be nurturing. It may not be comfortable to be authoritative and take charge. If the family member with Alzheimer's was always the one in control, taking charge and setting limits on behavior will be more difficult for a time. In the realm of Alzheimer's caregiving, developing this response will be necessary. It might help to think of it as a caregiver's version of tough love.

Caregivers may want to know what they can expect. How long will AD last? How long will they need to provide care? We have some guidelines about both, but since it is impossible to be exact about either, this information only gives families a general impression of what to expect. We know that caregivers spend an average of 60 hours a week in caregiving and will spend the next 6 to 8 years providing care. Alzheimer's is terminal. Knowing this doesn't help eliminate caregivers' uncertainties. Because their future is uncertain. Consider these words:

> All things may be endurable if the demands are finite in depth and time. But a future that offers no exit at all, even if the burden on a daily basis is not utterly overwhelming, can be an obvious source of sadness and depression. . . . No burden can be greater than trying to imagine how one can cope with a future that promises no relief. (Callahan, 1988)

Such a possibility does nothing to recommend caregiving.

Creating a Better Future

Caregivers can do some things to make their future a little more predictable and manageable, even though caregiving is burdensome and stressful. Caregivers must look beyond themselves and their own resources. They will need to identify and utilize other community services and resources, for example, respite, adult day care, support groups, assisted living situations, and supportive counseling. Caregivers can involve other family members who can either assist with caregiving activities or help caregivers with their other needs.

Most caregivers have most of these options. Service utilization, however, is quite low. It is clear that caregivers are able to care for loved ones. Their capacities to take care of loved ones is rarely an issue until their own health deteriorates. Then their capacity to continue in such a strenuous role is in doubt. Ample evidence shows that chronic stress has very deleterious effects on their physical and mental health. Under the circumstances, taking care of themselves is as great a challenge for caregivers as caring for loved ones. A future without relief is a real burden. When there is relief but it is not sought, a needless tragedy occurs.

Caregiving is the primary strategy for Alzheimer's care. Once family members have become caregivers, they rarely find it easy to relinquish responsibilities. Even though services and treatments exist that will help them manage their burden, less than 20 percent of family caregivers use these resources.

Caregiving is an ancient tradition. We could develop job responsibilities for a caregiver. It would describe what caregivers do. It does not convey the deeper meaning attached to caregiving.

A MAN WAS ASKED BY HIS FRIEND to tell him one more time what it was his wife had. The man told him she had something doctors called Alzheimer's.

They had known about it for a long time but didn't know anything that would help get rid of it. Then the friend asked what he did for her if there was nothing much doctors could do to help. The man said he just did what he could to take care of her. Now he spent most of his time caring for his wife. If he spent so much time caring for her, the friend thought there should be a special name for what he did. The man said he had heard it was called caregiving. The friend was still curious and wanted to know if there was a name for people who spent so much time doing caregiving. The man said he went to group meetings. Those people called each other caregivers. He guessed he must be one, too, because he did the same kinds of things for his wife that they did for their people. Yes, that was what he was. A caregiver. Well, then, how did he become a caregiver? Well, he just took care of everything that came up as best as he could. So how do you learn all that? Well, some things you learned from people helping you grow up. Some things you learned from other people. Like his wife took good care of the kids and him. And some things you already knew. Being patient, kind, loving, and forgiving helps. And being thankful.

Being a Caregiver

Caregiving is defined as much by the lives of people who become caregivers as by the things that they do. Although people may question how prepared or capable they are to be caregivers, few question whether they will do it. Although it is a very stressful experience, many caregivers report that it is personally meaningful and satisfying. These caregivers believe that their own personal growth has advanced as a result of the caregiving experience.

We first experienced caregiving when we were infants. The images, feelings, and values associated with this experience have been a model for how we respond to loved ones who are sick or unable to care for themselves. Our first caregiver nursed and cuddled us. She prepared our meals, made us rest, gave us medication, and helped us learn other activities. She empathized with our pain and frustrations. She comforted us. She would not allow us to do foolish things that endangered us.

These relationships helped us develop a sense of security and attachment. When something happened to us, we learned someone would be there to help us. We knew we would be loved and cared for whether we were naughty, nice, sick, or feeling down on our luck. Our response to caring for each other is shaped by these family experiences, values, and traditions.

This view of family caregiving is well suited for many of the situations in which family members have needed to help each other. We value this view of family care as much as we value the people who introduced us to it. But caring for a person with Alzheimer's disease will require more.

As a family caregiver, you are having a relationship with someone who can no longer have the same kind of relationship with you that he or she had before. And as hard as you try, you realize you cannot have the relationship you want. That makes being a caregiver even more challenging.

Differences in Alzheimer's Caregiving and Traditional Family Care

A Significant Expenditure of Time and Energy

Alzheimer's care calls for a commitment for an indefinite period of time. It may be necessary to suspend other activities, interests, and relationships. This is no small sacrifice.

Caregivers should plan for ways to find relief from their burden before the demands for energy exceed their personal resources. To manage competing demands, some caregivers find it helpful to prioritize their daily activities and maintain a routine. Order provides a sense of predictability and security. But caregivers can also become slaves to routine. At times it is more important to be more flexible. Prioritizing is a way to look at what is and what is not important. What can be done later? What really needs to be done now? What do you have to do? Are you sure? What do you want to do? What will be good for you? Some items don't even need to be on the list.

Caregivers need to build in opportunities for themselves so that they do not lose contact with the rest of the world and cut themselves off from the support and invigorating distractions that refresh them physically and mentally.

Changes in Level of Needs

Alzheimer's disease progresses and the care recipient requires increased involvement from the caregiver as needs change. The increasing needs of persons with AD compete with a caregiver's participation in other important areas of life. When caregiving is consuming, the caregiver is held captive by the role.

Type of Stress

The stress associated with Alzheimer's caregiving is chronic, severe, and perceived as being caused by multiple stressors. Different approaches are needed to cope with stressors that are diverse and changeable. Caregivers who use the same problem-solving approach to address problems that are quite different will not be effective. Stress and coping are handled extensively in Chapter 8.

Caregiving Role Unanticipated and/or Unwanted

No one can predict exactly how Alzheimer's caregiving will affect their life, but the impact will be significant. Major disruptions occur when Alzheimer's is not anticipated and when the caregiver still has significant responsibilities for work and family. Many of the early-onset Alzheimer's cases are found in people from 50 to 60 years of age. These families are still quite involved in raising children and making a living. Another dependent person without an income places a large burden on the spousal caregiver. A similar situation occurs when an adult child becomes the caregiver for a parent.

When unwanted role changes occur because of caregiving, adjusting to the role can be awkward, even demoralizing. Women who have been caregivers most of their lives may not welcome this role again. Women develop Alzheimer's more frequently than men. Husbands who had expected their wives to be caring for them must deal with this unexpected situation. However, research shows that men find this switch meaningful. Husbands use caregiving as a way to honor their wives for caring for the family. Some men may find the role stressful because they are not comfortable with the more intimate aspects of hands-on caregiving. Adult children may find themselves in a caregiving situation that involves more intimacy than some have ever had with the parent. Dealing with intimacy becomes worthwhile if caregivers grow closer to the care recipient and other family members in the process.

Some caregivers will be faced with caring for a person with whom they have had a difficult relationship. They may expect less support from other family members because of prior conflicts. The time has come to either put the conflicts aside or seek help for resolving the problems. Old issues that have been put aside may be resurrected by conflicts arising from the caregiving situation. These issues can exacerbate relationship problems. Caregivers must seriously consider counseling before relationship problems create major obstacles to helping.

Need for Increasing Assistance, Behavioral Problems, Personality Changes, and Reminders of Loss

Assisting a family member who has become completely dependent will be marked with frustration. The experience will also be filled with moments of grief or despair. Behavior problems and personality changes are reminders of the changes that eventually mark the loss of a loved one. Grief cannot be easily acknowledged in these situations. With so much to do, it is easy to stay busy and avoid these feelings. Caregivers need support for their grief experience. Opportunities for solitude are important. Family, friends, church or professional counselors can be helpful. Grief is present throughout the caregiving experience; support groups address it. Caregivers will benefit from learning more about the complications that Alzheimer's disease creates for mourning.

Unreciprocated Help

Caregiving in families without Alzheimer's provides abundant opportunities to help and be helped. When parents take care of their children, children are able to express their appreciation. Helping each other is an important part of being a family.

This family formula for helping goes through a disturbing change in Alzheimer's caregiving. The disease causes most of the change. The capacity to relate is compromised. People with Alzheimer's become more self-centered and less aware of others. They are less likely to state their appreciation for the things their caregivers do. Still caregivers are uplifted when they are acknowledged in some way. It may be a smile or a more peaceful countenance. Any positive feedback is encouraging. The absence of negative feedback is encouraging, too.

Caregivers need to be prepared for this change and not take it personally. The lack of positive feedback is distressing; negative feedback is discouraging, but neither of these responses is a reflection on the extraordinary help caregivers render to loved ones. To compensate for this lack of support, caregivers should look for other ways of evaluating and rewarding their efforts. For instance, they should talk to themselves positively after successfully completing a difficult task. Having several moments of quiet might be taken as a reward for how well they have managed. Smiles or other indications that a care recipient is feeling well can be counted as a blessing for that moment.

Coping with Problems Common to Chronic Disease

Families coping with chronic diseases experience common social and psychological problems (Strauss et al., 1984). Alzheimer's caregivers will encounter them as well. Caregivers who are able to anticipate these problems have a better opportunity to develop adaptive responses. This, in turn, gives family caregivers a better chance to cope with and prepare for what lies ahead.

The crises of Alzheimer's caregiving often involve behavioral problems and psychiatric symptoms. Hostile, aggressive behavior directed at the caregiver is an example. Insidious threats to the health and well-being of the caregiver can eventually have a serious impact on the caregiver's physical and mental health.

One key to crisis management in Alzheimer's care is learning to respond to problems while understanding how disease-related impairments affect how the person with AD interprets demands placed on him or her by caregivers. When caregivers learn to fine-tune their expectations to the degree of assistance needed by care recipients, there is a greater possibility that loved ones will be able to respond more appropriately. Likewise, caregivers need to reassess their expectations of themselves. Sometimes the crisis that needs to be managed does not involve the person with Alzheimer's. It involves the caregiver's appraisal of what is happening.

When experiencing persistent, high levels of stress, our understanding of what is or is not threatening becomes skewed and we may react to situations that are not as critical as we thought they were. This happens to caregivers for several reasons. They are confronted by situations that are unfamiliar to them and they do not know how to respond. Repetitive questions and being shadowed by care recipients are behaviors associated with impaired memory that may be annoying, and caregivers may overreact to them. Psychiatric symptoms and behavior problems may also qualify as misunderstood crises, although a real crisis exists where the care recipient becomes aggressive toward his caregiver.

Caregivers need to ask themselves what is critical and threatening about a situation before they respond to it as though it were an emergency. What will happen if they respond differently? Is it really necessary to respond immediately? Will their response to the perceived crisis help or hurt? Time pressures and the stress-related feelings of tension, anxiety, fear, dread, and anger may bring about the caregiver's sense of crisis.

The caregiver should remember that insisting the person with AD take a bath immediately can precipitate a behavioral crisis, whereas putting the task off for an hour or a day might be quite appropriate. Some caregivers may react to loved ones who refuse to change clothes. Requiring such behaviors to occur exactly as they did before AD is too much to expect. Time pressure creates more problems for the person with cognitive impairment. A caregiver who is trying to get someone to a doctor's appointment and who is in a hurry may be surprised when that person refuses to go.

A caregiver may be tired and want to give medications so that she can have some quiet time to herself. The care recipient's refusal to take the medication may cause the caregiver to become more forceful. Now the person with AD will become more agitated and uncooperative. The caregiver will be even more upset because it will be a long time before she will have time for herself. Again, caregivers must analyze their demands with these consequences in mind.

Caregivers will be confronted by serious crises. When the person with AD walks outside and gets lost, his attempts to get back home create more confusion and he is then further from home. This can be a real crisis. Caregivers can reduce the chance of such things happening if they prepare in advance for potential problems. One approach is to change their demands. Caregivers who modify their expectations of when, how quickly, and how well behaviors must occur will learn that some potential crises can be averted. Another important caregiver responsibility is to constantly review and take appropriate safety precautions.

Managing Symptoms and Behaviors

Medical conditions that cannot be cured are often treated symptomatically. When a patient complains of symptoms, medications or other treatments are administered to relieve symptoms or treat the condition causing them. Flu and viruses are treated symptomatically. Patients are given medications and other treatments to reduce body aches, diarrhea, fever, and other unpleasant symptoms. Symptoms may be our biggest concern, so we measure getting better by getting relief from the symptoms we associate with an illness or condition. Anyone who has had a bad case of flu feels better when his fever is down and the aches and pains have abated; people with allergies and respiratory viruses feel better when coughing, headaches, sneezing, and nasal congestion are reduced and they can breathe again.

When the underlying disease cannot be cured, symptom management becomes more important. Treating the symptoms of arthritis, asthma, or diabetes makes it possible for people to function better without as much pain, discomfort, or interference from other limitations imposed on them by their chronic health problems. For people who suffer depressive and anxiety disorders, experiencing relief from symptoms is almost like being cured, though their conditions may only be in remission. In Alzheimer's disease behaviors represent the symptoms that caregivers need to learn to manage. Managing behavior in Alzheimer's care is equivalent to the symptom management orientation we see with medically defined illnesses. Successful symptom management will benefit persons with the disease and their caregivers.

Caregivers need to examine what they believe about Alzheimer's-related behavior and why persons with AD act as they do. This may be challenging because our beliefs about behavior are often based on a strong belief that people should be responsible for their own actions. We also believe that people sometimes intend for their behavior to affect us the way it does, so persons with AD should be able to control their behavior. If they do not perform some activity appropriately, the result would improve if they put more effort into it and got focused on what they were doing. These beliefs are predicated on the idea that adults are capable of doing what they need to do; therefore they are responsible for their behavior and its consequences on others. No matter how great their desire, people with AD may not be able to do any better. When they are aware of their impaired functioning, they are often frustrated and embarrassed by their decreased capacity to perform in accordance with their previous standards of behavior.

Most caregivers realize they need to modify their old beliefs about family members' behavior. Developing realistic and compassionate perspectives on what loved ones are capable of doing allows caregivers to see their helping role in a different light. They recognize that they put loved ones with impaired brain function under considerable pressure when they expect too much of them. On the other hand, expecting too little of loved ones can be just as unrealistic and has the effect of disenfranchising them as persons of value. Caregivers need to look at the ways their own behavior affects loved ones' activities and interactions—positively and negatively. Deficits attributable to Alzheimer's are only one variable influencing how love ones act.

Caregivers need to develop new beliefs about behavior and its causes in order to appropriately manage Alzheimer's symptoms and behaviors. This may appear to be overwhelming at first, but caregivers can learn to manage behavior and symptoms just as they learned to handle challenges in traditional family caregiving. People are usually more comfortable taking care of family members who were ill after they learn how to do it. Alzheimer's caregivers have a rich backdrop of caregiving experiences from which to draw knowledge, motivation, and confidence. For instance, once we learned how to break a child's high fever, finding he has a temperature of 103 degrees two months later does not provoke the same alarm we first experienced. Dealing with behavior may be difficult for caregivers at first, but they can be more comfortable with their role in Alzheimer's care as they learn more about AD behaviors and behavior management.

Not all behavior is directly attributable to Alzheimer's disease or its symptoms. Part of being comfortable with behavior is learning to understand which behaviors are normal manifestations of the disease, which are intentional reactions, which mirror the personality and coping style of the person with the disease, and which represent a loved one's reaction to overwhelming cognitive and emotional demands. Caregivers need to realize that not all symptoms and behaviors are caused by Alzheimer's disease. A more inclusive perspective is needed, which will provide caregivers with more ways to understand problems and needs and, subsequently, to solve problems. The better your ability to interpret the meaning of behaviors from a broader perspective, the greater chance that the needs of the AD person can be met. Some behavioral changes can be signals of needs and not merely problems. For example, caregivers commonly confront agitation, combativeness, or uncooperativeness. Some people believe that the disease causes these behaviors. However, these behaviors are frequently responses to environmental and interpersonal stressors that the person with AD cannot manage. Maybe these behaviors are his way of adapting, or more likely our cue he needs more support and assistance from his environment and helpers. Agitation is also linked to medical problems and pain that persons with AD cannot express with verbal communication.

Symptoms and behaviors will be more meaningful if they can be understood in terms of the disease, its effect on the person, and enduring characteristics of the person with Alzheimer's. The physical, social, and psychological aspects of one's environment make demands that may exceed the capacity of the person with Alzheimer's to successfully cope. His response to implicit and explicit demands made of him is the resulting confluence of multiple factors: intelligence and adaptability before symptoms of the disease became apparent; the degree of brain impairment present; the effects of conditions such as depression or psychiatric symptoms that further compromise the integrity of one's response; the availability of compensatory support provided to the person by the environment; suitability of vision, hearing, and other sensory functions; and the pressures created by the demands made of the person. If the demands exceeded the person's ability to respond appropriately, the caregiver may see acting-out behaviors, agitation, anger, frustration, and other signs that indicate the person's emotional stability is threatened. Matching the level of demand to the capacity of the person with Alzheimer's to respond adequately will likely encourage more desirable behavior. Boredom and withdrawal result if demands are too meager, as is sometimes seen in persons manifesting earlier stages of AD.

Caregivers will encounter multiple behaviors and symptoms that are unfamiliar to them. It is helpful to consider these from three different frames of reference: symptoms of dementia, behavioral responses, and psychiatric symptoms. Examples of dementia symptoms are memory impairment, loss of executive functions such as impaired judgment and problem solving, and language difficulties. The reader will find it helpful to periodically review the dementia symptoms in Chapter 2. Medications that were developed to alter or improve the symptoms of Alzheimer's have not been as successful as hoped, but they have promoted some improvements in functioning. Behavioral and environmental approaches do not improve symptoms of the Alzheimer's disease, but they can reduce the negative impact of environment, making it possible for the person with AD to perform more in line with his functional capacity. We are not likely to look for any other way to understand or manage symptoms if we believe they are all caused by Alzheimer's disease or the person with the disease.

Behavioral changes that occur with Alzheimer's disease may be associated with the symptoms of the disease. For example, eating problems may occur because the individual does not remember to eat or is unable to make the motor movements required to grasp a fork or spoon, dip it in a plate of food, and raise the utensil to the mouth. These changes include loss of interest and initiative, wandering, sexual exposure, repetitive questioning/actions, and sleep problems. Withdrawal from activities and social interaction occur as well as problems with dressing and grooming. Losing or hiding things is a common behavior change. Some people become more dependent or clinging because their security has been eroded by loss of memory and cognitive skills. Some behavior changes become chronic disturbances such as confusion, forgetfulness and disorientation, night walking, and incontinence. This is true of disinhibition and sexual exposure as well. Agnosia, or the failure to recognize familiar places and things, is one symptom of AD that can be quite upsetting with it first occurs. Persons with AD are not able to recognize their homes or other persons who were quite familiar to them. Caregiver spouses may even be accused of being imposters.

Agitation, irritability, emotional outbursts, fearfulness, noisy behavior, over-activity, and catastrophic reactions represent acute behavioral disturbances. Fearfulness, paranoid reactions, anxiety, depression, violence, and aggression are also acute behavioral disturbances. Acute behavioral disturbances may be linked to situations that are stressful to persons with Alzheimer's or are reactions to perceived threats or overwhelming demands. These problems are usually prevented more easily than they can be managed after they have become more intense.

The nature of the relationship between the caregiver and person with AD may provide clues to some behavior problems. For example in relationships where the couples have always argued and reacted angrily, one would expect to observe more acute behavioral disturbances. These relationships can also have a very positive impact on the person with Alzheimer's.

Anger, agitation, and other acute disturbances can also be precipitated by demands that exceed the person's capacity to adapt and respond appropriately. Confrontation of the person's impairments or denial of impairment will often produce reactive behavior. Uncooperativeness, refusal to do tasks, and denial of problems suggest it is more difficult for the person to handle demands; the task may be incomprehensible, or time pressures may make it too unwieldy to perform. Sleep and appetite changes can be related to the disease but other explanations are appropriate. Depression and grief can account for significant changes in behavior. Psychiatric symptoms such as hallucinations and delusions can exacerbate insomnia and confusion at night, which can also contribute to anger and agitation.

Some behavior changes are caused by demands that exceed the capacity of the person with AD to adapt and are more likely to occur when the disease is more advanced. Caregivers need to modify their expectations according to the degree of disease-related impairment as well as the factors noted above. Behavior changes are sensitive to environmental factors, which can produce positive and negative changes in behavior—both desirable and undesirable. It will be easier to change the environment or the behavior of other persons involved than to change the behavior of the person with dementia.

Management of behavior problems with medications is not as effective as behavioral or environmental approaches. Behavioral problems may improve with changes in caregivers' interpersonal style and a reduction in environmental stressors and demands. Significant changes in behavior and behavioral problems may be a sign or depression. Caregivers should watch for any signs of depression and seek treatment. Treatment of depression will produce positive changes in behavior, and antidepressant medications can be helpful. Cholinesterase inhibitors such as Aricept (Donepezil) and Exelon (Rivastigmine) can also be helpful in reducing some behavior problems and promoting positive changes in behavior.

Psychiatric symptoms seen with AD include hallucinations and delusions. Depression or symptoms of depression are fairly common. Anxiety is a common reaction to memory loss. Psychiatric symptoms and conditions are associated with damage to specific areas of the brain and to heightened stress and losses. Some psychiatric symptoms are a reaction to disease-related symptoms. For example, one reaction to loss of short-term memory is the delusional belief that other people are stealing things. Personal items have not been misplaced or lost—someone has taken them. Caregivers are often quite uncomfortable dealing with psychiatric symptoms, but medications can be used to complement behavioral and environmental approaches to successfully treating psychiatric symptoms. Decreasing psychiatric symptoms helps to decrease the person's anxiety, fearfulness, and agitation. Sleep can be improved, which makes it possible for caregivers to get some sleep. With successful treatment of psychiatric symptoms, the person with Alzheimer's will interact more appropriately with the caregiver, reducing the caregiver's distress. In Alzheimer's care, small changes in symptoms and behavior can make a big difference.

Caregivers are often quite uncomfortable dealing with psychiatric symptoms, but they can be treated successfully. Medications may improve function and communication skills.

Managing Other Problems

Because of progressive brain impairment, a person with Alzheimer's does less for himself. Caregivers must assist with activities of daily living such as bathing, dressing, and toileting. Care recipients are not always cooperative, so caregivers need to look at these situations from different perspectives. Bathing must be done when the person is less angry or afraid, or a sponge bath can be given.

Psychiatric symptoms and behavioral problems can be precipitated by the caregiver's presentation of activities of daily living. Are you presenting demands too hastily? Pick a time when the person is calmer and more likely to cooperate with an activity. Focus on doing it together one step at a time. Make the task as pleasant as you can. One time of day may be better for one task than another. Problems outside the immediate caregiving situation may interfere. You will need to take care of these matters before you can carry out other activities.

Adjusting to Changes

Caregivers are confronted by scores of changes: their lifestyles, their relationships, their community and family involvement, and their health. Then there are the changes they witness in loved ones. The progression of changes provides time to learn how to cope and accept the things you cannot change.

Interpretation of some changes can be misleading. Good days raise hopes that more permanent improvement is taking place. Bad days suggest the disease is progressing. Good days and bad days don't necessarily mean there is deterioration or improvement. Variability in behavior and functioning is a common feature of AD. Factors such as mood and fatigue influence caregivers' perspectives of their situations.

Attempting to Continue Normal Interactions

Changes in how loved ones function and act are not always understood or tolerated well by other people. There is a chance that dementia-related behavior can carry the kind of stigma associated with psychiatric illnesses. This occurs in spite of the fact that Alzheimer's disease is a neurological disorder with psychiatric manifestations.

Before it has become too difficult for care recipients to participate in social interaction and activities outside of the protective setting of their home, caregivers may decrease the frequency of these social outings. They may worry about behavioral problems they would not be able to manage outside the home, or they may experience shame or embarrassment for their loved one's behavior. Hopefully, caregivers can develop reasonable expectations for social participation outside the home setting and not discontinue these events entirely.

Continued interaction with other family members and friends is crucial to the maintenance of a caregiver's identity, sense of self, and sense of belonging that extend well beyond the caregiving relationship. These relationships support the caregiver's adaptation to the disease and the promise of a future as a member of a larger community when caregiving is over. Caregivers who maintain normal social relationships with others and keep connections with their community do not become socially and psychologically isolated.

Managing Social Isolation

Social isolation is a result of several factors. It may seem too difficult to have contacts outside of the immediate care environment. Many caregivers are older. Health problems may further restrict the length and frequency of other social contact. Leaving the person with Alzheimer's alone is not an option; finding someone to stay with him or her is difficult. When caregivers are no longer able to go places and do things with loved ones, finding other alternatives for social contact and activity must be explored. Members of church or a support group offer other options for supportive relationships that could lessen the caregiver's sense of isolation.

Confronting Marital and Family Problems

Stress aggravates relationships. Some of the marital and family issues that surface during caregiving may relate to old conflicts. Others are precipitated by the caregiving experience. A familiar caregiver complaint is the lack of assistance and support received from other family members. The disruption of family relationships is another problem identified by caregivers.

Dealing with Alzheimer's may be the "last straw" for some families. For other families this crisis may represent a chance for resolution of longstanding problems. such a major threat to a family member may be reason enough to forgive hurts and resolve problems. Some may be able to put aside what they have been unable to forgive.

Marital or family problems negatively and directly affect the capacity of caregivers to administer their role. They cause enormous stress, which directly impacts the recipient of their care. These situations should to be confronted. The help of counselors and other health professionals may be necessary, and it should be sought before more hurt occurs.

Utilizing Resources to Fund the Costs of Care

Medicare, Medicaid, and private insurance provide coverage for some of the acute care needs of persons with Alzheimer's. For example, Medicare pays psychiatrists, clinical social workers, clinical psychologists, social workers, and physicians based on a fee schedule. The actual payment depends on whether the visit was for diagnosis or therapy. If the visit was to diagnosis AD, Medicare pays 80 percent of the Medicare-approved rate. If the visit was for a treatment of a mental illness, the Medicare payment is limited to 50 percent of the Medicare-approved rate. Under certain circumstances, Medicare will pay for the visit to a psychiatrist, clinical psychologist, or social worker. What and if it pays will be determined by codes the service provider uses in billing and whether Medicare views the service as appropriate. Frequently, payment for psychotherapy is denied because Medicare does not view Alzheimer's disease as a mental illness. Neither does Medicare see psychotherapy as medically necessary or reasonable when a person has dementia and significant cognitive impairment.

If the person with AD has depression, psychotherapy would be allowed if the provider gave depression as the primary reason for treatment. Family counseling would be reimbursed if the purpose was for the treatment of the person with Alzheimer's condition and treatment of a family member's problem.

Medicaid covers nursing home care for persons with Alzheimer's who qualify on the basis of medical need and financial status. Medicare does not cover adult day care but Medicaid does. Medicaid covers a specific number of medications a month, but Medicare does not yet cover medications. Medicare does not cover respite care for Alzheimer's disease except as described under the part A hospice benefit. Insurance coverage can be difficult to understand without the help of staff persons who are knowledgeable. Caregivers should not hesitate to check with these insurance staff when scheduling appointments for loved ones.

Long-term care constitutes the primary financial burden of Alzheimer's care. According to the Alzheimer's Association, more than 70 percent of people with AD are cared for in the home. Family and friends provide more than 75 percent of home care. Families cover home care at an average cost of $12,500 annually. If a family caregiver were paid the conservative amount $10 for each hour of home care services and worked an average 60 hours a week providing care for 1 year, this person would earn $31,200 a year.

The average cost of nursing home care per patient is $42,000 per year (in some areas the cost exceeds $70,000 a year). The average lifetime cost per patient—that is, the cost for the time in a facility until death—is estimated to be $174,000. Although the average person with AD lives 8 years after the onset of symptoms, some live as many as 20 years. The corresponding lifetime cost would be much greater, although much of the care would have been provided even longer in the home before admission to a nursing home. We fail to appreciate the involvement of caregivers in nursing home care and services. Often caregivers spend many hours with loved ones. They assist with dressing and meals. They may take clothes home to wash. They may choose to take loved ones to appointments with physicians. Their involvement and time in these activities represents another contribution of dollars that need not be spent by the government or insurance companies on Alzheimer's care.

Role and Lifestyle Changes

Role and lifestyle changes are significant stressors because they threaten the stability of a lifestyle that existed prior to the intrusion of a disease. Many caregivers have multiple family roles as spouse, parent, child, and in-law. They may have other roles in jobs or community activities. Multiple roles can bring about conflict because caregivers have less of themselves to give. Another family member may need to take on additional responsibilities. Other family members, for example, the young children of an adult child caring for a parent, may be able to assume additional responsibilities and feel satisfied because of their contribution to the family during a crisis. Alzheimer's doesn't happen to one person. It happens to a family. Families must deal realistically with each other regarding expectations they have and goals they hope to accomplish.

Caregiving restricts lifestyle by restricting important social and leisure activities. These restrictions are a concern because social and leisure activities are coping strategies. They offer caregivers a sense of play, exercise, and relaxation. They serve as pleasant distractions and offer a chance to interact socially, providing a brief respite from Alzheimer's care. Social activities provide important social contacts that keep caregivers anchored in their larger social community.

Being with a person who requires more and more of your presence creates a need for privacy. The person with Alzheimer's may be anxious and may follow you. Even when alone, caregivers may find it difficult to have a truly private moment because they are listening for distress signs from their loved one. This is a chance to slow down and look within, to consider what is important, to search for answers, to count blessings or face fears. Privacy and quiet are important ingredients in meditation, relaxation, prayer, and spiritual practices. Caregivers can use moments of privacy to restore themselves and focus on what lies ahead. Moments alone facilitate coping and survival.

Role Engulfment

Many Alzheimer's caregivers are engulfed by their role. Their thoughts are dominated by what needs to be done, watching loved ones and thinking about them, anticipating what will happen, and wondering how they can keep going. They even wish it were over.

Some caregivers will be more vulnerable to role engulfment. Some people identify too much with the caretaker aspect of caregiving. It becomes an overriding basis for identity, and when their involvement in the role is threatened, their identity is jeopardized because it is the sole self-defining activity of their life. People who have become compulsively involved in task-oriented activities may have more trouble keeping boundaries between the demands of caregiving and other important activities of living.

Caregiving can be a meaningful role, but it cannot take the place of the rest of one's life. Consumed by the activities and thoughts of caregiving, caregivers are separated from activities, roles, and relationships that connected them to a broader social world. This separation threatens the caregiver's social support and undercuts other important sources of self-esteem and identity. Severe role engulfment fostered by chronic caregiving can result in extreme social and psychological isolation. Preservation of meaningful roles, activities, and relationships can buffer caregivers from this kind of isolation.

Loss of Identity

Alzheimer's caregiving makes it difficult for caregivers to maintain contact with other sources of identity that help define who they are and give them a richer and broader base for their sense of self. The imminent loss of a family member and lifestyle that involves them are other threats. There is a qualitative aspect of identity that is threatened by caregiving for progressive, terminal conditions.

Our identity involves a concept of self—the way we see ourselves—and an evaluation of self. This process contributes to or takes away from our self-esteem, the way we feel about ourselves. Caregivers whose self-esteem and concept of self are too tightly bound to the person with Alzheimer's are at greater risk of self-loss and a weaker view of self

The person with AD may have directed the caregiver and may have been a source of security and esteem as well. The loss of this person represents a major threat. Caregivers can use this situation to develop other supportive relationships. Persons with AD become self-centered. They are unable to provide approval. No caregiver can beat Alzheimer's disease. Caregivers should not base their view of themselves on unrealistic expectations, but they should feel good about what they do to ease the existential pain of the one they honor with their care.

Lack of Sufficient Help from Health Professionals and Agencies

Family members often expect to receive assistance and services from physicians beyond the scope of what our present health care system provides. Treatments for Alzheimer's disease are very limited. Professional providers have made tremendous efforts to care for Alzheimer's patients who have needs in their areas of expertise.

Caregivers need to abandon the passive role they sometimes assume with physicians and other professionals. They need to express concerns they have about loved ones and themselves. Learning how to be a partner with the professional caregiver is important. When compared with the ways families commonly care for one another, Alzheimer's caregiving represents an extraordinary example of care.

Motivations for Helping

Motivations for helping have some effect on how much and how long people are able to cope with caregiving. When the need for care exceeds what caregivers have anticipated, their reasons for helping can revive their purpose and renew their resolve. Motivation and personal goals can make caregiving more meaningful and rewarding. Caregivers can develop a better understanding of their reasons for helping by considering these questions:

- What will caring for this person mean to me?
- How will it change my life?
- Is this something I want to do?
- Do I have doubts about becoming a caregiver?
- What are the personal gains I hope to accomplish as a caregiver?
- What does caregiving have to do with who I am and my values?

There are two general explanations for why people help each other. One is egoistic. Self-interest and serving the self are motivations for helping. With this orientation to helping, we expect some kind of a reward. And if we do not help, we expect some form of punishment. Self-oriented helping is not necessarily selfish. Self-generated rewards are supportive of personal goals. A caregiver who has not been satisfied with her ability to manage her husband has the opportunity for positive self-talk as she learns to manage Alzheimer's-related impairments.

The second explanation for helping involves empathy and altruism. In this case, the motivation for helping is guided by devotion to the welfare of others and a deep understanding of the situation of the person needing help. This other-oriented reason for helping may benefit the helper, but the primary goal is to benefit the other person.

Both types of motivations influence the helping behavior of caregivers. Caregivers with multiple motivations will have more than one reason to go on when they no longer believe they can continue to cope with a life of caregiving. If their belief in one motivation weakens and their resolve to continue declines, becoming aware of others restores their determination to continue.

The caregiving role may also provide the caregiver an opportunity to grow and develop as an individual. Caregivers can set goals for themselves that serve as measures for personal growth. For instance, some caregivers can gain self-confidence and become more self-reliant through the caregiving journey. Others may want to learn to be more accepting of others and themselves. Learning how to feel good about accepting help may be important. By accomplishing goals that reinforce their sense of worth and self-esteem, caregivers protect themselves from self-loss. Being able to solve problems from day to day, caregivers find the inspiration to overcome subsequent adversities.

A deeper connection with their reasons for helping confers a greater sense of meaning and purpose to caregivers. For example, family members might recognize that the caregiver role is a way for them to love, honor, and respect loved ones who have developed Alzheimer's disease. They can become closer to the person they are caring for, or they can develop closer relationships with other family members. Through others they encounter in their journey, caregivers find opportunities to know themselves through the eyes of these other people.

Below is a small variety of reasons for helping. Caregivers usually don't have that many motivations for helping when first asked. As they begin to discuss their reasons other possibilities surface.

- Expectation of some type of payment
- To see oneself as a good person, good daughter or son, and so forth
- To avoid guilt or shame
- To make up for failures or debts
- To give back what others have done or given
- To honor marriage vows
- To honor a relationship or the person
- Out of duty or obligation
- To get social approval
- To avoid the disapproval or criticism of others
- To honor longstanding promises
- To uphold personal or spiritual values
- To comply with social norms
- To comply with family or cultural values
- To express affection and love
- Empathy for the other
- Commitment to the welfare of others
- To avoid judgment and condemnation
- Out of self-reliance
- Atonement for sins and offenses against the person
- Emotional attachment and bonds to the person
- Identity and continuity of the relationship
- Fear of being alone in the world

8

Understanding Behavioral Changes

Over an indefinite period of time, Alzheimer's disease destroys many of the brain's billions of nerve cells. Another part of this process disrupts the brain's capacity to produce specialized chemicals that allow nerve cells to communicate information to each other. In the healthy brain, this unique system of nerve cells and their specialized chemical messengers enables us to think and reason, remember and be conscious of our experiences, feel and express emotion, learn and achieve goals, and relate these experiences to one another. Because of our brain, we are able to make adaptive changes in how or where we live.

From the moment a child is born, his development is carefully observed. His smiles suggest he is happy and willing to interact positively with his new world. The first steps or first words are hallmarks of development. We expect the child to grow and develop "normally," to learn and have knowledge. This knowledge, and his use of it, is a part of his identity. Memory allows him to store and retrieve this knowledge as it is needed. Sometimes he is more conscious of what he does than the way his thoughts influence his actions.

Later in his life, he will be asked a question, and if unable to answer it he will say, "Nothing comes to mind." All of us have had this experience many times. We can also recall those times we were under pressure to respond quickly to questions raised in a demanding situation. Much to our dismay, we remember thinking how our minds went blank. Situations like this are frustrating.

We suffer greater frustration when we realize it is a little harder to learn or remember something than it used to be. We may experience situations that exceed our ability to adapt to them. Despite the extreme stress or health problems we may be experiencing, we conclude our minds are not what they used to be. And if we continue to have experiences like these, we may translate our frustrations into a belief that imparts greater doubts and concerns. "I'm not what I used to be" or "I'm just not myself anymore." Something unique and treasured about us is threatened—the special relationship between our minds and who we are.

Early Threats to Who We Are

Alzheimer's disease directly affects the way the mind works. Family members become aware of difficulties with memory or changes in behavior long before they discover that these differences represent the beginnings of a disease process. It is normal for families to conclude that dramatic behavioral changes must have something to do with the personality or emotional state of their loved one. For whatever reason, that person's "uniqueness" has changed. That uniqueness is what makes one person different from another. The idea that individuals we intimately know essentially remain the same is important to our relationship. This uniformity persists regardless of age or other factors. Our uniqueness as individuals is more likely to be attributed to our personalities than to our minds. While Alzheimer's disease strips away the memories, behaviors, and abilities held in the mind, its assault on the personality is not so complete.

Glimmers of the Person

The personality of your loved one will change, but it will happen slowly. As caregiver, you have the chance to observe and relate to many parts of the person that remain unchanged. Even in the more advanced stages of Alzheimer's disease, there will be "glimmers" of the person that was and still is. These glimmers of the person may be sufficient to stimulate other memories: ways he or she was unique, and experiences you shared. These tenuous aspects of your loved one's personality and mind may help sustain you through the caregiving—even through the massive losses you must witness—because there is still evidence of the old self.

The Impact of Losses on Relating

Understanding the relationship between the brain and behavior can help caregivers respond more reasonably to the behavioral changes in their loved one, but not at the expense of their appreciation of what is unique about the person and his or her history. Patterns of behavior and personality characteristics that existed before this disease may continue. Their expression may not be as appropriate (Shomaker, 1987), or they may be more irritating than they used to be. They are not immediately erased.

Threats to Relationships

Over time Alzheimer's disease distinctly changes our relationship with the person who has developed this disease. Our personal loss is manifested in the series of losses we witness as our loved ones lose the ability to reason, think, remember, and behave in ways that were uniquely "their ways." Watching them behave differently, with the ability to do less and less for themselves, represents moments of grief for us and for them. In these moments, we realize we are not only losing the person, we are losing the relationship we had with this one we loved. This may be one reason it is so difficult for caregivers to deal with the behavioral changes associated with this disease.

New and Unexpected Demands to Change

As loved ones become less and less like themselves, and act in unusual and unexpected ways, caregivers are confronted by the growing awareness they are on unfamiliar ground. They found their way through uncharted territory before, for instance, when they were first left alone by their mothers at school, had their first date, got married, raised their first child, or started their first job. These experiences were anticipated. They had not occurred without warning. There had been opportunities to prepare for these experiences through education and learning. Caregivers have no preparation for the changes they experience.

Few family members who become caregivers are experienced in caring for persons who are affected by a progressive form of brain disease such as Alzheimer's. As they enter the process of providing care, it is much easier to relate to their loved ones as they always have rather than view their thoughts, behaviors, and moods as the result of brain impairment. It is difficult at first to appreciate how this applies to the caregiver situation and the problems with which caregivers, must contend. How much of what happens is related to disease? How much is related to personality, relationships, or the environment?

Attempts to Understand Behavior

People need to understand why things happen. They want to know what causes problems so that they can solve or prevent them. If your husband has always been reasonably responsive to doing the things you ask him to do, then this expectation does not immediately change just because he has Alzheimer's disease. If you ask him to get dressed and find he is still sitting on the bed 15 minutes later, you are inclined to think he is deliberately being uncooperative. If he says he can't dress himself, you may believe he is not trying hard enough. On the other hand, you might believe the problem has something to do with you, or what you have done. Maybe grandchildren are visiting and their excitement while they play is simply too much for your husband to handle.

Who Is to Blame

Some family caregivers have a tendency to blame the loved one for the agitation, uncooperativeness, and other behavioral problems that make it more difficult to care compassionately. Others blame themselves for the difficulties being experienced. In either case, caregivers occasionally feel frustration, anger, guilt, or hopelessness in caring for their afflicted relatives. But keep in mind that caregivers are attempting to relate to their loved one as though he were still the capable person he was before the effects of a disease began to undermine his ability to function without help.

Revising Your Expectations

If there is a specific problem in a caregiver relationship, several approaches to solving the problem naturally occur to us. First, we might expect the other person involved to change. We don't usually like to change ourselves. However, if it seems easier to own up to the problem than argue with the other person, we are more likely to agree to change. Sometimes it seems best to change what initially appeared to cause the problem rather than get the other person involved to act differently. For example, if we can't agree on what program to watch on television, we might just turn off the television. Other times, it's just easier to overlook the problem and attempt to do something else.

Changing Beliefs About Behavior

Alzheimer's caregivers will benefit if they revise the ways they think about problems and what causes them. Blaming the problems on the person affected by the disease, or on yourself is not likely to lead to a solution. It will simply intensify the unpleasant feelings associated with the situation. As caregivers, you must be able to see how the behavior of a loved one is influenced by your expectations. Do you expect too much or too little? Will you treat the person differently if you expect less of her? If you expect too much, will she always get upset?

Adults, Not Children

Caring for an adult who had been fully capable and who is now becoming progressively more dependent is not the same as caring for a dependent child who is becoming more capable and independent. It is reasonable to expect a child to change her behavior, whether it requires learning a new skill or simply choosing to behave in a more socially appropriate manner. As parents, we consider the child before expecting her to do something. Is she ready to handle this particular task or situation? What is deemed appropriate is measured by where the child is in her development.

Caring for adults with Alzheimer's disease requires caregivers to maintain a similar developmental point of view, but reverse the direction of their expectations. What these adults are capable of doing becomes a matter of what abilities still remain. Appropriate behavior must be defined by standards that acknowledge the effects of progressive damage to the brain. Since there is fluctuation in abilities and the degree of impairments, caregivers must be flexible enough to change expectations from one day to the next. Beliefs appropriate for Alzheimer's care must reflect these differences. People with this disease become less and less able to be responsible for their behavior. How well they act and what they are able to do depends in part on the success caregivers have in predicting what their loved one is capable of doing at different times, on different tasks, and in different environments.

Problems and the Disease

Years ago it seemed helpful to advise caregivers to attribute problems to the disease itself, and not blame themselves or their loved ones for what happened. If relatives behaved in ways that were uncharacteristic of them, then it was helpful to say that unusual behavior was caused by Alzheimer's disease. Without further explanation, this approach is not much different from the idea that since there is no cure, nothing can be done. Why try to manage behavior? Anything that happens is the result of a disease that cannot be cured. You can't stop it. Why try? Such a proposition would seem to strengthen the sense of helplessness and hopelessness.

People have different ways of dealing with the enormity of the disease. For example, recently I was meeting with people who were forming a new support group in a small rural city. One of the persons present had just heard that her father had been diagnosed with Alzheimer's disease. Her mother related to her that the neurologist said her dad had a "little bit" of Alzheimer's. I have no way of knowing what the neurologist actually said, but to this family the idea that a loved one had a "little bit" of Alzheimer's was much easier to acknowledge. One cannot have a little bit of Alzheimer's, although one case may be more advanced than another. Still, having a "touch of it" gives one more time to understand what that means.

Other Ways to View Problems

Attributing problems to the disease is similar to having a "little bit" of Alzheimer's. It is a point where caregivers begin to understand how to deal with the challenges that lie before them. To offset the impact of the disease's progression, caregivers must have the opportunity to learn other ways to view the problems they encounter. They need to go beyond an understanding that simply explains problems as the result of brain cells being destroyed. They need to feel they have more control over what happens. When they are helping a family member do what he or she used to do, they want to know how to determine if an approach will be successful or if it might cause greater problems.

Questioning Old Beliefs About Behavior

Behavior changes dramatically and unexpectedly with Alzheimer's disease. The ways victims behave seems to have no rhyme or reason. Some changes can indeed be attributed to the fact that Alzheimer's destroys the way the brain works. But what is responsible for the other changes that occur? How can family caregivers feel more assured they are responding to the need of their loved one in the best possible way?

These questions are difficult. Professionals who study behavior—the ways people act and what they do—appreciate the fact that we cannot always know why people behave as they do. It can be even more difficult to understand why individuals whose behavior is influenced by brain impairment act as they do. Why does Mary, who has Alzheimer's disease, explode in rage when her husband repeatedly asks her if she wants to go for a walk? Anthony, whose wife has the disease, is bewildered by her persistent allegations that he is having an affair. How could she accuse him of such a thing.? Joseph's wife continues to tear clothes out of the dresser drawer each time he puts them back. Is his wife trying to get back at him for something he has done? Do these persons intentionally do these things? Are persons with this disease just naturally mean and belligerent? Does the disease make them want to hurt the ones they love?

Intent of Behavior

Most of us assume that people intend to do whatever it is they do. From the time we were children, we have been taught to be responsible for our actions. We believe we will be held accountable for what we do. If we fail to do what is right or acceptable, it is likely we will be held responsible for our failures. Many of us are harsh judges of ourselves. On other occasions, we make excuses, saying we forgot to do something, or insisting that what happened was not what we intended. Others involved may be reluctant to accept these excuses because they, too, believe behavior is intentional.

It seems we are most convinced something was intentional when it hurts or angers us, makes our day longer or our life harder. When we believe the acts or words directed at us were intentional, we personalize them. They anger and hurt us more when they continue, because now it is clear the person has purposely planned what is happening. We are angry and hurt because that was the intended result of a premeditated plan. We can only accept so many "accidents" of behavior.

Stress from Intentional Beliefs

The idea that behavior is intentional becomes a source of stress in caregiving. This idea is not easy to abandon when family members are caregivers. Even professional caregivers may feel the behavioral problems that confront them are the result of well-planned and purposeful efforts cleverly designed to disrupt the care they are attempting to provide, or simply to get attention. Even in the later stages of the disease, these people with brain damage are credited with devising grand schemes to sabotage their care or create greater misery for their caregivers.

The following examples may remind caregivers of similar experiences. We use these examples as we discuss the effects of Alzheimer's disease.

Geneva was getting ready to go to church. Her husband, who she had just taken from the bathroom and seated so that he could watch television, stood up, dropped his pants, and promptly soiled himself and the area around him. He had effectively manipulated her into staying with him. She was angry and resentful of the control he still exerted over her life.

Angie, a nurse's aide for 8 months, worked with Alzheimer's patients daily. Today, while she was taking Mr. Knots into a day area, he became agitated and resistant. She had told him she had to hurry so that she could take her break. He started yelling "no" loudly and repeatedly, and soon other residents in the area became upset. By the time she and other staff had calmed everyone down, it was too late to take her break. When she gave Mr. Knots a resentful glance, he was looking at his feet laughing. What reason had she given him to act this way?

Madge had just finished dressing her husband. He looked nice, and she was excited that her sister would be dropping by shortly. She left her husband sitting in the living room. Even though he did not care for her sister, he had agreed to open the door so that Madge could get dressed herself. It wasn't until Madge came out of the bedroom that she saw her husband wasn't where she had left him. The front door was open. Maybe her sister and husband were outside. A quick glance revealed an empty yard. About that time, her sister drove up. Now, she and her sister would spend time looking for her husband.

Old Beliefs about Intent

As couples, relating to one another may have become second nature because you are so familiar with each other. You relate to each other as you do because you "know how the other person is." You know what to ask and how to ask it. You are familiar with what your spouse likes and what he despises. You know how to get him to do something and when it is useless to try. You know what he can do and if he will support what you do. You even have a reasonable idea of why he does things and feels the way he does. From this perspective, it is possible to believe behavior is intentional.

Dealing with the behavior changes associated with Alzheimer's disease challenges our beliefs about behavior being intentional and planned. Caregivers must reexamine the relationship they have had with persons now affected by the disease. This involves taking inventory of what you know about their behavior and preferences. It includes recalling how you have dealt with problems in the past that affected your relationship. Some upsetting behaviors may upset you more when you believe they result from personality and the way the person has commonly reacted to past difficulties. Both personality and old styles of coping play a role in the way brain-damaged individuals behave.

Simpler Coping Styles

Persons experiencing brain impairment tend to retain old coping styles. They are expressed as old habits, or strategies that are simple, straightforward, and more immediate (Mace, 1990). John had never liked to stay long at the doctor's office. Now he is even more restless if he must wait very long. Catherine had always been prone to get upset at the smallest thing going wrong. She is now difficult for her husband to manage. Instead of thinking about her husband's request to do something, Dorothy simply says no, or walks away from the situation.

In an earlier example, Geneva believed her husband had soiled himself to keep her from going to church. If he had often manipulated her in the past, she may have reason to believe this behavior was manipulative. However, he may not have been aware of his surroundings or that his social judgment was faulty. He solved his immediate problem by using the living room floor for a bathroom.

This knowledge about the established patterns of behavior and why it occurs is valuable, but the effects of this disease will begin to disturb these patterns. You will wonder what happened to the predictability you used to take for granted. Combined with a better understanding of how the disease is changing the way loved ones act, this knowledge of the predictable patterns enables caregivers to learn new ways to interpret the reasons for behavior and modify the ways they interact with their family members. But to be completely open to this view of behavior, it will be helpful to reconsider what is involved in behavior being intentional.

Intentional behavior is directed toward some specific goal or purpose. It may be part of a conscious plan designed to accomplish or achieve something.

The brain damage associated with Alzheimer's disease gradually reduces the capacity individuals have for reasoning, planning, and carrying out anything but the most basic demonstrations of goal-directed behavior. These individuals lose sight of the normal consequences of behavior. They can no longer appreciate how their behavior affects others. Because their memory is faulty, they cannot remember what they might have started out doing when you find them standing in the middle of the room looking lost. They are lost in the sense that their behavior has no goal or destination.

Victims of Beliefs

In the examples given earlier, the caregivers were victims of their own assumptions about intentional behavior. Since their own intentions were clear to them, they assumed their loved ones understood what was expected of them. Everything would go smoothly if everyone did their part. But Geneva's husband didn't use the bathroom when he was supposed to, or in the appropriate way or place. The patient Angie who was taking to the day area failed to understand the reason she was in a hurry. He probably sensed she was in a hurry as she rushed him into the confusing social situation represented by the day area. His laughter had no relationship to the frustration she was experiencing. Madge's husband probably simply forgot her sister was coming and wandered off after he opened the door. He was as likely to be in another room of the house as he was wandering down the street.

Admittedly, the intentions of all these caregivers had been disrupted, but not as the result of some willful, premeditated plan made and executed by persons with Alzheimer's disease. Their world of needs, and the behavior produced to satisfy these needs, is much more basic. They may express a desire for something but fail to appreciate that it is impractical, dangerous, or even impossible. They respond to the "small picture," not the "big picture." As a result, they fail to understand the consequences of what they want or do; what they refuse to do or will not accept. They may want to go home to a place that doesn't exist or refuse to allow you to change clothes they have been worn for several days. They may do something dangerous, but become angry when you remove them from the dangerous situation. Their behavior in this compressed world will reveal more dramatic examples of poor judgment that seem to have little to do with the reality perceived by caregivers.

Decreased Behavior Control

Another aspect of our beliefs about behavior affects caregiving and must be modified so that it can be more realistically applied to the caregiving situation. We believe that people should control their behavior. This expectation requires continual revision as the degree of impairment increases. Ultimately, caregivers must accept the fact loved ones cannot control what they do. Their behavior is progressively influenced more by the interactions of others and the environments in which they live.

Feeling the need to urinate will signal the need to use the bathroom, and finding the bathroom will usually not be a problem. Later the person may feel the need to go to the bathroom, but may need reminders or assistance to get to it. The bathroom itself may stimulate its appropriate use for a while. Later reminders or instructions to use the bathroom will be required even when the person has been seated on the commode. Scheduling of routine trips to the bathroom will prevent accidents. Finally, the individual will no longer understand what the physical signals of his body mean or recognize what should be done. He cannot control his bladder the way he used to.

In the past, we believed people with Alzheimer's could have tried harder if their level of effort was insufficient for accomplishing something or doing it better. Unfortunately, many caregivers still believe that if the person tries harder, he should be able to do things he used to do, or at least do better. This belief is fostered by the fact that behavior fluctuates in Alzheimer's victims. One moment they can do something; the next moment they can't—or won't. Assuming this is only a case of stubbornness, some caregivers insist that loved ones should try harder. Sometimes the person does better, reinforcing the caregivers' belief that trying harder works; however, trying harder is not always an option.

People with Alzheimer's may be overwhelmed by demands that become threatening to them. They may not be aware of or understand what is expected of them. They may not know what to do or how to do it today, even though they knew yesterday. The emotional message communicated by caregivers may upset and confuse them, and distract their attention from tasks at hand.

Resulting Confusion

Finally, individuals may not even be aware of their impairments. Their response to demands may be reduced to anger, tears, or even greater stubbornness. They may be confused because they don't understand the task or why they must do it. They may be able to sense the caregiver's frustration, yet not understand its source.

Even though you may be in doubt, it generally is best to assume loved ones are trying as hard as they can. There might be other ways to get them to complete a task or improve their behavior. There is a saying employers often share with employees who may be working furiously but failing to accomplish enough: "Work smarter, not harder." This can be applied to Alzheimer's care. Pressing the person to work harder may create a catastrophic reaction. As a caregiver, you can work smarter by trying other approaches, backing off for a while, or changing your mind about how important it is for this particular thing to be done right now.

Emotions and Alzheimer's Behavior

Caregivers often wonder how loved ones perceive emotions. The fact that their intellectual abilities are diminishing does not necessarily mean they cannot experience a wide range of emotions, or be aware of the emotional content of what you express to them. In many cases, they may be more sensitive to what is communicated emotionally. Their own emotional expressions may reflect their reactions to what is happening at a particular moment, or represent the more persistent feelings they experience from time to time, such as fear, anger, anxiety, embarrassment, or different faces of confusion.

Emotions Are Messages

Displays of negative emotions may be uncomfortable for you as the caregiver. They may signal that something you are doing is distressing, or that the person with Alzheimer's fails to comprehend what is expected of him. Negative emotions may suggest something unpleasant or stressful in your environment. For instance, it is too dark, too noisy, too cold, or too hot. Perhaps the normal daily routine has been changed. Furniture may have been moved, or something else may have changed in what had been a familiar place. This is disconcerting and creates a greater sense of insecurity for the person with Alzheimer's. Persons with brain impairment have greater difficulty adjusting to changes.

As caregivers become more familiar with how their own behaviors and certain aspects of the physical environment affect loved ones emotionally, they can change what and how things are being done. Perhaps they need to slow down and be more encouraging. The music that was enjoyable for a little while becomes irritating if it continues. Unpleasant activities like bathing may be difficult to get started. Once the resistance has faded, this type of activity can be positive. On the other hand, behavioral or emotional problems in loved ones can suggest something internal is bothering them that has nothing to do with you or the external environment.

Negative emotions might also indicate that loved ones are more aware of changes in themselves. At times, denial or being unaware of the changes protects them from what must be an awesome realization. When they recognize that they cannot remember well, are unable to do things right, or don't know what to do, their behavior and emotional reactions may be more negative. Their caregivers may be perplexed or frightened by these situations. They may feel helpless in knowing their loved ones are experiencing emotions that are the result of disturbing but inaccessible perceptions.

Emotions and Behaviors as Clues

These emotions may reflect loved ones' grief over the loss of their abilities and themselves. They may experience regret about their dependence upon you and the burden they have become. They may be fearful of being left alone to face a process they are quite unable to stop. Worst of all, those persons for whom caregivers have so much concern might be unable to verbalize their fears and confusion. The thoughts are locked in; caregivers are locked out. Therefore, the best clues in helping caregivers understand their loved ones are the emotions and behaviors they observe.

Not all emotional reactions are negative. Positive emotions are also experienced by your loved one. Many of the same activities and experiences that used to stimulate positive emotions may still produce pleasant reactions. Your wife or husband's emotional reaction to something still depends upon his or her perception and understanding of it. If we don't catch the humor in a joke someone tells us, we are not likely to laugh even though it is expected of us. If other people are laughing outrageously, we might chuckle, but we still don't understand what is so funny. In contrast, if some scene in a movie touches us in a sad way we might cry. Other people may not have perceived that scene the way we did. Their experiences may have been different, or they simply did not understand things the way we did.

Individual Emotional Factors

The emotional reactions of Alzheimer's victims are still influenced by their individual characteristics. Family members must remember that affected loved ones are no longer as perceptive and do not perceive many situations as clearly as they may have in the past. They are unable to understand what is happening as well. Instead of becoming more involved in activities or situations that were previously enjoyable, they might withdraw more as familiar situations become confusing.

Situational Influences

If—on the basis of their understanding of behavior—family members can accommodate relatives in activities, their brain-impaired relatives have a better chance of following what is happening. Simple and clearer explanations of what is going on and how it applies to them enhance their chances of enjoying situations. Expectations are more specific and attainable. People with Alzheimer's may not be able to perceive the whole situation, but they can at least feel more appropriately involved.

Social situations created by family get-togethers may produce overwhelming mental and emotional stimulation. Making such situations more comprehensible for your loved one also reduces his own emotional reactions to the behavior of others around him. For instance, when a caregiving daughter invites other family members to dinner, her father will probably relate better to this situation if she can intercede on his behalf. If two people are speaking to him at once, he will likely become more anxious and confused. Rather than be able to say, "I can't answer everybody at once," he may walk away or become more irritated than the situation would have normally suggested. He might tell everyone to leave. He could perceive he is doing something wrong. The person with Alzheimer's might seem more suspicious to family members unaccustomed to the changes he has undergone in their absence.

Emotions and Morale

Positive emotional expressions have very positive effects on caregivers. Laughter, smiles, responses of humor, and expressions of affection are always welcomed. For that matter, the absence of negative emotion is readily accepted. Positive emotions and the absence of negative emotions give us the impression that our loved one is feeling fine and not suffering so much. If those we care for are not distressed and seem satisfied with what is going on for the moment, our burdens are lightened a bit.

Caregivers cannot easily separate themselves from the emotional responses of their relatives. A relationship exists and many interactions are bound to it. We are sensitive to the emotional expressions of loved ones because they help us understand the relationship. Alzheimer's disease does more than affect one spouse or parent. It impacts all relationships. It affects everyone in the family. Just as patterns of behavior existed prior to Alzheimer's disease, patterns of emotional reactions also existed. Recognition of these patterns were an important means of knowing your loved one. For a time, these reactions can still be predicted because they are still a part of your loved one's personality.

The aspects of relationships that involve the intellect and thinking tend to diminish early in the disease process. Social aspects of relationships, particularly intimacy, are gradually lost. Caregivers often remain intensely involved in efforts to sustain some semblance of these relationships. Their efforts are constantly threatened by the person's behavioral changes, the presence of psychiatric symptoms such as delusions, angry or hostile behavior directed at them, and the discouraging advice of others. The absence of encouragement and appreciation from their relative is all too obvious.

Emotional and Behavioral Communication

All of us like to know that what we do is appreciated. We all benefit from encouragement, especially when the challenge maybe greater than our physical and emotional resources. Caregivers must expect less encouragement and appreciation from loved ones affected by Alzheimer's, since their world is being diminished by loss of memory, the capacity to think, and the ability to relate to others as appropriately as they had before the disease became more pronounced. These changes in brain function ultimately contribute to severe errors of social judgment. These errors are not the result of ill intentions, although they may appear so at times.

Feedback as Aid to Communication

When we interact with people, it's helpful to know how effectively we are communicating with them. Feedback tells us how the other person is receiving what we are saying or doing: Does he understand what you mean? Does she like what you are doing? Emotional expressions, the way the person acts, or what the person says are all sources of feedback. We can modify what we say or do on the basis of this information. He or she will be less likely to give you much verbal information unless you ask questions. You may be able to get some type of yes or no response to simple questions if what you are asking is understood by your family member. These responses may add to your confusion, rather than your understanding of what did or did not happen. Since verbal behavior becomes less reliable and understandable in Alzheimer's patients, caregivers must rely on other aspects of communication for feedback.

Emotional reactions and behavior of those for whom we care become important sources of feedback for caregivers. Negative emotional reactions may tell you that you are asking too much, or expecting it too quickly. Anxious or agitated behavior suggests your loved ones may become more upset unless you modify your expectations and become more supportive and encouraging. When your husband passively resists a request to get up and go to the kitchen, he may not understand your request or be sure how to get to the kitchen. He might feel ashamed about this and depend on you to guide him to the kitchen. Emotional and behavioral messages provide caregivers with important clues for managing behavior. Caregivers who fail to recognize and interpret these clues appropriately may be inviting the occurrence of a catastrophic reaction. This failure is common in brain-damaged individuals and is predicted by specific emotional and behavioral signs. We will consider this phenomenon shortly.

There is a scene in the video production of *Caregiving with Grace* (Cohen and Whiteford, 1987) that illustrates our points about behavior, emotional reactions to experiences, the effects of the disease on relationships, and the need caregivers have for some small signs of appreciation. *Caregiving with Grace* reflects the changes in Grace's behavior and abilities about 10 years after Alzheimer's had been diagnosed. Her husband, Glen, demonstrates how he interacts and works with his wife when providing the assistance necessary for activities of daily living to be completed. Rather than simply doing these activities for Grace, Glen tries to involve her in some part of the task.

Glen is painting his wife's fingernails. Though Glen is a model caregiver with an exemplary understanding of the disease's effects on Grace's behavior, he has related the frustrations he experiences daily. He recognizes the fact that Grace cannot be expected to express her gratitude for what he does. In fact, her emotional expressions seem anxious and tense during this experience of having her fingernails painted. Glen is not just painting her fingernails; he is repeatedly encouraging Grace to participate in this activity in small but significant ways. "Hold still." "Give me this hand." He also gives Grace feedback about how she is doing and how nice she looks with her fingernails painted. Finally, his task is done, and he both asks and shows Grace how to wave her hands in the air so that they will dry quicker.

Grace looks pleased and relieved. Perhaps she is pleased with how her fingernails look and that she had some involvement in the completion of this activity. They completed something as a couple. She is certainly relieved by the decrease of demands on her. Then Glen invites her to thank him for what he has done. She appears a little perplexed. Maybe she thought everything was finished, yet now she must say "thank you" when she had not uttered a word all day. Glen persists with encouragement. The emotional expressions on her face indicate she is trying. She makes sounds that are a closer approximation of frustration than "thank you." Suddenly the viewer witnesses a victory. The words come forth. Her facial expressions suggest she has accomplished something. Despite the fact that it was solicited, she gave something to her husband—something that suggests more about a relationship than it does the completion of a task.

Behavior and Stress

Caregivers less familiar with how to perform an activity with a relative whose impaired memory creates deficits in behavior might have been more reluctant than Glen to continue. Without understanding why, they could have anticipated the situation to worsen. Instead of completing the desired task, they could have been confronted by more difficult behavioral problems. Both the caregiver and the person with Alzheimer's would then be involved in a progressively more sensitive and stressful situation. Some activities of daily living, for example, dressing, bathing, eating, and toileting, need to be completed. One time may be better than another, but people with Alzheimer's eventually do not remember why these things must be done. Caregivers experience a good deal of stress from the anticipated behavioral and emotional reactions loved ones might exhibit when they are trying to finish simple activities of daily living.

Stress as Predictor of Problems

Glen was very attentive to Grace's behavior and emotional expressions. They were good measures of how stressful having her fingernails painted was for her. Glen gauged how firm and encouraging he needed to be on the basis of behavioral and emotional clues. He did not require too much of Grace, though at times she became more anxious. His own emotional reaction was calm, which matched the content of his verbal encouragement. His approach prevented her from overreacting to minor stressors.

The stress experienced by persons with Alzheimer's and the way they behave and function is closely related. Their anxiety will serve as a fairly reliable indicator of how much activity and stimulation they can tolerate. They are quite responsive to reductions of stress in their environments; the more impaired they are, the more strongly their environments influence the outcomes of their interactions (Lawton, 1989). In this sense, environment is more than the physical setting in which these persons live. Environment involves their interactions with people and things, and even their responses to their own thoughts.

Multiple and simultaneous messages or distractions are two examples of stressors that people with Alzheimer's experience. Nonverbal messages that pressure them to hurry are stressful, as are commands that carry the same message. Any demands that are placed on areas of impaired cognitive functioning will increase their experience of stress. Other sources of stress include pressure to perform tasks that are complex because they have multiple steps, illness, not being understood or being able to understand, fatigue, frustration, fear, anxiety, or perceiving nonverbal negative messages. Receiving negative verbal messages can be stressful and demoralizing to these individuals. Their own awareness of their mistakes and impairments is probably a fairly persistent source of stress.

Stress Reduction as a Tool

Caregivers need to pay careful attention to other sources of stress that individuals experience and remove or diminish the strength of such stressors. Brain damage itself does not sufficiently explain many of the behavior difficulties you and your loved one experience. Situations that are overly stressful can have much to do with these problems. If you minimize stressors, you reduce the possibility of more severe behavioral and emotional outbursts.

Catastrophic Reactions

Stress, fear, fatigue, and anxiety are common experiences for people with Alzheimer's disease. Everyone of us has a breaking point. We are already dealing with more stress than we thought we could handle. It only takes another small demand on us and we explode. From one day to the next, that breaking point may change, depending on how much stress we are under at the time. Brain-damaged individuals cannot tolerate the amount of stress they used to handle. Small things can become big things. When brain-damaged individuals overreact to minor stressors, they exhibit catastrophic reactions. Little things are overwhelming.

What is meant by catastrophic reactions has already been shown in the examples in this chapter. They include behaviors and emotional reactions that are as common as they are disturbing. Catastrophic reactions are manifested as angry outbursts, refusals to do something, agitation, pacing, more intense anxiety, tearfulness, whining, mumbling, or even crying. In more extreme cases, catastrophic reactions may include hitting or striking out.

Too often the assertion that persons with Alzheimer's disease are aggressive results from a poor understanding of catastrophic reactions. Persons with Alzheimer's disease are already overwhelmed and their choices of protective responses are reduced to basic fight or flight. If they are cornered during catastrophic reactions, these individuals often try to withdraw. Their other response to these feelings is likely to be defensive, but it is labeled aggressive by those who misinterpret it, thus making it worse.

The behavioral and emotional changes associated with catastrophic reactions usually build in intensity, but they can appear suddenly and be quite intense. Catastrophic reactions may occur infrequently and seem to be unpredictable and sporadic. They may also occur almost continuously, and environmental or interpersonal factors that encourage them can be identified. Some sources may be very simple, such as asking a person to do more than he is capable of doing or asking too many questions. A new situation, person, or environment can precipitate catastrophic reactions. Some source of confusion or insecurity is often involved. It may take a combination of factors to precipitate these reactions one day, and many fewer factors the next. The reactions are largely beyond the control of the person exhibiting them.

Easier to Prevent Than Stop

Alzheimer's caregivers need to attend to potential sources of anxiety, fear, fatigue, and stress since it is much easier to prevent catastrophic reactions than to stop them in progress (Mace, 1990). While catastrophic reactions are common with this disease, their sources are often a function of the individual preferences of the person experiencing them. An activity or situation may be comfortable for one individual but become quite threatening to another. For example, some persons can tolerate being alone; others cling to caregivers whenever there is an indication they might be left alone.

Excess Disability

Caregivers may notice that loved ones are not functioning as well as they could realistically expect. Some fluctuations in behavior can be anticipated because of the progressive but sometimes unpredictable progression of this disease. However, some impairment or disability may not be attributable to the disease. This problem has been called excess disability and has many potential sources during the course of this disease.

In Alzheimer's disease, excess disability can commonly be attributed to the presence of other illnesses, medications, psychiatric symptoms related to the disease, sensory impairments such as poor vision and hearing, stress, fatigue, and anxiety (Mace, 1990). Care environments that encourage unnecessary dependency foster excess disability. Social or physical environments that have too little stimulation have the same result. Caregivers must take the presence of excess disability very seriously and see that it is eliminated or reduced. This may require professional assistance whenever possible. The result is certainly worthwhile. Loved ones might be able to function better and more appropriately. This in turn reduces the additional stress you as a caregiver experience, and those for who you care might feel better about themselves.

Summary

Behavioral changes associated with the experience of Alzheimer's disease have many sources. Brain damage is only one source of change in behavior and the behavior management problems caregivers must face. Understanding the changes that occur through the stages of the disease process might help family caregivers appreciate some of the changes they may encounter. Like so many aspects of Alzheimer's disease, stages are a rough guide. They map how behavior might change, providing a general sense of what you can expect, but you must be ready to respond to changes when the map is wrong. Behavior is the result of a dynamic pattern of responses to stimuli that produce action, feelings, and thoughts. Individual personality, the severity of brain impairment, the physical and interpersonal environment, and many other factors influence how people perceive and respond to stimulation outside themselves.

Beliefs about Behavior

Emotional and behavioral reactions can be traced to the thoughts and feelings that relatives experience. Many of the ideas we have considered have application to the behavior of caregivers; themselves. Beliefs that caregivers have about behavior influence their own understanding and reactions to it. It will be necessary to change beliefs that fail to account for the impact of brain damage on behavior. It is important to better understand the relationship between behavior and brain damage.

Brain damage influences the ways persons with Alzheimer's disease understand and perceive things. It affects how these individuals act and react. Their behavior and emotional reactions to experiences will gradually suggest more of the impact of the disease, and both will provide clues that suggest how the caregiver can manage the situation. They provide the caregiver with information about what to do and not to do. Recognizing this helps prevent a catastrophic reaction and reduce the stress of the situation.

Emotions—negative and positive—influence behavior and the way afflicted people can think and remember. Their behavior and personality will fit together in less predictable ways as Alzheimer's advances. These changes will have dramatic effects on what they can do and what they require of you.

Environments play a key role in the way people with Alzheimer's function. Physical and social environments must be adapted so that they are less confusing and overwhelming, more secure and familiar. The environment must be comfortable and supportive of caregiving and daily living. Although these environments should provide stimulation, they should not provide so much that they significantly exceed the coping abilities of loved ones. The behavior and emotional reactions of loved ones progressively become determined more by their environments and the persons in those environments.

Excess disabilities created by such conditions as depression and other health problems must be addressed so that the functioning of individuals experiencing the mental, emotional, and eventually physical manifestations of this disease is not further compromised.

Within these changes, there are many losses. But these losses cannot be experienced only as losses of behavior. They represent the losses of relationships, the losses of persons you love. Caregivers are compelled to care for someone they love with very little encouragement. The more they care for the person, the more they realize that the person is leaving. This departure seems never to be finished and one feels suspended in a moment of grief that constantly repeats itself.

Glimpses of the Person

Understanding behavioral changes helps caregivers appreciate those small glimmers of the old personality that appear through the long days of caring. Someone is still there and must be trying just as you are trying. A small step is not much, but it might remind you of a moment when you were walking together, and the relationship you once had is again present. Little things can make a big difference.

As a relative who has become the caregiver for someone with Alzheimer's disease, you will be tempted to feel solely responsible for all of the problems that arise during the course of the disease. We must not forget that loved ones, too, are often struggling to do something about what is happening to them. The changes that you may witness that are unacceptable and cause greater concern may represent another glimmer of personality. They may represent the efforts of loved ones to adapt to what is so difficult to understand and accept. When that is the case, it is something you share. You are both trying to understand and accept the changes.

Acceptance

You have Alzheimer's disease
and you're losing the power
to remember—to reason—to understand,
to do the simple tasks
we take for granted:
to put on a shoe—
to button a shirt—
to read a book—
to remember a face or name.

It's a hard thing to understand—
to accept . . .
Perhaps it's been the hardest for me,
for I've lived with you—
but I know—you can't help it—
can't act otherwise . . .

I must take you as you are
and expect—not more—but less
as the disease continues to progress.

Maude S. Newton

9

Stages of Family Adjustment

Accepting the Disease

Adjusting to the reality of Alzheimer's disease in a loved one is a complex and difficult process. Yet we must find a way to reconcile ourselves to the disease as best we can, for accepting the disease makes it easier to handle the emotional and physical strains that Alzheimer's brings. If we continue to deny the disease and its implications, we risk denying both the person with Alzheimer's and ourselves the support and care that are needed.

Adjusting to Alzheimer's Like Adjusting to a Death.

Because Alzheimer's is a fatal disease and one that often involves a lingering death, the stages of grief that family members go through are very similar to the stages of adjustment to death described by Dr. Elizabeth Kübler-Ross in her 1969 book, *On Death and Dying*. It is useful to understand these stages, both as they correspond to one's own psychological adjustment to the disease and for the light they may shed on the reactions of other family members.

Not everyone will go through these stages in the same way, of course, and some family members will find it easier to accept the disease than others. Each individual will probably find that she can reconcile herself to what is happening at some times better than others. Often we may misinterpret the reactions of those around us or wish they would adjust differently. If family members accept the idea that each person must face up to the disease in his own way, however, the family can serve as a strong support system throughout the adjustment process.

In one family, for example, a mother and her son may react very differently to the illness of the father. The mother may feel a helpless anger and

134

compensate by becoming overly involved with the illness, shutting out her son. The son may feel abandoned by his father and snubbed by his mother, and may lash out in frustration when she refuses to let him help. Rather than make things more difficult for each other, both mother and son must work to understand the other's adjustment process and to accept it, as long as serious questions of sufficient care or the caregiver's health are not involved.

In considering the family's stages of acceptance, it is important to remember the following facts:

- Each family member must have the chance to work through the stages of grief to final acceptance of the disease. This does not mean that encouragement and support are not needed, or that professional help is not indicated.

- What family members are willing to do about the loved one's needs and their own is influenced by where they are in the adjustment process. Caregiving is not simply a mechanical experience; it also involves thoughts and feelings.

- The adjustment process does not always occur in clearly defined stages. Longstanding conflicts and repressed feelings may need resolving before acceptance can be reached. In such cases, professional counseling may be advisable.

Kübler-Ross's Stages of Acceptance

The following are Dr. Kübler-Ross's stages of adjustment to death.

1. **Denial and isolation.** The person experiences shocked disbelief when faced with imminent death. She thinks: "No, this can't happen to me . . . it can't be true!"

2. **Anger and resentment.** The person's thoughts revolve around "Why me?" and "What have I done to deserve this?" She feels anger and bitterness toward others, the world, and even herself

3. **Bargaining.** In her mind, the person tries to buy back her life with some promise or action. "I'll do anything if you'll give me another day, a year, five years," she may think. God may be called on in the bargaining to heal the person and restore life.

4. **Depression.** The person despairingly gives in to death because it cannot be stopped. "What's the use?" she thinks. "Why go on fighting?"

5. **Acceptance.** The person withdraws into peace and a final rest.

While these reactions are generally experienced by the dying person, family members may experience them as well.

The stages defined by Kübler-Ross, do not entail all that is involved in one's acceptance of death. Some persons may never accept death. They may die still angry that life has cheated them. A spouse may be depressed for months after the death and remain angry even longer.

Perception of Loss an Individual Experience

It is not appropriate to compare one family's loss with the losses of others. However, some families may be affected by the following factors that make their loss especially difficult to accept:

1. **The age of the person when Alzheimer's is diagnosed.** Younger people with Alzheimer's forced to leave their jobs must contend with loss of income and insurance benefits. The healthy spouse may still be working, which makes arranging for caregiving more difficult.

2. **The general health of the victim.** When the person with Alzheimer's is in otherwise good health, the feeling of being cheated by life may be more intense. A person may have been prepared for cancer or heart disease but not a mysterious illness like Alzheimer's.

3. **The length of the illness.** The emotional strains of extended caregiving, along with its physical and financial costs, may intensify the family's feeling of abandonment and loss.

4. **The family's expectations.** Alzheimer's disease may be nothing like the family imagined, or the family may feel disappointed in the response of health professionals to their loved one's condition.

5. **The family's emotional closeness.** The afflicted person's loss of social and intellectual capabilities creates tremendous barriers to communication, and some families may not be able to counteract their sense of separation and isolation from the person.

6. **Preexisting family roles.** The spouse affected by Alzheimer's may have been responsible for managing most, if not all, of the family's affairs. The manifestations of the illness create a greater threat to the spouse-caregiver when she must assume the new duties of family management plus caregiving.

Adjustment to the Disease Usually Includes Five Stages

The following stages of family adjustment are based upon the stages identified by Kübler-Ross but have been modified by Paul Teusink and Susan Mahler (1984) to reflect the normal series of responses that families go through when confronted by Alzheimer's disease:

1. **Denial.** Reflects the initial response that nothing is wrong

2. **Overinvolvement.** Similar to bargaining; represents an attempt to compensate for the illness and associated impairments
3. **Anger.** Follows when the family realizes that compensation has failed
4. **Guilt.** Develops out of the anger and "what ifs" precipitated by looking back
5. **Acceptance.** Resolution or acceptance of the problems

Each of these stages is treated in depth.

1. Denial

Denial is the most common and frequently used defense, and it comes into play from the beginning. Beliefs about senility and old age lead the family to excuse the person's forgetfulness and thus help to sustain denial. Family members really may not feel certain that anything serious is wrong.

Denial Can Create Dangerous Situations

Denying the problem allows family members to postpone action. When the person lives alone, children may resist evaluating what is happening. Neighbors or friends may call to report some concerns; children may visit the parent to check these reports. However, their own denial prevents them from doing more than visiting more frequently or encouraging the parent to get out and do more.

The denial also prevents the family from adequately recognizing or facing the extent of the impairment and its consequences. The family's failure to understand such consequences places the loved one in a higher-risk situation, particularly if she is living alone.

Denial Can Create Family Conflict

Some family members may recognize that action needs to be taken but encounter denial from other family members. If a family leader is denying the problem, it can be more difficult for the others to get professional help for the affected relative.

Denying symptoms is a normal defense against threats to one's well-being. It is normal and necessary to gradually adjust to the implications of the disease. The slow progression of the illness provides time for the family to make this adjustment and to accept what is happening.

Excessive denial can be quite destructive, however. It blocks help and any movement toward acceptance. Plans for care cannot be made until a realistic assessment of the patient's and the family's needs is made.

Moving Past Denial

The following steps can help families to move past denial:

- Seeking and receiving information about Alzheimer's disease and the family experience
- Getting a professional evaluation of the person's degree of impairment
- Understanding the consequences of the impairment and, with professional assistance, becoming sensitive to the patient's reactions to the illness
- Seeking counseling with a professional if denial is excessive
- Addressing issues emerging from the denial with personal, family, and professional support

A Thorough Evaluation Involves Numerous Health Professionals

During the actual evaluation process, it is quite appropriate for families to seek a second opinion. However, seeking many opinions can indicate desperate denial. In most situations, the Alzheimer's diagnosis already involves several opinions. For example, the following evaluative process is used at DePaul Center, a psychiatric hospital in Waco, Texas. Such a process addresses the need for a comprehensive evaluation to effectively plan activities involving the patient, family, and community resources.

Medical evaluation.   Includes basic tests (e.g., blood chemistry, chest X-ray, electrocardiogram, etc.) and specified elective tests (e.g., EEG or brain scan). Additionally, a neurologist or other specialists may be consulted.

Psychiatric evaluation.   Assesses the presence of other psychiatric illnesses consistent with symptoms, such as severe depression; considers effects and utilization of medications as well as other medical findings.

Social history.   Includes psychosocial history and assessment of the family system, resources available, and resources needed.

Psychological/Neuropsychological testing.   Assists in differentiating strengths and weaknesses related to dementia and a person's emotional reactions to it; identifies actual deficits related to impaired brain function or other psychiatric disorders.

Therapy evaluation.   A physical therapist and occupational therapist evaluate functioning and determine rehabilitation needs and potential.

Even when family members seem to accept the diagnosis of Alzheimer's disease, denial may leave them vulnerable to shopping for cures or believing that medication prescribed to manage symptoms will cure the disease.

False Hopes

Sometimes, denial reemerges when there seem to be fluctuations in the person's condition. Good days seem to promise the person is improving. Bad days intensify the family's worries that the person is deteriorating rapid can profit most by getting off the emotional roller coaster of alternati and despair, while making the most of the good days.

2. Overinvolvement

The primary caregiver may try to meet every need of the affected person, become severely isolated, and refuse assistance or support from any source. Often, the individual demonstrating overinvolvement is a spouse, although families as a whole can be overinvolved as well.

Overinvolvement Seeks to Counter the Impact of the Illness

Once family members overcome the denial stage and admit to themselves that the illness exists, they naturally want to take action. For the family of an Alzheimer's patient, active involvement with this person represents a way to attempt to counteract the effects of the illness and compensate for their relative's losses. The impact of the illness can be made less noticeable when the family is covering for the relative in all areas.

A family's overinvolvement can become a tool for providing the best possible care to the afflicted relative. As this stage begins, the family can plan their involvement in the overall care. Particular attention should be paid to support for the person with Alzheimer's and her spouse, who very likely will become overinvolved. Overinvolvement is a form of bargaining. When compensations fail, other strong emotions emerge.

Overinvolvement Can Create Barriers to Asking for Help

Overinvolvement becomes dangerous, however, when it reaches extreme proportions. Many persons who become overinvolved fail to seek help when they should. Loyalty, duty, family, and cultural values, combined with a strong sense of obligation, reinforce the view that the caregiver must handle the illness alone. Nonetheless, such individuals reach a point when they are more open to help, even though they may not ask for it directly.

Extreme overinvolvement can lead to greater isolation and to the caregiver's sacrificing herself to the illness. Examples of caregivers who have experienced major health problems, such as high blood pressure and stress-related illnesses, are common.

Help for the Overinvolved Caregiver

The following is an outline to follow in helping the overinvolved caregiver:

- Explore and discuss available options. A caregiver may accept the need for help in the home before she can consider institutionalization.
- Involve other family members and friends in different aspects of the care situation.

relinquish the burden of guilt by pointing out that
ave surpassed the resources of any one person.

that the type of care needed cannot successfully be
me setting.

r to realize that her overinvolvement is hurting both
erself, and is likely creating problems for the rest of the

- Sugg-   ssening the spouse's care load may improve the quality of
time she spends with the loved one.

3. Anger

The third stage of the acceptance process is anger, which can stem from the added physical and emotional burden caused by continued deterioration in the person and the caregiving situation. The caregiver's dedication and sacrifices may not seem to have made any difference. Also, the resources needed may not be available or may cost more than the family can afford.

Angry Reactions Cause Guilt

Caregivers who have been tolerant of their relative's embarrassing behavior may begin to get angry as the behavior moves beyond their control. In turn, the loss of control may precipitate guilt. Unfortunately, some family members lose even more control under intense stress and verbally and/or physically abuse the loved one.

Anger Can Stem from Feelings of Abandonment

The family can feel angry about being abandoned by the clearly dysfunctional relative, which can be further complicated by longstanding interpersonal problems. Whether justified or not, a caregiver may be hostile toward family and friends. Feelings of being left alone and having to make all the decisions alone can intensify anger. However, angry outbursts should be avoided, as they can alienate family members from one another. The anger stage of acceptance may leave the primary caregiver and others in the family quite sensitive to critical remarks about the care decisions they have made.

Misdirected Anger Common

While a person is in the anger stage, her reactions can touch others who have been less directly involved with in-home caregiving. Staff members in long-term care facilities need to recognize that anger is a part of the road to acceptance. However, family members should recognize and address its real source. Otherwise, it can be misdirected toward persons who are crucial to the loved one's care or others who play vital roles in supporting the family.

4. Guilt

Guilt is a normal reaction to Alzheimer's. However, those involved must take care that the powerful combination of unresolved anger and guilt they feel does not become overwhelming and develop into serious depression (see Chapter 3). Caregivers may need professional help to resolve unrelenting feelings of anger and guilt.

Guilt Can Arise from Old Conflicts

Much guilt can arise from family conflicts left unresolved over the years. Family members may dwell on past regrets, wishing they could only do things over. Relatives may find themselves dwelling on such questions as "What if an evaluation had been done a year sooner?" or "What if we had seen another doctor?" They may think "We should have done more for her and spent more time with her while she was healthy." But the family must eventually put aside such thoughts, forgive themselves, and go on living.

Guilt about the Wish for Death

It is not uncommon for family members to wish that their loved one would die and then feel guilty about that wish. As hard as it is to lose someone, most persons can view death in the last stage of Alzheimer's disease as a real blessing for their loved one and for those who cared so much for so long.

Regrets Can Become Overwhelming

Guilt also can be triggered by the caregiver's angry acts or imagined omissions. Perhaps she did not do enough, or perhaps she lashed out at her relative in frustration. But the caregiver must not let regrets and guilt overwhelm her, it is only human to occasionally lose control under such stressful circumstances.

Other Sources of Guilt

Family members often find themselves giving their relative with Alzheimer's information that is not completely true. They may tell their relative they are taking her to the store, when the destination is really the doctor's office. They may not be truthful about the purpose of a medication for delusions or agitation. These "white lies" are sometimes a source of guilt because family members believe they are being dishonest with their loved one, tricking her or lying to her. It is best to remember the motivations behind these actions.

Half-Truths and Caring

Half-truths may be necessary for appropriate care or to help families manage their affected relatives. Persons with Alzheimer's disease fail to understand the logic behind many actions as their illness progresses. Attempts to reason with them will only make matters worse in many cases. If they become extremely agitated and resistant, taking medication or trips to the doctor can become major caregiving stressors. Family members need not feel guilty about many of the half-truths they use to care for their loved ones.

Tough Decisions Can Create Guilt

Decisions made against the wishes of the patient can leave the caregiver struggling with feelings of guilt. If a spouse or child forced the visit to the doctor, she may feel guilt after the evaluation confirming the diagnosis of Alzheimer's. Likewise, placing her loved one in a nursing home or another institution can raise doubts and feelings of guilt. Hopefully, this conflict can be handled by realizing that the loved one's needs cannot be provided for at home. Most likely, the caregiver did all she could and gave much more of herself than she would have thought possible.

5. Acceptance

The Fight Is Over

Acceptance, the final stage of a family's response to Alzheimer's disease, is possible when the process of the disease and its effect on others is fully understood. It is easier once the family members have found within themselves the resources to cope with Alzheimer's. Resources in the community become a part of their strength and are accepted in turn once they fully comprehend the impact of the illness.

The anger and guilt associated with each person's adjustment is now behind her, and she can see each stage's place in moving toward a more peaceful acceptance of fate. She can recognize, without reservation, that her loved one is no longer the person she once knew.

New situations can precipitate a return or regression to earlier stages of adjustment. The need to let go of unfinished plans or dreams, or the comments of friends and family, may trigger a temporary setback. The caregiver should understand that such experiences are simply brief detours rather than roadblocks in the adjustment process.

10

Family Responses to Care

The experience of grief is a significant part of the family adjustment to Alzheimer's disease. Victims of the disease know something bad is happening. Our understanding of how these persons grieve is imperfect. Some behavioral and emotional problems may be manifestations of their grief. The family caregiver and other relatives experience stress and strain that directly relate to the grief experience. They also experience stress resulting from failure of the family to support the tasks of caregiving—the interactions that provide for the needs of the chronically affected relative on an unrelenting, daily basis. Alzheimer's disease creates a crisis in a family.

The losses that reflect the progressive deterioration of an individual suggest the loss of the family as it was known. Gradually it becomes apparent that the roles played by the relative with Alzheimer's disease can no longer be managed by that individual. Other family members must assume some of these responsibilities. The wife, for example, may find herself responsible for decisions that her husband would ordinarily have made. Even though she may now make these decisions, his influence may still be considerable. In more extreme cases, the Alzheimer's spouse—even while suffering the more advanced manifestations of the disease—may actually be involved in decision making.

Need for Family Support

The influence of other family members and friends will be critical in helping caregivers to take over and control activities such as driving and making financial decisions. Often, the family caregiver will not prevent the loved one with Alzheimer's from driving, carelessly paying bills, or making extravagant purchases. In other families, the children will prevent opportunities for the afflicted person to drive or handle money. Their response might be so forceful that it causes more emotional difficulties in the family. One child might be willing to intervene in certain family matters, but stay away from other situations. Another child may choose to stay away from family interactions altogether.

Changing Roles

Part of the family adjustment to the crisis of Alzheimer's disease involves changes in normal family roles. Preexisting patterns of interacting and communicating will have considerable influence on how families address these changes. They can be quite difficult or even impossible to make. In other families, they seem to be made with relative ease. Families are unique. In some families, changes are too unsettling, even when they would support the stability of the family and the needs of the affected relative and his caregiver.

More directly than other family members, the primary family caregiver will experience the successes and failures of family responses to the needs created by Alzheimer's disease. Expectations of family members need to be tempered with an understanding of how they have responded to previous crises in the family. Consider the various roles different family members have assumed, the quality of their support, and their willingness to be involved. In short, family members need to reevaluate how they interact with one another. When all family members are together, the atmosphere and quality of the interaction may be quite different.

There are several ways family interactions can be considered during times of crises. We examine some characteristics of different family interactions (Blazer, 1984). The quality of interactions in these descriptions of family characteristics varies considerably. Several characteristics apply to families and influence their effectiveness in dealing with the stress of caregiving as a healthy family unit.

Compatible vs. Conflictual Families

Family interactions are compatible when members usually agree with one another. Small differences can exist but are usually reconciled without much apparent disagreement. Interactions that reveal conflict and more obvious differences are more likely to impede family attempts to develop clear, unified responses to problems. Some conflict may be desirable. An extremely compatible family may be afraid of conflict. To avoid conflict, major issues may be ignored. Compatible family interactions are likely to promote a more relaxed atmosphere that further fosters working together; highly conflictual family interactions create an atmosphere of tension, anxiety, anger, and hurt. The tasks of caregiving are frustrated by interpersonal conflicts.

Crises such as Alzheimer's disease have the capacity to stimulate conflict. All family members are affected. The future of the family and its members may become uncertain. Such a situation affects relationships and changes them. These changes among parents and children have been referred to as "rejoining" (Blazer, 1984). Rejoining parents and children can be difficult because of some of the conflicts that arise. There are three types of conflict that can occur when a crisis affects changes in the parent/child relationship during rejoining: continuing, new, and reactivated.

Continuing Conflicts

Continuing conflicts have always been present between parents and their children. When Alzheimer's disease develops, new problems face the family. Adult daughters may feel compelled to become more involved than their own immediate family responsibilities would seem to allow. However, their reason for declining the responsibility of hands-on care for a parent may be supported by old, unresolved conflicts. Perhaps the parent with Alzheimer's disease was the parent who drank too much and was abusive. Continuing conflicts that involve a history of abuse can predict risks in Alzheimer's caregiving when the abused child is faced with caring for the abusive parent. The expectation of reasonable give-and-take between parents and children might have been violated and might represent the source of continuing conflict.

Continuing conflicts may interfere with new problems being addressed in Alzheimer's care. The unfinished business they reflect needs to be resolved if at all possible. If it involves the parent now afflicted with Alzheimer's, it needs to be completed before the intellectual impairment surpasses the person's capacity to participate in the problem-solving process. Alzheimer's disease can affect all family members in continuing conflicts.

New Conflicts

New conflicts may develop in families confronted by Alzheimer's disease and reflect issues that never required attention before. These crises are normal for well-adjusted families (Blazer, 1984) and relate to issues concerning nursing home placement, death and dying, living arrangements, the type of professional help that might be needed, and the distribution of family resources and responsibilities. These issues may be difficult to address. Conflicting views may be intense and divergent, but well-adjusted families have a healthy foundation for addressing them. The capability to resolve conflicts and solve problems gives family members confidence and restores hope.

Reactivated Conflicts

Sometimes old conflicts appear to have been resolved in families. This may turn out to be an illusion. The conflicts may have been buried or avoided so successfully they were forgotten. Family members may be shocked and dismayed when they realize the new conflict they experience is an old conflict that has been reactivated by a new situation. *Reactivated* conflicts in the family tend to focus on issues of independence and dependence, acceptance and rejection, and sibling rivalries that had become more obscure (Siegler and Hyer, 1984).

When adult children assume the responsibility of caring for a parent, they commonly assume roles that would have been naturally associated with the parent. The parent tends to be viewed as less capable in some areas of functioning, perhaps acting less like an adult. Alzheimer's disease affects adults in this manner. As children take care of their parent, the roles are reversed. At times they may view the parent's behavior as childish. Some children view the parent as a child and treat him or her as they would a child, perhaps the way they remember being treated as children. Within the reactivated conflict, old feelings surface. Role reversals may reactivate conflicts experienced by families involved in the care of persons with Alzheimer's.

Dependent Needs Change

An adult child who had depended upon the parent affected by Alzheimer's disease, may resent the disease and the parent because his or her source of dependency is severely threatened. Continued demands of the parent will produce problems in coping with the illness for both the parent and the adult child. For the adult child, time to establish a more independent lifestyle is quickly running out. If the parent recognizes this, dealing with Alzheimer's disease is complicated by concerns for the welfare of the adult child. In cases where the dependent adult child is the primary source of support, there may be additional concerns about that individual's capacity to provide what will be needed. These family members are likely to become so bonded to one another that it may be difficult for other family members to effectively assist with the needed care.

The caregiver spouse may find it necessary to seek the assistance of children who have been rejected by the other parent. As these children become involved, the behavior of the parent—even though it may be influenced by brain damage and a disease process—may be looked upon as a manifestation of earlier rejection. At first, a child may refuse to help because it is awkward to manage the parent's behavior. The real reason may be related to feelings associated with an old conflict that has been reactivated.

The increased dependence of parents and resolution of old conflicts represents a *filial* crisis that faces all adult children (Blenkner, 1965). In order for adult children to resolve the conflicts associated with this crisis, they must accept the dependencies of their parents. This involves clarifying the confusion associated with new roles that develop between children and their parents. Parents, from whom adult children had sought support in times of emotional trouble and economic pressure, now need the comfort and support of their children.

New Views of Parent

The acceptance of this role requires adult children to develop a vastly different view of the relationship they have with their parents. Through this view, children recognize and accept the interdependent future of parents without ignoring or invalidating their independent past (Eyde and Rich, 1983). They mature into a role that is supportive of the potential for remaining independent and responsive to developing dependencies. This is superior to the idea of simple role reversal because it integrates the image of who parents were with who they are. Alzheimer's disease changes what a parent can do. This threatens our view of who they were. Our responses to their needs must support their dignity and not ignore the memory of who they were. The mature child has resolved the conflicts of the filial crisis or refuses to allow them to interfere with his or her ability to respond positively and effectively to the needs of an afflicted parent.

Cohesive vs. Fragmented Families

Some families become closer during crises. Individual members are concerned about the views of other family members. Cohesive families function as a unit rather than as isolated individuals. This provides a sense of belonging and a stronger impression that it is the family addressing a crisis, not separate individuals who cannot stick together. Even families who experience a good deal of conflict can prove to be cohesive (Blazer, 1984). More fragmented families are likely to experience more tension than cohesive families. This leaves them with less energy available to address the challenges posed by caregiving.

Relating to Outside Help

Professionals involved in Alzheimer's care will find it easier to develop alliances with more cohesive families. If your family is quite fragmented, professionals may encounter a string of different individuals. When the style of family interactions is also conflictual, professional alliances may be more difficult to maintain. A fragmented and conflictual family, over time, jeopardizes the professional affiliations that would be supportive of the family's responses.

Productive vs. Nonproductive Families

Families who can work together in providing care are more likely to be productive. Families who cannot work together are less likely to be productive.

Productivity is not simply a matter of working together, since it involves the ability of families to plan, organize, and delegate responsibilities and activities. Some families have the potential to be productive, but if the person who had mobilized the family is stricken by Alzheimer's disease, new leadership needs to develop. Different types of family styles have different responses to this need. The fact that the spouse or daughter is most likely to become the primary provider of care also influences the development of new roles in the family.

Degree of Involvement

Often it seems the primary caregiver is the only family member involved in the caregiving. This person is unable or unwilling to involve other family members in some aspect of responding to enormous demands. In such cases, the potential productivity of the family's response to care is greatly reduced.

This may occur for several reasons. The involvement of some family members may increase conflict. A source of potential conflict is eliminated when these members are absent. Geographical or emotional distance between family members may separate them from the hands-on caregiving. There may be no other family members. In order to preserve their relationships with the person with Alzheimer's, caregivers become extremely attached to the loved one. This emotional attachment may push other family members away. It is a source of frustration and reduced family productivity when other members could help and want to help.

Caregivers of persons with Alzheimer's disease must manage incredible stress. The daily care takes its toll on their physical, emotional, and mental resources. They are involved in a progressive, incomplete loss. The burdens of care pile up, and their productivity is threatened. Hope fades and caregivers resign themselves to what cannot be changed.

Fragile vs. Stable Families

The fragile versus stable characteristics of families affect the functioning of the family over time, not just at the moment of crisis. Since a family unit consists of individuals, the stability of those individuals must also be considered. Families who face Alzheimer's disease have faced crises before. It is helpful to examine the ways these crises were handled, and how the family was affected by them. For example, if a family member experienced a fairly significant health problem in the past, how supportive were other members of the family? Did they temporarily assume responsibilities or roles that had been associated with this individual? Were their expectations of recovery reasonable? Did the family unite to deal with the crisis or were they remarkably unconcerned?

Families facing Alzheimer's disease are not addressing problems and needs that can be quickly handled or easily dismissed. Caregiving will last a long time. Family members will be required to contend with unfamiliar and unpredictable situations. A stable family will be better prepared to address these situations over time; a fragile family will have greater difficulty providing sufficient support unless a healthier member assumes the primary role.

The members of a stable family are likely to be stable as individuals. If difficulties in relationships develop, they are resolved in reasonable ways without the family being disabled. The history of family relationships and interactions is not riddled with recurrent problems and longstanding conflicts. Support from children can be counted on because they are not continually absorbed by their emotional or relational problems.

Alzheimer's disease may develop in a family that has been characteristically stable, but as a result of the health problems the stability of the family itself has been threatened. Alzheimer's is more likely to develop in older family members. Potentially supportive siblings and children may be older themselves. The spouse who becomes the caregiver may have chronic health problems that are magnified by stress and less attention to his or her own needs for care.

Energy Drain

Tension is always seen in fragile and fragmented families. This reduces the energy available for being productive and may support the need for greater utilization of resources in the community. Families who have successfully met prior crises and maintained healthy interactions and productivity still have a good chance of meeting the caregiver's challenge if they can be flexible enough to involve other sources of support.

Family Roles and Rules

If the person affected by Alzheimer's disease had been the one who provided leadership and stability to the family, any type of family will experience the impact of his or her loss. Some families will be more adept than others in filling this gradually increasing void. Other family members must become available to assume this role or parts of it. They must be willing to accept the role, and the family must be open to this kind of change. Some families may have such rigid roles that other family members would be reluctant to assume the responsibilities. The roles within the family may be so unclear or mixed that the need for a designated leader might not at first be apparent.

Some families have very clear procedures or rules for responding to problems. A family hierarchy may exist that dictates in advance how changes in leadership should be handled. Even these may not sufficiently address how other family members assume new roles until the family comprehends what Alzheimer's does to the abilities of the affected person. The family's sensitivity to this person's remaining capabilities and wishes also influences how new roles of leadership are developed. In addition, cultural differences influence how rigid or flexible families can be in changing roles within the family

Flexible Responses

The presence of Alzheimer's disease in a family demands a family response. The flexibility of the family in responding to a situation that requires change in leadership is critical. Flexibility enables them to adapt and change, regroup and develop new patterns in any established hierarchy so that the family can care for the relative who is impaired (Blazer, 1984). A family characterized by flexibility is less likely to be burdened by the weight of resigned or pessimistic attitudes.

Guides for Relating

The quality of family interactions influences family communication and problem solving. It is also helpful to examine the factors in family relationships that influence the degree to which family members are involved with one another. Invisible boundaries exist in families. These boundaries act like rules that suggest how closely family members should be involved in each other's lives (Miller, 1982). In some families, these boundaries are very clear so that interactions within the family are neither too involved nor too distant. Children have supportive alliances with each other, and the boundaries that characterize their involvement with parents are clear. The response of this type of family to the problems and needs created by Alzheimer's disease will be more readily defined. Issues concerning how involved each member is to become are not so confusing.

Disengaged Families

There are other families where the boundaries influencing the usual degree of involvement result in too little or too much response. The degree of involvement tends to be consistent whether the family issues have major or minor significance. Disengaged families are at one extreme end of the continuum of involvement. Boundaries in these families are quite rigid. This rigidity inhibits communication. The elderly in this type of family are likely to be emotionally isolated from both their children and their siblings. If the diagnosis of Alzheimer's is made, the spouse is unlikely to request help from her family unless the level of her stress becomes quite extreme. Even in this situation, she would be hesitant to share many of her thoughts or feelings with her family (Miller, 1982). Alzheimer's care in this family is likely to be a solitary activity. The likelihood of the caregiver to become overwhelmed would appear to be high unless other supportive resources are developed outside the home.

Enmeshed Families

At the other extreme of the continuum of involvement, the enmeshed family is characterized as being so close that its members lose their own sense of autonomy. Members of this family will have a very strong sense of belonging but a very low sense of their own ability in mastering skills, or appreciating the individually determined abilities they may have acquired. Individuals in the enmeshed family are not given the opportunity to solve problems in their own way and own time, so it would have been difficult to learn and grow from any stressful experiences that preceded the crisis of Alzheimer's disease. The excessive concern and involvement characteristic of enmeshed families produces intense overreactions, particularly during periods of stress (Miller, 1982). What is stressful to these families may not be that stressful to other families. While the person with Alzheimer's in this family will have physical and other concrete needs met, these needs will be met at the expense of the person's self-worth and individuality. Parents and children can be so overinvolved in each other's lives that when one member is down or depressed, they all tend to suffer.

The overinvolvement that characterizes the enmeshed family can produce overload during Alzheimer's caregiving. As time passes, the energy for mutual support may have been expended on minor details, so the family as a whole has less to give. Fortunately, most families are not characteristically either enmeshed or disengaged. Styles that are more prominently enmeshed or disengaged may inhibit individuals providing Alzheimer's care; they need not prohibit it. When family problems persist that do interfere with care, professional help should be sought.

Family Roles During Crisis

Individuals in a family may take on different roles to cope with the situations and demands associated with Alzheimer's disease. Generally these roles are supportive of the impaired person and enable the family to cope adequately. Different roles may be assumed by different family members at various times. Several roles may be assumed by the same family member.

The Role of Facilitator

The stability of the family is the most important thing to the facilitator. Although other members of a family will support the involvement of a professional to determine what is wrong with a family member, the facilitator will oppose this suggestion. This family member will probably obstruct other family efforts to get help for the impaired person, for example, getting second opinions or seeking psychiatric treatment for the psychiatric manifestations of the disease. Facilitators believe, consciously or unconsciously, that all members of the family, including themselves, are best served by keeping the relatives in a sick or more dependent role. Thus, they facilitate and encourage the illness and the problems associated with it. If the diagnosis has been made, the facilitator may oppose it being made known if he or she perceives it as a threat to the equilibrium of the family.

Other care-related decisions may involve additional family members in the facilitator role. The family stability may return once family members have had the chance to adjust and make the necessary changes in their lifestyles. Family members become more resistant to changes once things have settled down. They probably realize that changes in routine can be unsettling to everyone. If a support group member encourages a family member to explore adult day care or respite care, the suggestion might threaten the stability the family has achieved in its present response to a loved one's needs. The stress of the caregiver or the deteriorating status of the person with Alzheimer's are not considered. It is better to maintain the perceived stability of the family than upset this balance, as fragile as it might be.

The Role of Victim
The victim is the individual in the family who is most likely to have the most contact with other family members. He or she is quite likely to also have the most contact with professionals. There may be one or more victims in a family. Different family members at different times may assume the victim role. The victim views Alzheimer's as a direct and personal threat for a number of reasons. If he or she has been dependent upon the stricken individual, his or her own well-being, particularly in the future, might be at stake. Spouses may feel at risk since their relationship and marriage is threatened by the disease. Other family members are victims because their future with a loved one has been dramatically changed. The genetic fears of Alzheimer's families certainly contribute to the perception of the victim role. The frequency of family interactions may be reduced for all family members, but the caregiver spouse may also become isolated from friends. The disease threatens relationships. The victim would feel less threatened if someone could reverse the course that Alzheimer's disease has taken. Professionals working with victims in a family may receive more criticism because they are unable to remove the ultimate personal threat, death.

The Role of Manager
When a family crisis occurs, one family member often takes charge. He or she is calm during the crisis and can be a stabilizing force. Emotions are usually contained and this person may be somewhat intellectual in contacts with professionals. The explanations given to family members by the "manager" will be more intellectual than emotional in content. He may not be able to give as much emotional support, but he plays a key role in organizing the family's response to what needs to be done. The family member can be an important liaison with professionals who become involved in caring for the needs of the affected family member and the primary family caregiver. The family manager is not usually as involved in the intimate aspects of care and may maintain

some distance from family members who are. Family members who live some distance from where the care is provided to loved ones can assume some part of this family role. Their assistance with practical problem solving is supportive to an emotionally drained caregiver. Providing practical assistance supports the family manager's sense of being a part of the family as they deal with AD.

The Role of Caretaker

Caretakers have a deep desire to nurture the sick. They may have assumed this role in the family or chosen a profession that supports the fulfillment of this need. Many caretakers may be women who assume this role because of an innate need or give in to social pressures that assign this role to them. Husbands are thought to suffer less stress as Alzheimer's caregivers because it gives them the opportunity to reciprocate in kind to wives who nurtured them and their children.

The caregivers' need to nurture may obscure their need to care for themselves. When they view their relative as a helpless child, there is a good chance their nurturing tendencies will re-create a relationship with the spouse or parent that resembles the relationship they would have with a child. This reinforces a rebonding process that may lead to an inseparable bond. The relationship becomes resistant to any threat of separation. Caretakers frequently avoid opportunities for respite. As a result, they frequently wear themselves out to the point that they have no desire for any useful or meaningful activity. Their life is singularly consumed by caring for a loved one. Any other family attempting to separate them from this consuming activity will be resisted because it is "all they can do" for the loved one.

The caretaker role may be motivated by guilt. It corresponds to the over-involvement stage of grief during family adjustment. Caretakers may remain stuck at this stage because the role itself seems to encourage overinvolvement. When the Alzheimer's patient dies, the person who has become entrenched in the caretaker role can suffer a tremendous void. She has not only lost a loved one—she has lost a role that sustained her. Caretakers may experience a severe and prolonged grief reaction.

Escapee

Escapees may be found in many types of families, but they are more frequently found in families characterized by intense conflict. Some escapees may have left severely enmeshed families in order to find autonomy as worthwhile individuals. The escapee has withdrawn from the usual interactions in the family. He is often blamed for not showing up in the Alzheimer's crisis. He is criticized for failing to show more concern.

Absence Protects.   It is not unusual for escapees to have moved some distance from the family and become involved in activities that are more rewarding and appreciative of them as worthwhile persons. They try to compensate for past relationships and interactions that had been unhealthy. Their withdrawal from their families is self-protective. While they may function well outside of their family, they seem to realize they cannot tolerate reinvolvement in a highly stressed and conflictual family (Blazer, 1984), even if a parent is dying with Alzheimer's disease. They would rather leave the terrible business of the past unfinished. Their absence may be quite acceptable to some family members. However, the parent who becomes the caregiver might wish that old matters could be put aside to allow the family to be together during a time of crisis.

The Role of Patient

The person with Alzheimer's disease is the patient. He or she has the problem that clearly precipitated the crisis for the family. This problem then creates further stresses on the emotional, physical, mental, spiritual, and financial resources available to the family as a whole. As the patient, the person with Alzheimer's will be the focus of these resources. However, other family members may assume the role of a "hidden patient" when they seek professional help for a loved one. They use their relationship and helping role with the patient to get their own needs addressed. Contact with a professional also affords them the opportunity to bring up old issues and problems. These problems may not be directly related to Alzheimer's disease but may influence the ability of family members to provide care, support one another, and generally participate in caregiving. Some issues may directly relate to family issues that still affect the family's ability to work together productively.

Hidden Patient.   The needs of these family members seem to be in competition with the relative who has Alzheimer's disease. They have legitimate needs that warrant professional attention. Uncomfortable in seeking help directly for themselves, they seize the opportunity on the coattails of the relative. No other disease has given so much credence to the idea that the needs of caregivers are as legitimate as the needs of the person identified as the patient. Unfortunately, family members who are caretakers may not be able to balance meeting their needs and the needs of loved ones. They should consider professional help. The needs of the caregiver and patient must be addressed with more balanced responses from the professionals and health care system.

Caregivers and Caregiving

The need to care for people who are vulnerable or needy in some way is a strong social value. Some people make a profession out of taking care of people who have problems and needs of one kind or another. Some caregivers are strongly motivated by the need to nurture, but not all caregivers are caretakers. Different approaches to caregiving can be influenced by the roles just discussed. Since caregiving occurs within a family and a relationship, these relational factors further characterize the process. What we call *caregiving* involves an attitude of caring and the expression of this attitude through actions. In such cases, professionals must quickly recognize that the needs of caregivers are as significant as the patients.

Taking care of people we love can be viewed as an obligation or expectation of families. As much as 80 percent of the care elderly persons receive is provided by family members who become caregivers. But it is more difficult to care for members of our families if our motivation is solely a sense of duty or obligation. Resentment and similar feelings breed more readily when care is performed out of a sense of family obligation. There must be other reasons for caring.

Several years ago I had the opportunity to speak at two consecutive conferences, one in El Paso and another in Baltimore. Both were sponsored by the Alzheimer's organization in those cities. At that time, the sponsors were extremely concerned about the difficulties support groups had in reaching many of the family caregivers who had become isolated and overinvolved. They were equally concerned in reaching caregivers who had become so overwhelmed that their physical and mental health had been jeopardized. Offers of help had been rejected, and these caregivers continued along a path that would surely lead to greater risks for themselves and their loved ones. By this time, there were a number of very helpful books available to caregivers. Social research had inundated journals with studies concerning caregiver stresses, strains, and burdens. Although very little research had addressed how persons with the disease coped, research had begun to look more carefully at how caregivers coped with stress. The impact of grief on caregivers and loved ones losing themselves to a disease was beginning to receive more attention.

In one sense, caregiving was a job. A job description would be appropriate to introduce caregivers to the job they had accepted. In some cases, it had been accepted out of choice; in other cases, there may not have been a choice. It needed to be done. And despite the fact that most family caregivers did not have the prerequisite skills, they had performed the job as well as anyone. It had been difficult, but they learned to manage strange behaviors, adjust to a more rigid routine, and solve problems without the benefit of reasoning. Some had even learned a few things that would benefit nurses, psychiatrists, and neurologists. Others had acquired a rudimentary knowledge of family law. Some were proud of the fact that they had learned to do the things their spouses had claimed they would never be able to do. Let's look back at the job description more closely.

Caregivers work with virtually no supervision. They are their own supervisors with a staff of one who has some trouble performing his or her job according to expectations. For a job that is performed without a salary, some type of benefits could be expected. A few days off would be a good start. A good physical or mental health day sure wouldn't hurt. Unfortunately, the benefits look suspiciously like a plan for growth and development. For example, any decent job should increase your self-esteem. This one expects you to accept your life and recognize how it is still meaningful. Worst of all, it would be disgraceful to quit even if you didn't like the job. When you accept the job, things are a little confusing. Come to think of it, there was something else mentioned in the job description about confusion. But it is clearer now what "risk of isolation" means. And the warnings about the job creating high levels of stress are not exaggerated.

Becoming a caregiver is a little like starting a new job. At least you know the person you work for, and you have known him for a long time. Much of what you know about him is still helpful. Like other bosses, he gives you more feedback about your performance when you first start than later when you might need it more. When you do something wrong, this boss is more likely to act differently rather than tell you what you need to change. Other family members act like they are in the workplace. They are not really your supervisor, but they always know what you should do.

More than a Job

Becoming a caregiver involves much more than performing job duties, because what you do happens within an established relationship that is one among many others in a family. Caregiving is not really a role, but it refers to the care that is given within established roles like husband-wife, parent-child (Pearlin et al., 1990). When this care is given out of affection, it is more positively meaningful than similar actions resulting from a sense of duty and obligation.

Caring Involves Feelings

Caring is the part of our commitment to the welfare of other persons that involves our feelings about them and our emotional reactions to experiences involving them. Caregiving is the behavioral expression of this commitment (Pearlin et al., 1990). Giving care to a parent, spouse, or sibling is an extension of caring about that person. Both caring and caregiving are present in all relationships where people attempt to protect and enhance each other's well-being. When family members become caregivers, their commitments require that they do something different for the person who needs their care. The experiences involved in caregiving will be new, and these may produce emotional reactions that are different in kind or intensity from those produced by previous experiences.

Alzheimer's disease inevitably leads to greater impairment. The progressively increasing dependency resulting from this impairment demands more caregiving activity. This, in turn, leads to profound changes in the relationship in which caregiving occurs. The give and take in the relationship had flowed back and forth. As the needs and dependencies of relatives become greater, the *give* flows in one direction. Caregiving may expand so that it occupies virtually the whole relationship. The affection that was originally associated with caring flows but does not come back. Ultimately, a cherished relationship comprised of two people is transformed into one in which one person is caregiving for the other. This dramatic and involuntary transformation is itself a major source of stress.

Caring for Caregiver

Family caregivers directly face this transformation of a relationship. Other family members experience it as well, but are not confronted by it daily. The caring part of the family caregiver receives less and less encouragement from the loved one to whom he or she gives care. As concerned as family members and friends may be about the relative who is being transformed by Alzheimer's disease, their concern about the relative who is the caregiver may seem greater. Their concerns may be interpreted as comments about the quality of caregiving, even though these messages are really about caring. Their behavior is their own attempt *to be* a caregiver *for* a caregiver. They may be attempting to increase the diminishing flow of assistance and affection.

Caring about Caregiving

Sometimes the giving attempts of other family members indicate frustration, and the caregiver believes these same family members may not care. When you are losing a relationship and a person, you do not stop giving care. The part of you that is caring may need to be nurtured, but your expression of caring seems to be reduced to caregiving. Your reactions to the experience of caregiving begin to involve feelings that are inconsistent with the caring part of you. Anger toward your loved one leads to guilt. You may wish the caregiving would end, but that would mean the relationship would end. It would be nice to have help and take a break, but what if something happened while you were gone? You have needs, too. You feel drained and empty, but what are these feelings when they are compared to what your loved one feels? Whenever caregivers begin to respond to their own needs, they are reminded of the conflicts that seem to be inherent in caring simultaneously for two persons. It is always easier to give into the voice that says the other's needs are greater when you are too tired to be sure anymore.

Providing for the needs of two people was not as difficult when both people could speak for themselves. You knew each other well enough to know the preferences of the other. But in time, the other person can no longer speak for himself. Then it becomes questionable whether preferences make that much difference. Alzheimer's—must it change everything? How can I separate myself from its grip? How can I feel that I am part of a family again? How do I know when it is okay to be myself in other ways again? When am I no longer just a caregiver?

Care for Self

Caregivers reach a point where it is important to them to be whole individuals again. They want more of life, even in the face of the losses they endure. Some recognize this after the mourning becomes less intense and they decide to go on living. Some grow and develop during this experience. But the social and personal injunctions to care are very powerful. Caregivers need something to guide them in making choices that help them care for themselves. They need something that suggests it is their moral and ethical right to consider their own needs. They need something to empower them to take care of themselves. In Alzheimer's family support groups caregivers see that dilemmas are the same for virtually all caregivers. These support groups often develop a Caregivers' Bill of Rights (Gwyther, 1990).

The idea of a formalized bill of rights is healthy. It provides some balance to offset the moral and social injunctions caregivers sense from society, family, and their respective cultures. It also asserts that individuals and families are more important than the unrelenting tasks of caregiving itself. The idea of sacrificing our life for another may be viewed as heroic and noble when we are fully conscious of what we are doing. Otherwise, it is self-destructive and unnecessary. Caregivers do not willingly embrace this idea of sacrificing their life.

The sample Caregivers' Bill of Rights that follows can help caregivers find the balance that supports their value and the value of those for whom they care. It also encourages caregivers to exercise these rights for the sake of their health and the health of loved ones. Some of these loved ones are people with Alzheimer's disease. Others are family members with whom relationships will still exist when caregiving has ended.

These rights apply to the life of the family as aptly as they do to the life of the family caregiver. For many caregivers, learning to become a part of their families again is as worthy a goal as establishing their own separate identities once caregiving has ended and the presence of grief has become more pronounced.

Caregivers' Bill of Rights

Inasmuch as WE, THE CAREGIVERS, devote both ourselves and our resources to the care, maintenance, and support of loved ones with Alzheimer's disease, we affirm that we have basic and inalienable rights.

We affirm that we are not alone in the challenge to maintain a dignified and humane lifestyle for ourselves and the loved ones for whom we care. Furthermore, we recognize that we are not alone in seeking better ways to accomplish this goal for loved ones and ourselves, and respect those who join us in this endeavor. As a result of the responsibility we knowingly accept for our loved ones, we must also accept responsibility for ourselves. We declare the following individual rights:

- The right to make decisions on behalf of loved ones and ourselves that support what is best for both of us

- The right to have time and activities for ourselves without guilt, fear, or criticism

- The right to have feelings that are inherently a part of losing someone we love

- The right to deal with what we can alone, and the right to ask about what we do not understand

- The right to seek options that reasonably accommodate our needs and the needs of our loved ones

- The right to be treated with respect by those from whom we seek advice and assistance; the right to expect our loved ones to be treated in the same manner

- The right to make mistakes and be forgiven

- The right to be accepted as a vital and valued member of our families even when our views are different

- The right to love ourselves and accept that we have done what was humanly possible

- The right to learn what we can do and the time to learn it

- The right to say goodbye before we must finally let go of the one we love

- The right to be free from feelings and thoughts that are negative, destructive, and unfounded; and to work through feelings that are hard to understand

- The right to develop our lives again before our endeavor of love is complete

11

Values, Beliefs, and the Caregiver Experience

Expectations Influence Our Feelings and Reactions

It is not an easy job to change our expectations or image of a person we have known for years. However, an examination of our beliefs about the behavior of the person with Alzheimer's can give caregivers new insights into interacting with loved ones. Using this revised perspective, the caregiver can gain more control of the situation and can help the person with Alzheimer's to retain his capacity to reason, understand, and act appropriately as long as possible.

Taking Forgetfulness Personally

What the caregiver believes about the behavior of the person with Alzheimer's definitely influences what he feels and how he reacts. If he believes the loved one is asking the same questions over and over just to annoy him and thus becomes irritated, this irritation will be obvious to the person with Alzheimer's, even though he probably will not understand what he has done to annoy the caregiver. Such needless irritation is stressful for the caregiver, and it can have an emotionally unsettling effect on the person with Alzheimer's, leading to more complicated problems. It is therefore important that each caregiver learns not to take his loved one's behavior personally.

Unrealistic Expectations

A caregiver's expectations of himself also affect how he cares for a loved one. Many caregivers put great pressure on themselves. Lacking a full understanding of the physical causes of the illness and its impact on the person's functional capabilities, they hold themselves responsible for their relative's problems and failures. Anger, guilt, frustration, and similar feelings push caregivers beyond their limits. Caregivers must realistically assess their limitations plus the resources available. Otherwise, the stress of caregiving can lead to desperation and fatigue.

Previous Adjustments to Illness and Loss Can Predict Our Adjustment to Alzheimer's

Caregivers must learn to solicit and accept the help of others during the course of the illness. Those of us who find this difficult should examine our beliefs. Do we believe it is our sole responsibility to provide for all the person's needs, or is it a responsibility to be shared by other family members? Also to be considered is how well we tend to take care of ourselves. In the past, have we become so consumed by the needs of our family and others that we neglected our own needs? In the caregiving role, how are we responding to the needs of our loved one? What beliefs do we have about our role? These questions are critical to the basic pattern of our caregiving.

The Caregiver Should Allow the Patient to Remain as Independent as Possible

As the disease progresses, the caregiver will find himself shouldering increased responsibility for the patient. In particular, a child may find himself caring for a parent with Alzheimer's in ways that the parent once cared for him. This phenomenon is known as role reversal. It is very important, however, not to speed up this reversal process any sooner than is absolutely necessary. Alzheimer's disease is a gradually progressive illness, which means that a person does not lose all capabilities suddenly and simultaneously, nor does his family need to take over his total care all at once. The caregiver can best help the Alzheimer's patient by allowing him to remain as independent as possible for as long as possible. When the person providing care attempts to take control over all areas of the person's life simultaneously, some very unfortunate consequences such as the following may result:

- The person refuses to admit he needs any help at all and rejects all aid.
- The adult relationship between the caregiver and the afflicted person is severed prematurely.
- The self-concept of the person with Alzheimer's is eroded by doubts about his existing abilities.
- The person with Alzheimer's becomes prematurely dependent.
- The caregiver becomes overwhelmed by the unnecessary burden created.

Caregivers must therefore monitor themselves to make sure that, in their desire to be helpful, they do not hasten the end of the loved one's self-sufficient life.

Changes Not Always Obvious

In contrast, family members may overlook symptoms of the disease and therefore fail to provide aid soon enough. If contact with the person is only occasional, they may have no reason to suspect that a medical condition is responsible for subtle changes in the person's grooming, dress, speech, or behavior.

When changes occur, particularly in a spouse, we tend to ignore them, if possible, or to attribute them to temporary circumstances. It is often easier to dismiss things that irritate or bother us than it is to deal with them, especially when they do not seem to be cause for alarm. If the spouse continues to have problems, we may still feel hesitant to get a professional opinion.

Each Member of the Family Adjusts Differently.

If the severity of the problems is more apparent to some family members than to others, conflict may arise about the best course of action. For example, Betty may want to play down her husband John's increasing problems with memory and suspicious ideas. When her son and daughter insist that she take their father to a doctor, Betty may deny that a problem exists, leading her son and daughter to become as distressed by their mother's behavior as by their father's. Betty is in conflict; her denial suggests she is having trouble thinking about the frightening possibilities. Additionally, there is the issue of convincing John to see a professional about problems he blames on her and others. Betty may believe that the family holds her responsible for what her husband is doing and what might be happening to him.

Examining Beliefs

It is natural at times to have counterproductive reactions to the problems of Alzheimer's disease. It can be a very difficult balancing act to determine what caregivers can and cannot expect, how much assistance should be offered, and how much is too much. The point is that caregivers should not blame themselves or their loved one, but they should examine how their beliefs influence their thinking, the way they act and react, and the emotions they experience and express. Such a self-examination will help caregivers to respond more constructively as they begin to care for a family member who is affected by a disease that significantly changes his behavior and character before it changes his health.

Beliefs Influence Actions

The following personalized example will help to illustrate how a caregiver's beliefs can influence his reactions to a typical problem arising from the Alzheimer's condition of a spouse.

Problem:

Helen is yelling at her husband Tom. From the bedroom she screams, "Come here! You never come fast enough when I need you!" Then she bursts into tears.

Belief:

Tom believes that his wife Helen depends on him too much and should do more for herself. He knows she has Alzheimer's, but he feels she is being lazy. He has always felt she was a demanding person. When he hears her crying, he thinks to himself that it is just like her to get hysterical about nothing.

What Beliefs Relate to Tom's Thoughts and Feelings?

Because he thinks Helen is just being lazy, Tom feels aggravated. This feeling grows as he considers how often she depends on him to do things that she really could do for herself. He is already washing dishes, which is not his job. Her crying irritates him more than it frightens or concerns him; he believes she cries to get what she wants. Because he feels manipulated, he becomes angrier.

Tom's Reaction:

"Helen, shut up! I'll be there in a minute, or you can come in here." Tom is too angry to ask her what she needs or to go to the bedroom immediately. He disregards the fact that his wife now has difficulties in clearly expressing her needs.

Helen's Problem:

Actually, Helen has slipped out of the chair in her bedroom. She is not hurt, but she is frightened and upset. She has made statements in the past about her husband not coming to her when she asked, even before the Alzheimer's condition, and that almost habitual response has slipped out when, in a panic, she cannot describe what has really happened. The disease has affected her coordination, and in her fright, she cannot organize her movements to pull herself up. She is crying out of fear and frustration.

Tom is reluctant to respond to the initial yelling because of past experiences. He still does not understand the impact of the illness well enough to appreciate how it is eroding his wife's ability to manage for herself. Neither does he understand the insecurity created by the illness.

With more knowledge of Helen's limitations, Tom might ask her if something is wrong or simply walk into the bedroom. He has probably gotten tired of taking care of his wife and feels frustrated and angry. These reactions are intensified by feeling unappreciated. His irritation has delayed his response to Helen.

Caregivers can respond more appropriately to problems when they identify the various reasons for their reactions. The previous illustration shows that the perceived problem is not always the real problem, and that beliefs and feelings about a problem can lead to interpretations, judgments, and reactions that can prevent caregivers from successfully handling the situation.

12

How to Respond Positively to Alzheimer's Behaviors

In Chapter 2, we discuss the symptoms of Alzheimer's disease. Even when we recognize a disturbing behavior on the part of our loved one as an Alzheimer's symptom, it is not always easy to know what the appropriate response should be. Unaccustomed to our loved one's new impairment, we naturally tend to respond to the behavior as we would have in the past when the person was healthy. Unfortunately, this often means responding with annoyance, frustration, and anger—which, as we have seen, is not helpful either for us or the person with Alzheimer's.

This chapter suggests more productive ways to respond to common disturbing behaviors exhibited by Alzheimer's patients. After listing the behavior, we first identify the common immediate reactions. Usually this is an interpretation and response that would be appropriate if we were responding to a healthy person's behavior, but it is not a useful response to behavior by an Alzheimer's patient. We then guide the reader through a better interpretation of the behavior, based on an understanding of the brain impairment produced by Alzheimer's disease. Finally, we offer specific suggestions for productive ways of responding to the problem.

Our goal is to create an accurate and practical guide to caring for Alzheimer's patients that will help both caregivers and patients enjoy the good days and minimize the bad days. Our examples cannot possibly cover all situations. However, when caregivers, learn this approach, they can use it with different situations and in different care settings.

Behavior *1. The person asks the same questions over and over.*

Common responses.   The person is not listening or trying to remember, she wants attention or is trying to annoy you; she should be able to control this.

Alzheimer's interpretation.   The person is suffering memory loss, which in turn creates a strong sense of insecurity and uncertainty. She may be asking the same questions repeatedly because she seeks reassurance and security, or perhaps your earlier answers seemed vague or unclear. She may sense you are avoiding the answer, which could heighten her sense of insecurity.

In more advanced stages, memory impairment may be so severe that she does not recall asking the question, or she may feel threatened by your earlier answer. For example, if she asks repeatedly when she is going to the doctor, the doctor may be a source of insecurity for her.

Helpful Responses

- Respond clearly, slowly, and concretely to questions.
- Have the person repeat what you say.
- If you suspect that your earlier answer disturbed the person, provide reassurance and/or factual information that will set her mind at rest.
- Distract the person into other activities or other topics of discussion and ignore further questions.
- Avoid arguing or responding with anger, do not rebuke the person for the memory problem.
- Write down the information in question for the person who can still read.

Behavior *2. The person's personality appears to have changed.*

Common responses.   He is going crazy or having a nervous breakdown; he has lost all self-respect and pride.

Alzheimer's interpretation.   Personality changes are characteristic symptoms of Alzheimer's. Often, these changes are observed prior to any clear impairment of memory or intellectual abilities. Brain impairment associated with Alzheimer's can radically change the way the person acts. Additionally, personality characteristics can be exaggerated in early phases of the illness.

Subtle changes in personality can represent an early signal that a problem exists. If the person realizes that he is acting in ways that are not like him, he may fear that he is having a nervous breakdown or losing his mind.

Eventually the brain impairment erases most traits of individuality. Some examples of personality changes follow:

Normal Personality	*New Traits*
Socially active	Socially withdrawn
Calm, easygoing	Worried, easily upset
Kind, understanding	Selfish, demanding
Relaxed	Paranoid
Emotionally controlled	Excessively emotional
Careful, cautious	Careless
Good judgment	Poor judgment
Sexually sensitive	Sexually demanding
Friendly	Unfriendly, hostile
Honest	Dishonest
Flexible	Rigid
Loving	Uncaring

Helpful Responses

- Accept personality changes as results of, or reactions to, brain impairment.
- Try to satisfy the needs underlying behavior, such as the person's need for security, self-esteem, dignity, and love.

Behavior 3. *The person does not do what she says she will or leaves a task uncompleted.*

Common responses.   She is lazy and not really trying; she is lying to you; she wants your help with everything.

Alzheimer's interpretation.   Memory impairment makes it more difficult to do something that was agreed upon. For example, seeing a shirt laid on the bed may no longer trigger the idea that the person should put it on. Memory abilities cannot be separated from intellectual abilities, such as reasoning, and both faculties are being lost.

Helpful Responses

- Use reminders and memory lists.
- Maintain a routine for daily activities.
- Make requests close to the time the task is to be completed.
- Provide step-by-step assistance for more complicated tasks.
- Always request the desired behavior in the same setting (e.g., eating in the kitchen or dining room, dressing in the bedroom or bathroom).

- Provide verbal assistance if the person seems to have forgotten how to complete parts of the task or has forgotten what she is doing.

Behavior 4. *The person denies his memory problems and makes excuses for mistakes, blames others, or seems unaware of the problem.*

Common responses.   The person is not being honest; he should face the problem and accept responsibility for his own mistakes; he is just getting old and senile.

Alzheimer's interpretation.   Denial of memory problems is a very common response to Alzheimer's. Initially, denial is a necessary defense. It protects the person from frightening changes that are difficult to accept. If he makes excuses or blames others, he may be desperately trying to explain the memory impairment without directly confronting the problem.

Helpful Responses
- Avoid forcing the person to face up to the memory problems.
- Provide reminders or suggest checklists as ways to aid memory.
- Be understanding of the threat that memory impairment poses for your relative.
- Arrange for the person to talk to a professional if he seems troubled but cannot admit the problem to his family.

Behavior 5. *The person insists she does not need help because she has always done things for herself; she becomes angry when you offer assistance.*

Common responses.   She is stubborn and unreasonable; she is rejecting you personally; her anger is unfair.

Alzheimer's interpretation.   The person's refusal of help is an effort to maintain independence. Anger directed toward you may really be caused by her frustration with the illness. Her self-worth and self-esteem are threatened. Later, such denial may show she has lost a grasp of her own needs and problems.

Helpful Responses
- Determine what help is needed and provide it in a kind manner.
- Realize that the person may genuinely lack awareness of her needs and problems.
- Provide encouragement and reinforcement for even the smallest successes and for acceptance of your help.

- Avoid overemphasizing the person's weaknesses or communicating disgust.
- Avoid confronting problems too directly if you suspect the confrontation could provoke strong emotional reactions.

Behavior   6. *A spouse's sexual interests and demands are higher than normal or more difficult for you to satisfy.*

Common responses.   A sexual relationship is inappropriate in light of the illness. How could he enjoy sexual activity at such a time?

Alzheimer's interpretation.   Brain damage can increase a person's desire for sexual activity. It also can decrease his sexual inhibitions, create difficulties in relating sexually, and reduce sensitivity to his partner. Alzheimer's can threaten a person's sexual identity and self-esteem.

The loss of intimacy that occurs as the disease gradually diminishes the person's personality may make it difficult for the caregiver spouse to sustain a sexual relationship. The affected person may continue to find sexual satisfaction, but the spouse may suffer a loss of emotional satisfaction.

Despite these problems, sexual relations can continue to be important, and they are a matter of personal choice. The person with Alzheimer's needs to feel wanted and loved. Adjustments in relating sexually may be necessary.

Helpful Responses

- Understand changing sexual interests and demands in the context of both the illness and your prior sexual relationship.
- Rely upon touching, being caressed, and nonverbal relating as substitutes for the sex act.
- Talk with a physician or counselor if the sexual problems persist.

Behavior   7. *The person mishandles her money and monthly bills; she accuses you and others of stealing her money; she claims her banker is handling money matters.*

Common responses.   She is inconsiderate and irresponsible; she is unfair and will not face the facts; she is lying and avoiding the issue.

Alzheimer's interpretation.   Having and handling money is one of the symbols of a person's independence and competence. The person may blame others for her mistakes because she is trying to protect her self-esteem and maintain her independence.

Early problems with memory and reasoning abilities make it difficult to handle more complex financial matters. Trying to perform calculations, even on paper, becomes frustrating. Accusing others of taking money is one way in which the person fills the gaps in her memory and protects her self-esteem.

Helpful Responses

- Be sure there is no truth to accusations of theft, particularly when the person lives alone and is vulnerable.
- Let the spouse or adult child assume the responsibility for financial matters.
- Monitor the person's monthly bills and contact creditors about questionable charges.
- Be sensitive to the person's insecurity and fears when discussing financial matters.
- Allow the person to have some cash on hand to enable an easier adjustment to alternative financial arrangements.
- Consider legal arrangements such as power of attorney and guardianship as means of protecting the person's financial security.

Behavior 8. *The person tells ridiculous stories or says unusual things.*

Common responses.   He is lying or being mean; he is going crazy or getting senile.

Alzheimer's interpretation.   Such stories are easy to take personally, but they are rarely malicious. As memory and reasoning abilities continue to decline, larger gaps are left in the person's perception of reality. It is harder for him to explain or understand what is happening because his grasp of logic is deteriorating. Ridiculous stories and obvious untruths may be attempts to fill in the blanks, to explain what he cannot understand.

If the person believes his own stories, the things he says may cause real agitation, anger, and fearfulness. If his stories place blame on others, he may be trying to defend his self-respect and integrity.

Some of the unusual things a person says may also represent difficulties in speech. Finding words to explain things or even name things correctly becomes difficult as the disease develops. The person may be able to manage only fragmentary ideas or statements.

Helpful Responses

- Clarify and correct the person's understanding of events.
- Respond sensitively to underlying feelings of insecurity, fear, or frustration.
- Avoid overreacting to stories or allowing an argument to start.

- Distract the person with conversation about other things.
- If the person is upset, give him a chance to calm down.

Behavior 9. *The person wants things to be done immediately; she wants you to do everything.*

Common responses.   The person is being inconsiderate; she is acting childish and overly dependent; she is attempting to control you.

Alzheimer's interpretation.   If the person was demanding before the brain impairment, the disease could accentuate such traits. In addition, her loss of memory may have triggered anxiety and panic, and her demanding or overly dependent behavior may be an attempt to gain control. Her anger may mask fear.

Helpful Responses

- Remind yourself that there is no point in becoming frustrated and angry.
- Respond calmly.
- Let the person know what is going on and being done.
- Do something with the person, even if it is not what the person asks.
- Talk to other people about your frustrations.

Behavior 10. *The person repeatedly talks about experiences from the past.*

Common responses.   He is living in the past; he does not want to relate to the present.

Alzheimer's interpretation.   Although the brain-impaired person's ability to recall recent experiences is becoming less reliable, he still may remember more remote material from the past. This material remains accessible to the person longer and can provide a more meaningful basis for self-esteem and identity. The present has become more threatening and difficult to accept emotionally. The person may also be losing his ability to relate to time and may be confused about the relation of past to present.

Helpful Responses

- Use past memories to make activities in the present more meaningful.
- Provide concrete information that distinguishes the present from the past; for example, contrast pictures of grown-up grandchildren with their childhood pictures.
- Set aside time for reminiscing.
- Patiently and supportively orient the person to the present when confusion is apparent.

Behavior   *11. The person's abilities fluctuate from day to day or hour to hour, she remembers some things but not others.*

Common responses.   She remembers what she wants to; she is not trying to remember; she must be getting old and senile.

Alzheimer's interpretation.   It is normal for the memory of all Alzheimer's patients to fluctuate in this fashion. It is a mistake to believe that improved memory on a given day means the condition is improving, however. Some information or events may be easier to remember. Material that is unpleasant or threatening may be more easily forgotten.

Helpful Responses
- Make the most of good days.
- Determine the kinds of information more easily recalled.
- Note if a certain manner of presenting information improves some kinds of memory.
- Realize that the person will tend to remember more under relaxed and quiet circumstances.

Behavior   *12. The person continues to drive the car despite safety problems.*

Common responses.   He is being stubborn and showing poor judgment; he should give up driving.

Alzheimer's interpretation.   Driving gives a person freedom and control of his daily life. Denying he is lost or confused, despite obvious problems, is his way of defending his self-esteem and independence. Confronting him about mistakes may produce more vigorous denial and angry reactions.

Despite resistance, family members must limit and eventually eliminate the person's driving opportunities. Even during the early stages of the illness, the person is vulnerable in situations requiring quick decisions because his reaction time is impaired. Alzheimer's also affects visual perception, including perception of distance.

Concentration difficulties will eventually erode the person's ability to drive safely. For example, if the traffic light before him changes to green but a car on the intersecting street is going through the red light, the brain-impaired person may be unable to decide which change is the most important. Too many things are happening at once, and his problem-solving abilities become overwhelmed.

Giving up driving is very difficult for most people with Alzheimer's. They may be more willing to stop driving if another health problem, such as visual impairment, is cited as the reason. Most caregivers will want a loved one to stop driving long before the affected person is ready.

Helpful Responses

- Enlist the support of other family members in convincing the person to stop driving.
- Enlist the help of the person's physician, attorney, insurance agent, mental health professional, or trusted friend; the instructions of authority figures may be followed more closely.
- Discuss the problem with your insurance representative.
- Contact your police department or department of public safety and inquire about license nonrenewal, suspension, or restrictions and other procedures to ground an unsafe driver.
- Remove keys or dismantle the car's starter as a last resort.
- Understand the person's anger and resentment about such a loss and avoid confrontations about driving difficulties.
- Remember that removal of driving responsibilities eliminates the possibility of an unfortunate accident.

Behavior   *13. The person accuses you, family, and friends of doing things or makes up stories about you.*

Common responses.   She is becoming paranoid, losing her mind, being unfair, becoming unmanageable, or trying to hurt or embarrass you; she is getting senile.

Alzheimer's interpretation.   Such problems are other ways in which brain impaired persons react to the insecurity created by memory loss. In this case, the problem more directly involves the caregiver, since the person with Alzheimer's is most likely to accuse her spouse and other close family members.

Arguments tend to reinforce beliefs. Confrontations and other negative approaches tend to worsen the situation rather than help it.

Helpful Responses

- Avoid contradicting the person directly, as this may only make her angry and confused.
- Avoid highlighting mistakes and give calm and reasonable explanations; communicate a sense that things are all right or will improve.
- If something is lost, offer to help find it or suggest specific places it could be found.

Behavior   *14. The person has hallucinations or bizarre and frightening delusions.*

Common responses.   The person is mentally ill; Alzheimer's is getting worse.

Alzheimer's interpretation.   Progressive brain impairment affects an individual's ability to interpret information accurately. Hallucinations are often misinterpretations of real sights and sounds. Delusional beliefs represent an attempt to fill in gaps of information and explain what happened. For example, if the person says someone is knocking on the walls and is trying to break into his house, he may really have heard a tree branch rubbing against the house. Insecurity, so often associated with progressive brain impairment, leads the person to interpret events from a fearful and threatening perspective. Suspiciousness is a common response to a person's diminishing control of her world.

When a person seems to be talking with someone who is not present, he may not actually see or hear the person, but he may be involved in a delusional belief, such as thinking a deceased person is alive, or talking to a child who lives 400 miles away.

A number of other problems contribute to hallucinations and delusional beliefs. These include medical problems such as infections, changes in diabetic conditions, or pernicious anemia. Medications also must be evaluated.

Other conditions that impair a person's ability to receive information can contribute to hallucinations or delusional beliefs. Hearing or visual impairment are examples.

Helpful Responses

- When delusions or hallucinations are observed, consult a physician.
- Provide the person with concrete information.
- Show support for the feeling of the experience, responding with reassurance.
- Avoid arguing or disagreeing with the person, as that will only upset him more.
- Try to distract the person, move him to another room, or talk about something comforting.

Behavior *15. The person becomes disinterested and withdrawn in social situations.*

Common responses.   She does not care about friends or people anymore; she wants you to stay home all the time.

Alzheimer's interpretation.   The person's cognitive and memory deficits are making it very difficult to follow social conversations and interact appropriately. This inability leads to frustration and anxiety in social situations, thus prompting her to withdraw.

This withdrawal may be preceded by restlessness, tension, and agitation. If the demands on the person are not decreased, she may become more upset or even rude to uninformed observers.

Helpful Responses

- Provide emotional support and verbal assistance in demanding social situations and observe obvious changes in the person's anxiety level.
- When the person becomes nervous, encourage her to simply withdraw from the social situation for a while.
- Anticipate the more demanding situations before they become uncomfortable.
- Inform friends about her behavior and how they can make her participation easier.
- Search for social situations that are less demanding.

Behavior   *16. The person is very restless, cannot stay still, or is easily agitated.*

Common responses.   Something is bothering him; he does not have anything to do.

Alzheimer's interpretation.   As the disease progresses, agitation and restlessness commonly accompany the insecurity created by the person's diminishing abilities to cope. Denial and rationalization, which previously helped to block out awareness of functional losses, become less successful protective devices as his problems become more pronounced.

Some restlessness may suggest anxiety and underlying fears, though the person cannot always explain these feelings. Too much stimulation can contribute to anxious and agitated behavior. Medication given to control these symptoms should be carefully monitored, as it can sometimes intensify the symptoms it was prescribed to decrease.

Helpful Responses

- Use a calm, reassuring approach that supports his feelings, even when the underlying source is not apparent.
- If he can say what is bothering him, try to eliminate the source of trouble; if he cannot, avoid pressing for explanations.
- Reduce noise and activity levels.
- Ask the physician if the agitation can be decreased with medication or if medication might be creating the undesired effects.
- Involve the person in an activity that helps burn off excess energy.

Behavior   *17. The person constantly watches you and follows you around.*

Common responses.   She wants too much attention; she is overly dependent; she will not entertain herself, she is suspicious and distrustful of you.

Alzheimer's interpretation.   This problem develops from the fear and insecurity caused by the person's memory impairment; watching or following the caregiver provides greater security. Such behavior also promotes her sense of belonging and alleviates her sense of isolation, which might otherwise intensify anxiety and fear.

Mistrust or suspiciousness may develop because the person is less sure of what is happening. Her interpretations of information and her reasoning capabilities are less reliable. Some persons develop paranoia or more intense suspiciousness because they feel threatened.

Helpful Responses

- Understand such behaviors as a search for security.
- Identify and alleviate specific fears that are creating insecurity, for example, the fear that you are leaving the house.
- Orient her as to what is happening and clarify what you are doing.
- Spend time with the person.
- Engage her in constructive activity; ask her to do some supervised things with you.
- Avoid dramatic changes in routine.

Behavior   *18. The person's moods change for no apparent reason. He gets upset and even aggressive if cornered.*

Common responses.   The changes are related to medication, changes in his condition, or something you've done; he is losing his mind and cannot control his emotions.

Alzheimer's interpretation.   Such mood swings are often related to changes in the body and brain as the disease progresses. The mood swings also can be precipitated by thoughts and ideas the person has but is unable or unwilling to express.

The person may also be experiencing a catastrophic reaction, which means that he is overwhelmed by too much happening too quickly, has become extremely upset by his confusion and loss of control, and cannot respond adequately to the situation.

Helpful Responses

- Consult a physician if significant mood swings occur without cause or are increasing in intensity.

- Remove the person from the upsetting situation slowly and quietly.
- Be realistic in your expectations and avoid pushing.
- Reduce outside stimulants.
- Avoid expressing anger and frustration.
- Avoid reasoning or arguing, and use nonverbal support such as holding hands in a calming fashion.

Behavior *19. The person refuses to bathe and groom; she says she has already done so.*

Common responses.   She does not care about her personal appearance; she is being stubborn and uncooperative; she is lying.

Alzheimer's interpretation.   Regular bathing and attention to personal hygiene lose their social significance for persons with brain impairment. Social judgment and awareness diminish. Since taking care of personal hygiene is the most basic sign of independence, however, it becomes threatening to adults to become dependent upon someone's help for bathing and grooming.

Bathing can become embarrassing to the brain-impaired person. Being nude, closed in, and helpless in a bathtub or shower creates a sense of vulnerability that may be frightening. Because the person is accustomed to bathing regularly, it may make perfect sense in her mind to claim she has bathed.

Helpful Responses
- Maintain bathing and grooming at regularly scheduled times.
- Make bathing and grooming comfortable and relaxing experiences; for example, offer a warm bath and relaxing back massage.
- Be aware of potential fears such as anxiety about falling or water that is too hot.

Behavior *20. The person fails to recognize familiar persons, places, and things.*

Common responses.   He is getting much worse and is terribly confused.

Alzheimer's interpretation.   Due to a kind of brain impairment known as agnosia, the person is gradually losing his function of recognition. What his eyes see no longer can be put together into the previously meaningful and understandable picture. Thus, people, places, and things he has been around all of his life now truly appear unfamiliar.

Helpful Responses
- Avoid arguing, as conflict will increase the person's confusion and fear.

- Agree that things look different and calmly indicate who you are or identify the thing in question.
- Bring specific and recognizable things to the person's attention to help reestablish contact with the past.
- Avoid rushing the person.

Behavior 21. *The person wanders around at night or seems to be looking for something.*

Common responses.   She is confused and does not know what she is doing; she is being inconsiderate.

Alzheimer's interpretation.   Wandering may occur when the person is disoriented in the middle of the night and has forgotten her reason for awakening. The sleeping difficulties may be caused by frightening noises, hallucinations, or nightmares. When there is a lack of structured daily routine, the difference between night and day is less pronounced.

Helpful Responses
- Reorient the person when she is wandering in the household.
- Reassure the person that she can look for whatever she wants tomorrow, after a good night's sleep.
- Keep a light on in the bathroom.
- Consult a physician if sleeping difficulties persist.
- Increase the person's level of activity during the day.

Behavior 22. *The person refuses to eat, or he eats very little.*

Common responses.   He has a poor appetite; he is too picky about food; he needs to be more active.

Alzheimer's interpretation.   As Alzheimer's progresses, it is common for decreases in appetite to occur. Eating binges and a desire for sweets also occur, but greater concerns are created by the refusal to eat. Often persons fail to eat because they believe they have already eaten or because they simply forget what they are doing. This is more likely to occur with those who live alone or in situations without a daily routine.

Brain impairment also contributes to difficulties in using eating utensils. Swallowing can be difficult.

Helpful Responses
- Minimize between-meal snacks.
- Maintain as high a level of physical activity as possible.

- Provide regular meals that follow a routine.
- Eat with the person.
- Prepare familiar and favorite foods.
- Be sure food can be easily chewed and swallowed.
- Cut meat as necessary; use utensils that are easy to hold.
- As coordination deteriorates, offer direct assistance.
- Consider using vitamins or food supplements.
- Avoid overemphasizing neat eating habits.
- Give the person more time to eat.

Behavior   23. *The person does not seem to care for you anymore, and she says you do not love or care about her.*

Common responses.   She no longer loves and appreciates you.

Alzheimer's interpretation.   As brain impairment progresses, the person's awareness of the people around her naturally diminishes. She becomes less expressive and makes fewer gestures of appreciation. When she questions whether you love or care about her, she may be seeking reassurance to counteract her sense that she is losing you due to her diminishing abilities.

Helpful Responses
- Reassure her that you care, without taking offense at her questions.
- Provide as much involvement as possible with other individuals and supporting influences, such as an Alzheimer's family support group.

Behavior   24. *The person's hands and arms shake, he stumbles and is unsteady when he walks.*

Common responses.   He is nervous; he has visual problems; his arthritis is getting worse.

Alzheimer's interpretation.   While nervousness may be responsible for some of the shaking, other causes also should be considered. Side effects of medications prescribed for severe agitation, delusions, hallucinations, and sleeping problems may be the source. Stiffness also could be caused by these medications.

In other cases, tremors may be directly related to the brain impairment. Rapid jerking movements of the limbs or even the body can occur. These are called myoclonic jerks and should be evaluated by a physician.

Loss of mobility and coordination of large (gross) and small (fine) movements occurs with the disease. These coordination problems contribute to difficulties with all motor skills. Weakness, poor balance, and stooped posture make walking difficult; likewise, difficulty in getting up from a chair leads to long periods of sitting. Prompt medical attention should be sought as these conditions escalate.

Some persons with Alzheimer's may exhibit symptoms suggestive of Parkinson's disease. This neurological disorder can coexist with Alzheimer's, but it is difficult to differentiate when Alzheimer's is in its advanced stages.

Helpful Responses
- Check to be sure that poor vision or other impairments do not restrict the person's mobility.
- Change furniture, lighting, throw rugs, and so forth to promote safety at home.
- Provide the person with ample opportunities for exercise to prevent premature weakness and loss of coordination.
- Avoid rushing the person, provide assistance when required, and encourage him to carry out tasks one step at a time.
- Consult a physician when dramatic deterioration in motor skills occurs.

Behavior 25. *The person sits doing nothing for long periods of time.*

Common responses. She should be doing something worthwhile; she should be more active; she is bored, lazy, or depressed.

Alzheimer's interpretation. As brain impairment affects memory and intellectual abilities, spontaneous and self-initiated activity diminishes. Apathy and a lack of interest in what is going on develops because the person's ability to partake in daily life is compromised. Her abilities to plan and carry out purposeful activity are likewise affected by diminished cognitive abilities. Later, she may develop problems with walking and standing. More positively, sitting quietly may be a welcomed relief for her from the increasingly stressful demands of daily life.

Helpful Responses
- Develop daily routines that include enjoyable activities which require minimal concentration.
- Encourage and assist the person's participation in shared activities.
- Walk and exercise with the person to encourage muscle strength and coordination.
- Realize the person may be enjoying the chance to relax and be free of stressful activities.
- Use music and some television to add stimulation to time spent sitting.

Behavior *26. The person wets or soils himself.*

Common responses.   He is not trying to control his bodily functions and does not care anymore; he wants your attention; he is trying to get back at you for something.

Alzheimer's interpretation.   These problems are not uncommon in more advanced stages of Alzheimer's. The person is less aware of the need to relieve himself and does not associate this need with the bathroom.

Memory problems and perceptual difficulties make it more difficult for the person to find the bathroom. At night, disorientation and confusion make it more difficult to use the bathroom.

Helpful Responses

- Assist the person in maintaining regularly scheduled trips to the bathroom.
- Leave a night light on in the bathroom.
- Consider reducing the intake of liquids in the evening.
- Label the bathroom door and help the person practice finding it.
- Be understanding of bladder and bowel accidents, which are quite embarrassing to the individual.
- Have a doctor examine the person for other underlying medical problems.

Behavior *27. The person wanders aimlessly.*

Common responses.   She is disoriented and lost; she does not have anything to do.

Alzheimer's interpretation.   Wandering is a problem for people who have brain damage. It has potentially dangerous outcomes. The person could fall or become lost in the neighborhood. (We have considered some aspects of wandering in Behavior 16, restlessness/agitation and Behavior 21, nocturnal confusion.)

Wandering cannot be easily understood if one sees it as aimless. In fact, what appears to be aimless wandering is not an aimless activity at all in many cases. A brain damaged by Alzheimer's disease merely has difficulty determining the purpose or goal of such activity. The impaired person may not be able to communicate. In such cases, the caregiver may find that the purpose of the wandering becomes clearer through observation. Often people who are thought to be wandering aimlessly follow the same path repeatedly. This may be more evident in institutional settings. Along that path are sources of positive stimulation (outside views, water, coffee, social contact). Wandering can also be an effort to avoid or escape adversive situations, such as dark or noisy areas and more isolated spots, which create a strong sense of insecurity. Other explanations for what appears to be wandering behavior include the following possibilities:

1. The person is looking for something she has lost.

2. The person does not recognize her surroundings and may be looking for something familiar. (This may be an example of agnosia—failure to recognize familiar persons, things, places—or a reaction to a new or changed physical environment.)

3. The person is more confused, restless, or agitated as a reaction to tranquilizers or other medication.

4. The person may be more confused during certain parts of the day, for example, early morning or late evening.

5. The person may be confused as a result of sensory impairment. Because she hears or sees poorly, she cannot comprehend sights and sounds accurately. These types of impairments can also result from brain damage. In this case, the individual cannot process visual and auditory information correctly, and her perceptions are distorted.

6. The person may wander as a response to stress. She may walk away from upsetting situations and then become lost. A catastrophic reaction may precede the wandering behavior. Some persons may have always gotten upset easily by a stressful situation and walked away from it.

Helpful Responses

- First, determine the type of wandering. Is it really aimless, or is the wandering goal-directed?.
- Then, determine if the wandering is an attempt to gain something (stimulation, food, drink, security, or physical activity because of restlessness).
- Remember that restlessness and pacing are common during some phases of Alzheimer's disease. Supervise this activity constructively. Walk with the person in a safe and stimulating area. (Too much stimulation can be overwhelming at times.)
- Determine if the wandering behavior is a response to stressful environmental factors. For example, too much noise or demands placed on the person too quickly and forcefully may precipitate behavior that results in wandering and getting lost.
- Determine if the person's apparent wandering is a reaction to fear. Has the individual misinterpreted sights or sounds? Are these delusions or

hallucinations? Is she trying to get away from something that frightens her? If so, wandering may be her attempt to seek security and safety. Relate to this need.

- At night, leave some lights on and the door to the bathroom open so that the person does not get lost on the way to the bathroom.
- If you believe the wandering is created by medications, consult the physician for a medications review.
- Place locks on outside doors that cannot be undone by the impaired person but can be opened easily by you.
- Utilize the Alzheimer's Association Safe Return Program. This nationwide program assists with the identification and safe return of persons with AD and related conditions who have become lost as a result of wandering or driving. It includes identification products such as jewelry, wallet cards, and clothing labels. Safe Return has a national photo/information database along with a 24-hour toll-free crisis line. For more information, the reader should contact the local Alzheimer's Association chapter, or call 888-572-8566 to register by phone. Have a credit card handy. There is a registration fee of $40 and caregiver jewelry is $5. Scholarships may be available through your local Alzheimer's Association chapter.
- If wandering continues to be difficult to manage, consult a physician or mental health professional.

Wandering is a major source of stress to most caregivers. Understandably they worry because of its potential harmful outcomes. Caregivers should take action to deal with this problem, or it will create more stress and heighten the need for supervision considerably. If the memory-impaired person does wander away from home, notify the police department immediately. Having pictures of the person along with an accurate description of such characteristics as hair color, height, weight, and other identifiers will increase the chances of the person's being found quickly. Be sure to tell the police that the person is memory impaired, confused, and so forth. You may offer suggestions on how the person may best be approached. If you know, tell police about the status of the person when she left. Was she upset and angry? It may be better for the caregiver to remain home and have family or friends assist with the search so that someone is at the home should the patient return there.

When the person returns home, it will be better to relate positively to the return. Your anger or scolding will only make matters worse. The person will probably be frightened anyway.

13

Depression and the Alzheimer's Caregiver

Family caregivers are the most important people in the lives of persons who have Alzheimer's disease. With their help a diagnosis was sought. Persons with Alzheimer's began to adapt to their condition with their support. Because of their involvement, people with Alzheimer's have had a chance to remain in a familiar setting much longer. When the need for more assistance with tasks such as driving, taking medications, and managing a checkbook became evident, family caregivers intervened. When assistance with personal needs such as bathing and grooming was necessary, caregivers added these responsibilities to their growing list of things to do. After the person moved to a nursing home, caregivers followed to look after him. They remained with loved ones for the entire journey. They were not the same people when their journey ended. Some felt they had grown individually; some were glad they were able to complete this labor of love. Others suffered from the chronic stress and completed the journey with poorer health and depressive disorders. A few caregivers ended the journey prematurely. Major health problems caused their death. Caring for family members with Alzheimer's disease is not to be taken lightly.

Caregiving is associated with conditions that foster the development of depression and significant levels of stress. Caregiving duties and responsibilities increase in proportion to the increasing dependency of loved ones. Caregivers who care for family members in their home spend an average of 60 hours per week on these responsibilities (Haley et al., 1995). They spend an average of 6½ years providing in-home care before placing loved ones in a nursing home (Aneshensel et al., 1995). Caregivers spend 3,120 hours a year in caregiving. In 6½ years, they have given a total of 20,280 hours to caregiving. They spend an average of another 2½ years looking after loved ones in nursing homes, where they spend even more hours providing hands-on assistance or monitoring care.

Three conditions threaten the mental and physical well-being of caregivers: chronic stress, depression, and loss of physical health. The presence of one condition increases the chances that another will develop or worsen. For instance, chronic stress contributes to the development of depression. Physical health problems can precipitate or worsen caregiver depression. Any of these conditions can jeopardize a family member's involvement in the caregiver role.

If caregivers were able to recognize signs of depression, chronic stress, or health problems, they would be able to respond more appropriately to them. Early symptoms of all three suggest normal reactions to caregiving stress, which makes it easy to overlook the significance of these symptoms. Thinking they are just experiencing more stress when symptoms progress, caregivers often try to tolerate them.

Recognizing the possibility that depression is developing is the first step toward treatment. But depression is not that easy to recognize. Often seriously depressed people don't know they are depressed. Symptoms that suggest a diagnosis of depression are identified in this chapter so that caregivers can seek the appropriate help. Persons suspecting they might be depressed, however, do not always seek help, and some caregivers are at greater risk.

This chapter gives ways that caregivers might minimize some of the risks for depression. Risks include gender, age, health status, cultural affiliation, and lack of social support, as well as certain characteristics of the person with Alzheimer's. Behavior problems can be sources of greater stress and depression. The need for greater assistance with activities of daily living can be another trigger for stress and depression, often because these activities precipitate behavior problems.

How Common Is Caregiver Depression?

Caregivers of people with Alzheimer's disease have a substantial risk for depression. Estimates of caregiver depression vary considerably. Caregiving research indicates that from 14 to 81 percent of caregivers are affected by depression (Bodnar and Kiecolt-Glaser, 1994). One study found that 23 percent of spousal caregivers had symptoms of depressive disorders, and very few of these caregivers had any prior history of depression (Haley, 1997). Another study indicated that 70 percent of caregivers had depressive disorders (Terri, 1994). Several studies indicated that from 30 to 55 percent of Alzheimer's caregivers had clinically significant depression (Schulz et al., 1995; Haley et al., 1995). Differences in the percentages of caregivers reported to be depressed vary considerably because of different characteristics of caregivers (e.g., personality, health, education), care recipients (e.g., types and seriousness of behavior problems), and the circumstances under which care is provided. The coping style of some caregivers is more likely to foster depression.

Reasons We Fail to Recognize Depression

When people think of depression as being just sad and blue, they expect to get over it pretty quickly and move on. Brief episodes of being down are a normal part of life and they often follow upsetting situations. Once the situation changes or we find an effective way to deal with it, our feelings change. However, clinical depression is not determined by situations alone. And its symptoms go beyond feeling sad or hurt. Unlike short-lived symptoms related to upsetting situations, symptoms of depression persist. Caregivers who can recognize the difference between being down in the dumps and being really depressed are in a better position to get the help they need.

Caregivers experience grief. Distinguishing depression from grief can be difficult since they share some symptoms. However, some symptoms of depression—especially worthlessness, low self-esteem, hopelessness and helplessness, and excessive and inappropriate guilt—help distinguish it from grief.

People experience depressive symptoms differently. All depressed people do not experience sadness. Some describe a pervasive emptiness; some wish they could cry; some feel nervous or more irritable; some feel tired and lack energy. People with serious depression may not be able to say much at all about how they are feeling. Some depressed people mask depressive symptoms with physical symptoms and seem less aware of the emotional features.

Depression is a self-limiting condition. It's difficult for people who are depressed to care for themselves. Depressed caregivers may use virtually all of their physical and emotional reserves to care for loved ones. Depression stalls problem solving. Frequently, depressed persons say they don't want help because they don't believe anything will help, or they aren't worth helping. Depression causes a collapse in our ability to think and act. Depressed caregivers that recognize they are depressed may have trouble making the effort to act on this information.

Depression is a form of mental illness. Unfortunately, stigmas of mental illness are still prevalent. Mistaken beliefs about mental illnesses and prejudice against mentally ill persons prevent some people from seeking treatment. They feel embarrassed or ashamed when they recognize they have symptoms of mental illness. But these psychiatric disorders are diseases like diabetes or cancer. People no more want to be depressed than they want to have a heart attack or stroke. Depression is the most common psychiatric disorder. Approximately 10 million Americans suffer from a major depressive disorder. Nevertheless, depressed caregivers may resist seeking treatment because of their concerns about being labeled mentally ill or crazy, or losing control of their life because they seek psychiatric help.

People have other beliefs that create barriers to getting help. Some believe that depression is a sign of personal or moral weakness. They fear that if they get help their weaknesses will be exposed and they will be vulnerable to the judgment of others. The majority of caregivers, however, become depressed because of factors associated with the caregiving situation, chronic stress, and the same human limitations all of us have. Caregiver depression has nothing to do with physical, emotional, or moral weakness.

Avoidance and denial may prevent caregivers from acknowledging signs of depression or seeking help when they suspect depression. The use of psychological defenses helps soften the painful reality of some situations. As temporary defenses, they support adjustment. However, continuous use of denial and avoidance is not adaptive. These coping mechanisms are associated with an increase in caregiver depression.

In addition to creating barriers to getting help for depression, caregiver denial or avoidance can take many forms that create obstacles for other kinds of help. Caregivers may be defensive and refuse to acknowledge or discuss other problems. Some individuals try to cover the depressive symptoms by using alcohol, drugs, or other substances to feel better. Some caregivers may fear depressive symptoms are being caused by something worse than depression. Perhaps the symptoms are caused by a major medical problem. Although health problems may be aggravated by caregiving, depression is more likely the source of the person's pain and misery.

Some caregivers acknowledge symptoms yet minimize their significance. They try to justify depressive symptoms by normalizing them. The symptoms are caused by caregiving. Anyone doing what they are doing, dealing with the problems they are facing, would feel like they feel. The problem is not depression. They're just constantly exhausted. This reframing of the problem makes the symptoms temporarily more tolerable. When the symptoms don't improve, and in fact worsen, caregivers need to face the fact that they have a problem. Without treatment, caregiver depression does not improve.

Depressive Disorders

Caregivers, who have experienced either depressive disorders or other mental health disorders may become more vulnerable to these conditions because of chronic caregiver stress. It is wise to contact the health care professional who treated the disorder before. Because of the stressful nature of caregiving, it is important to closely monitor any symptoms that would suggest a recurrence of the disorder.

Caregivers may develop one of several depressive disorders: adjustment disorder with depressed mood, dysthymic disorder, or major depressive disorder. It is also possible that caregivers could develop a mood disorder due to a general medical condition. These conditions are discussed in terms of general diagnostic criteria consistent with the *Diagnostic and Statistical Manual of the American Psychiatric Association* (DSM-IV). My purpose in discussing symptoms and diagnostic criteria is to provide some guidelines to recognize and respond to symptoms that suggest a caregiver might have a depressive illness. The diagnostic criteria are not comprehensive, because if caregivers are experiencing depressive symptoms they need professional help to diagnose their illness and develop an individual treatment plan. It is not my intent that caregivers, family members, or friends use these guidelines to diagnosis their condition. Again, diagnosis and treatment are to be arranged with physicians or mental health professionals.

Major Depressive Disorder

A major depressive disorder is often described as a biological depression. Its origin is linked to neurotransmitters and other aspects of brain chemistry. That doesn't mean that this type of depression is unaffected by the stressful events that confront caregivers. The caregiver with a major depressive disorder must consistently have symptoms of either a depressed mood or a loss of interest or pleasure in daily activities for at least 2 weeks. The depressed mood must reflect a change from the person's normal mood. Because of the depressed mood, a caregiver's functioning in social, occupational, and educational areas is impaired. Other areas of impaired functioning can involve difficulties with caregiving tasks and not wanting to make social contacts or to be involved in activities outside the home.

This disorder is further characterized by the presence of the majority of these symptoms:

- Depression is evident most of the time as indicated by the caregiver's awareness of feeling sad or empty, or being tearful.

- Interest or pleasure in nearly all activities is markedly diminished most of the time.

- Significant weight loss or weight gain, or decrease or increase in appetite, occurs nearly every day without the caregiver dieting.

- The caregiver has difficulty getting to sleep and/or staying asleep, or sleeps too much.

- Nearly every day, psychomotor agitation (agitated movement, restlessness) or retardation (slowed movement and ponderous responses) is evident to others.

- Fatigue or loss of energy is present almost daily.

- Feelings of worthlessness or excessive or inappropriate guilt occur nearly every day.

- Ability to think or concentrate is diminished, or the caregiver is indecisive.

- The caregiver has recurrent thoughts of death (not just fear of dying), has recurrent ideas about suicide with or without a specific plan, or has attempted suicide.

Symptoms are not the result of medication or general medical condition. After loss of a loved one, bereavement does not account for these symptoms that have persisted for longer than two months and are characterized by considerable functional impairment, morbid preoccupation with one's worthlessness, suicidal ideation, psychotic symptoms, or psychomotor retardation. A major depressive episode is a very serious illness. Without treatment it will have serious consequences for caregivers and those who benefit from their care.

Dysthymic Disorder

This disorder represents a chronic state of depression. Origins of dysthymic disorder relate more to a caregiver's personality, coping and problem-solving abilities, and interpersonal skills than brain chemistry. Situational stressors may cause a worsening of symptoms. Caregivers with this disorder must have had a depressed mood for at least the majority of the past two years. They would not have been free from a depressed mood, and would have experienced two or more of the following symptoms for more than two months:

- Poor appetite or overeating
- Insomnia (trouble sleeping) or hypersomnia (sleeping excessively)
- Fatigue or low energy
- Low self-esteem
- Poor concentration or difficulty making decisions
- Feelings of hopelessness

These symptoms must cause significant distress or impairment in social, occupational, educational, or other important areas of a caregiver's functioning.

Mood Disorder Due to General Medical Condition

Symptoms of a mood disorder can be caused by medical problems. Caregivers with a mood disturbance caused by medical problems are more likely to have depressive symptoms, but symptoms of an elevated, expansive, or irritable mood might occur as well. Stress may indirectly contribute to the development of this type of mood disorder. We know, for instance, that the chronic stress of caregiving is a risk factor for declining health and the development of significant health problems. Many caregivers are older and are more likely to have chronic medical conditions. Even without the threat of chronic stress, these conditions make them more susceptible to stress-related decline. They also take more medications. Some medications have the potential to induce symptoms of a mood disorder.

A variety of medical conditions are linked to mood disorders, including degenerative neurological conditions such as Parkinson's disease. Cerebrovascular disease such as stroke can cause mood disorders. Diabetes that is poorly controlled can cause depression. Other medical conditions that may cause mood disorders are vitamin B_{12} deficiency, hypo- and hyperthyroidism, systemic lupus, hepatitis, and certain cancers. Caregivers may be tempted to attribute symptoms of mood disorders to stress alone. It is essential that they seek a medical opinion.

Adjustment Disorder

Caregivers can experience serious depressive symptoms and symptoms such as anxiety and anger that don't fit the types of depression already mentioned. The symptoms are reactions to specific situational stressors frequently related to caregiving, and they represent an adjustment disorder.

Adjustment disorders represent the development of emotional or behavioral symptoms that are a response to an identifiable stressor(s). The symptoms develop within 3 months of when the stressor(s) occurred. Within this time frame caregivers experience several emotional or behavioral symptoms. Either of the following may be observed:

- Marked distress in excess of what would be expected from exposure to the stressor
- Significant impairment in social, occupational, or educational functioning

This disorder will benefit from a variety of coping approaches. For example, if caregivers can learn to see the problem (stressor) in different ways, it might be possible to manage it effectively.

Generalized Anxiety Disorder

Anxiety is a feature of daily life, and some anxiety is certainly normal. Like stress, anxiety indicates we sense a threat or demand. If we take care of these situations, feelings of anxiety subside. Symptoms of anxiety may persist and become extremely disturbing. We do not always know why we continue to feel anxious. Sometimes we perceive threats that don't really exist, but because we have not evaluated the situation, we react as though the danger were quite real. Caregivers face unfamiliar and unpredictable situations, which heightens stress and anxiety. Anxiety may be increased by behavioral problems of care recipients who cannot be successfully managed on a consistent basis.

Anxiety is associated with depression, stress, and some medical problems. It is also associated with a number of conditions called anxiety disorders. Caregivers are more likely to experience one of these, generalized anxiety disorder.

Persons with this disorder have excessive anxiety and worry about a number of events or activities (such as caregiving tasks and management of behavior). Caregivers have these symptoms most of the time over a period of at least 6 months and find it difficult to control their worries. Worry and other manifestations of anxiety cause individuals significant distress or impairment in areas essential to their functioning as caregivers: maintaining supportive relationships and being involved with their families and friends.

Anxiety and worry are associated with three (or more) of the following symptoms:

- Restlessness or feeling keyed up or on edge
- Fatigue
- Difficulty concentrating or mind going blank
- Irritability
- Muscle tension
- Sleep disturbances (difficulty falling or staying asleep, or restless and unsatisfying sleep)

Anxiety, like depression, can result from underlying medical conditions or medications, and the caregiver's medical status should be assessed. Most anxiety disorders have psychological origins.

A number of medications are available to treat anxiety, and this approach to treatment is an important consideration. However, caregivers need to have the opportunity to learn more effective ways of coping with stress. If they can learn new ways to cope, they can reduce anxiety and their reliance on treatments that just manage their symptoms. Symptoms can be a manifestation of depression.

Risk Factors for Caregiver Depression

Personal and Family History of Depression

We might expect that a high percentage of depressed caregivers have had a personal or family history of depression. This assumption is wrong. While having suffered a previous episode of depression or having a family history of depression may increase the caregiver's risk for depression, these factors fail to explain the majority of caregiver depression. Most depressed caregivers have no prior personal or family history of this illness. Its onset is linked to the chronic strains of caregiving (Bodnar and Kiecolt-Glaser, 1994).

Behavioral Problems

Many people believe that the impaired memory and cognitive functions of the person with Alzheimer's are a major source of caregiver stress and depression. However, there is now overwhelming support that more behavior problems are associated with higher levels of caregiver depression (Clyburn et al., 2000). Functional impairment is beginning to be viewed as a more significant force in the development of caregiver depression, particularly as it corresponds to the need for assistance with activities of daily living. Caregivers are frequently faced with problem behaviors in activities of daily living as the dementia progresses. Thus, they must learn to understand and manage behavior in order to help themselves as well as the recipients of their care.

Chronic and Unique Stress

Caring for a person with Alzheimer's disease is thought to be more stressful than caring for persons with other conditions. Because of the types of experiences caregivers face during the difficult and prolonged period of caregiving, stress becomes chronic.

One of the strongest findings of current research is that clinical depression in most family caregivers results from the unique and chronic stressor of caring for an impaired older person (Steffen et al., 1998). One of the studies addressing caregiver depression has shown that 30 percent of spouses who assumed the role of caregiving became depressed compared to only 1 percent of persons like themselves who were not providing care (Dura et al., 1990). To put it another way, spousal caregivers were 30 times more likely to suffer depression than persons very similar to them who were not providing care. The depression suffered by Alzheimer's caregivers appears to be largely situational. We need to remember, however, that different people cope differently with comparable stressful situations.

Caregiver Burden

Burden is a risk factor for depression. It is one way to identify the negative aspects of caregiving such as cost, time, energy, anxiety, health problems, and the social and psychological impact of caregiving on the caregiver. Higher levels of caregiver burden increase the risk for depression. One study (Haley et al., 1987) found that caregivers with high levels of burden had poorer social, psychological, and physical health when compared to persons like themselves who were not caregivers. These caregivers experienced more depression and were less satisfied with their life. Their social activity was more limited and daily functioning was significantly compromised.

A positive outlook on life and the use of effective coping strategies are associated with less distress and burden, and consequently less risk of depression. Confidence in problem-solving ability, seeing a problem in different ways, and seeking spiritual support are coping strategies that have been associated with lower burden. Social support is also important, including backup for caregiving, close social contacts, and the presence of extended family.

Passive coping styles have been associated with greater burden. Persons who use an escape-avoidance type of coping are known to have more depression and interpersonal conflicts (Vitaliano et al., 1991). Coping is discussed thoroughly in Chapter 14.

Gender and Relationships

Depression is the major mental health problem in those caring for a spouse with dementia. Spousal caregivers are more likely to have depressive symptoms. They are also more likely than nonspousal caregivers to experience poor health and limited social activities (Clyburn et al., 2000). Female caregivers are likely to experience more frequent depression and to be more depressed than men (Knop et al., 1998). Women tend to show signs of depression earlier in the caregiver experience (Schulz and Williamson, 1991). Men tend to rely on problem-focused coping strategies that are particularly responsive to the earlier problems faced in caregiving. These strategies may not be as helpful further into the caregiver journey. By this time, chronic stress becomes more difficult to manage.

Depression in older male caregivers is of special concern. Depressed elderly white males have a high rate of suicide. Some have been involved in homicide-suicide pacts with spouses. The husband kills the wife so that she doesn't have to suffer. Then he kills himself.

Several factors place female caregivers at risk for depression. Persons closer to the dementia patient are more likely to experience stress or strain. The more closely related the caregiver is to the person with Alzheimer's, the greater stress and strain she will likely experience. A daughter caring for her mother is particularly vulnerable since she is both a female and a close blood relative. The combination of declining performance of activities of daily living and behavior problems represents a formidable stressor for caregivers, particularly spouses.

Caregivers who have had good marital relationships are more likely to find greater meaning and personal gratification caring for spouses with Alzheimer's disease. They will be distressed by the loss of their relationship, but through caregiving they can honor the bond they have had with their spouse. In contrast, where unresolved issues and discord already exist in marital relationships, the increasing dependency of the spouse with Alzheimer's and related behavioral problems will increase tension and conflict. The loss of the marital relationship is a real threat to caregivers, which can lead to sorrow, guilt, anger, resentment, and even hostility (Knop et al., 1998).

The caregiving relationship that adult children have with a parent is affected by some of the same relationship factors. Caregiving is an opportunity to honor their relationship with a parent. But if this relationship has been difficult, children may be placing themselves in a situation with the potential for stress, anxiety, anger, guilt, and depression. Caregiving may not be the best situation for their healing.

Nevertheless, some adult children use caregiving as a means to gain the approval or acceptance of the parent. They are not always aware that illness-related factors alone make it quite unlikely that they will ever receive the approval they have yearned for. They will have a better chance of healing their wounds if they look within themselves for reconciliation without expecting the disapproving parent to participate in the process. Caregivers do sometimes report some unexpected changes, but relationships that were very difficult before the onset of dementia are not likely to improve as the symptoms of dementia worsen.

Relationship difficulties trigger depressive disorders. If these problems existed before dementia developed, it is possible that depressive symptoms experienced by caregivers will worsen and develop into a depressive disorder. It is important for these individuals to address depression as soon as they can. Caregivers need to explore other avenues of reconciliation and support with professional counselors or spiritual mentors. Such steps might save caregivers from deeper pain, guilt, and resentment later when this chance to move on past old hurts has passed or has been lost in the weight of increasing stress. Sliding into a serious depressive illness precipitated by feelings of rejection, abandonment, and another serious blow to their self-worth can be prevented. Caregivers—not the Alzheimer's patient—can set themselves free.

Ethnic and Cultural Factors

Ethnicity has substantial impact on the caregiving experience. Several reports indicate that African American caregivers have lower rates of depression and burden than Caucasian Americans (Haley, 1997). This may be due to African American caregivers appraising caregiving activities as less stressful and themselves as more effective in the caregiving role. Differences in their expectations about caregiving and their previous experiences with adversity also seem to account for the lower rates.

One study (www.depression.com/news/19990722-353.html) looked at rates of depression in caregiver spouses from four ethnic groups. Mexican

American spouses had higher rates of depression than other ethnic groups. Clinically significant depressive symptoms were found in spouses from all ethnic groups: 89 percent of Mexican Americans, 78 percent of Japanese Americans, 66 percent of Caucasian Americans, and 57 percent of African Americans. The higher rate of depression in Mexican American spouses may be related to their higher perception of less support. And their actual social support was lower. This finding is surprising for an ethnic group known for the involvement of extended family in caregiving. Mexican American caregivers were most distressed when spouses had dementia-type behaviors. Obstacles in dealing with behavior problems have been identified as a risk for caregiver depression, which may be another factor in the level of depression found in this study.

White caregivers expressed increased levels of distress when spouses exhibited a decrease in cognitive abilities such as memory and learning. African American caregivers generally had more success coping with this problem. Mexican American caregivers suffered more even though they used religious, spiritual, and positive coping approaches. Spousal caregivers from all ethnic groups reported more distress when they used avoidance coping styles.

Other studies are needed to verify these findings. The study does show the importance in ethnic differences in identifying what is more distressing to one group of caregivers than another. Some differences in coping styles exist among ethnic groups as well. These groups need to be involved in developing care systems more appropriate to their needs.

Social Support

Spouses have often been the primary source of emotional closeness and support. Since a spouse is likely to be the person with whom one's most intimate thoughts and feelings have been shared, the caregiver is losing a valuable confidant and intimate companion when that person has Alzheimer's disease. This relationship may have been an important part of the caregiver's social support. Caregivers need to develop other avenues of social support.

Social support refers to the aspects of relationships that are positive and potentially stress-reducing. It involves receiving from others the care and concern that we associate with close, positive relationships. It reinforces our belief that others care about us. Persons in our support networks provide us with ideas about what we can do to manage different aspects of our life. We can talk with them and receive valuable feedback. Social support maintains the perception that we are connected to a bigger world. There is evidence that social support plays a key role in maintaining the well-being of caregivers. Those who perceive they have greater social support experience less depression (Clyburn et al., 2000).

Mexican American spousal caregivers who perceived little social support had a higher rate of depression (Clyburn et al., 2000). Caregivers who experienced this lack of support were found to have an increase in depression in other research (Mittelman et al., 1995).

The importance of social support in mediating the caregiver's vulnerability to depression is also supported by the fact that strong social ties are valuable mediators of caregiver depression (Bodnar and Kiecolt-Glaser, 1994). Caregivers with strong social ties are not as vulnerable to depression as caregivers who are socially isolated. The perception of social support is more important than the number of people who are actually counted as being part of it.

Family conflicts interfere with social support. If family members drop out of the social support role, it may be difficult to replace them. Nevertheless, because of the very negative impact some family members have on caregivers, the caregiver will function more effectively without their negative presence manifested as critical remarks and a judgmental attitude. Next to the caregiving strain, caregivers have cited family conflict as the most frequent problem. Family conflict has been identified as a very significant stressor underlying both depression and anger in Alzheimer's caregivers. Conflict involving family members' attitudes and behaviors toward the caregiver has been found to be closely associated with caregiver depression (Semple, 1992).

Social support has other important functions. In their social support system, caregivers may find out about services from people who have used them before in situations similar to their own. They can learn that the ways they feel about things are normal responses and these responses may be self-defeating. For example, caregiver guilt is common. The basis for this guilt is not always rational. Mediators from caregivers' social support networks can provide them with emotional support and help them overcome their guilt. Hearing other points of view about caregiving feelings and situations may produce a change of heart that leads to healthier caregiver choices.

Contacts with professional helpers may function as social support. If the family doctor has administered care over a long period of time, the caregiver may perceive the physician to be an important source of social support. Encouragement and guidance offered by the physician may be perceived to be as valuable as medical advice.

The patient with Alzheimer's disease may live from 11 to 15 years (Garity, 1997). The more involved caregivers become, the less social support they perceive they have. Sometimes caregivers who perceive they have little support may be reacting based on the pressures of caregiving rather than the actual status of social support. If they have more support than they perceive, they are reacting negatively to a stressor that has not been appraised correctly.

Friends and family become more invisible to caregivers as a result of the greater demands, stresses, and burden of caregiving.

Of course, lack of social support is also a real fact and stressor of caregiving. Caregivers were found to receive less social support (Thompson et al., 1993) when this need was increasing. This loss weakens caregiver resiliency. Resiliency can be likened to emotional stamina, which enables us to continue to adapt to life's misfortunes and the stress associated with them. When the going gets tough, we are able to carry on because we are resilient. Close and confiding relationships are important in developing and maintaining resiliency (Garity, 1997).

Choices and Control

People faced with situations over which they feel they have no control will generally find it more difficult to adapt. They lose their coping resiliency, thus encouraging the development of depression. Caregivers who perceive they have choices about caregiving will have more success adapting to the Alzheimer's experience than caregivers who see no choices. Caregivers who provide care because they have to or because they feel obligated to do so are more susceptible to depression, anger, and resentment. Unlike those who provide care out of affection, they may feel trapped by the role of caregiving. Without the perception of choice, caregivers are less likely to believe they have any control or mastery of the situation.

Choices about caregiving increase our adaptability to difficult situations. Caregivers who assume this role voluntarily and are dedicated to that person are likely to endure the caregiver role longer. They have fewer negative mental health consequences such as depression (Knop et al., 1998). Caregivers who provide more extensive care have been found to be especially susceptible to stress and depression (Mittelman et al., 1995). These people may feel they have no choice but to endure the persistent strains of caregiving .

Health Factors

Caring for family members with dementia has a greater impact on the caregiver's mental and physical health than caring for a family member who is physically impaired. Health problems are linked to an increased risk of depression. Men and women who suffer depression have greater cardiovascular risks. Men have a greater risk of having a fatal heart attack. Depressive symptoms should be brought to the attention of a physician.

Many caregivers do not pay sufficient attention to their needs for a healthy diet, sufficient sleep, and regular exercise. These practices are also important for successful stress management. They have a protective role in reducing the risk of depression and other health problems.

Caregivers use more psychotropic medications to manage symptoms of anxiety, tension, depression, and sleep problems compared with the general population, and they perceive their health to be poorer. When involved in caregiving tasks, caregivers may have high blood pressure, but it may be within the normal range when not involved in caregiving tasks. Caregivers who use avoidant coping styles or who have problems controlling their anger have significantly altered plasma lipid levels, which increases their risk of heart attack (Haley, 1997).

The immune systems of spousal caregivers are more likely to be impaired (Kiecolt-Glaser et al., 1991). In one study, ill effects persisted for up to 4 years after the death of the Alzheimer's patient. The immune system changes have been linked to increased rates of respiratory illnesses, decreased responses to vaccines for influenza, and slower healing of wounds.

Caregivers who do not attend to their own health needs have a greater chance of developing health problems, which leads to an increased risk of depression. The presence of depression should raise concerns about health problems and vice versa.

Role Engulfment and Loss of Self

Loss of self is associated with caregiver depression. To understand loss of self, we must first look at the term *self*. It describes our nature—the things about us that remain the same over time and make us unique. Self is who we are.

Relationships and the things we do are important sources of our identity. Both provide us with a broader sense of our world and ourselves. Before becoming a caregiver, you may have found that spending time with friends, working in the yard, teaching Sunday school, participating in social groups, going to the movies, traveling, and being involved with grandchildren were vital parts of your life. You realize their importance when you can no longer be involved in them.

Relationships continually provide us with important information about who we are and help us see our value as persons. We are challenged by relationships. When we are hurt and in despair, our relationships are like a loving blanket of comfort and encouragement. When cut off from important relationships during extremely stressful times, we are missing from a vital source of support for coping. It is important to maintain relationships during periods of extreme stress. Under stress we are prone to lose touch with who we are and where we are in the world.

Relationships, roles, and activities activate experiences that define us. We construct from them an image of self. In them we find meaning and purpose and are able to develop a sense of self that is more resilient and less vulnerable to losses. Life is diminished when our social involvement is severely restricted.

Caregivers face three processes that lead to loss of self: chronic stress, role engulfment, and the loss of the Alzheimer's patient. Role engulfment is common because caregivers no longer have the time or energy to engage in other activities. Before caregiving restricted their social contacts, these activities had been important sources of supportive and informative feedback. This feedback was a source of self-validation.

This validation is an important reference point for caregivers. They can gauge how well they are doing and gain different perspectives of their situations and themselves as well as new ideas that may be helpful. Loss of feedback makes it more difficult to maintain a healthy perspective about themselves and caregiving situations.

Caregivers who are involved in other self-affirming activities, as well as the relationship they have with the patient, are less vulnerable to self-loss. When their sense of self is threatened by the loss of loved ones, it is affirmed and renewed by the other activities and relationships. Self-loss occurs when they derive most of their identity from being a couple. The couple identity is lost with the progressive deterioration of the patient.

Caregivers with the following characteristics are more vulnerable to loss of self (Skaff and Pearlin, 1992) and subsequent depression. Spouses are at greater risk than adult children because of the differences in the intimacy of the relationship and the fact that adult children have other activities, roles, and relationships that support their identity. Women, who usually have more social contact outside of marriage than men, stand to lose more self-affirming aspects of their life as a result of role engulfment. Unlike men, who may approach caregiving as another job, women may view caregiving as an unwanted role they resent because they have been doing it all of their life.

Age is a factor. Younger adult children and spouses may have other priorities that compete with caregiving, for example, the need to care for children and other family members, keep a job, or go back to school. Younger caregivers are more likely to be caught in a conflict between what they want to do and feel they should do. Caregiving threatens the chance for younger caregivers to work toward other goals appropriate for this period of life. Single adult children who are caregivers, especially those with children, have competing demands that create a greater chance for role engulfment.

Two characteristics of the caregiving situation predict self-loss. Both restrict opportunities that allow caregivers to experience self-perpetuating activities. Problem behaviors predict self-loss because they require considerable vigilance and energy, leaving little motivation for caregivers to seek out other activities. The degree of assistance with the patient's activities of daily living such as bathing, dressing, and feeding is associated with self-loss when the vigilance and energy required to address these needs approaches that necessary to manage behavioral problems.

More identities provide caregivers with more potential sources of positive self-evaluation and feedback (Skaff and Pearlin, 1992). Being married, having children, and being employed offers adult children protection from loss of self.

Since employment occurs outside of the caregiving situation, it offers the caregiver a separate identity, another source of self-esteem, and a haven from caregiving stressors. Caregivers whose spouses are in nursing homes are finding that volunteer roles are rewarding. They say that volunteering helps them get their minds off of caregiving. It restores that part of themselves that may have been left dormant by caregiving— relating to adults other than the person for whom they have been caring for so long. Contact with friends provides protection against self-loss, especially for spouses and single adult children. Caregivers are protected from self-loss when they maintain activities and relationships that are supportive of those aspects of self that would otherwise be engulfed by caregiving and lost with the deterioration of the patient.

Caregivers cannot expect the caregiving role to take the place of everything they have given up. Certainly for some caregivers it threatens to take more from their life than it gives back to them. Loss of a loved one represents a substantial threat to caregivers. Those with few other self-sustaining relationships or activities may experience a greater threat to identity. Whatever the reasons for self-loss, caregivers need to look for ways to maintain important connections to the rest of their life. If they lose less of themselves to caregiving, they will have less of themselves to recover when caregiving ends.

14

Coping with Ongoing
Caregiving Stress

Learning to Analyze and Manage Change

Family caregivers are the mainstays of Alzheimer's care. Because of the chronic and deteriorating course of Alzheimer's disease (AD), the career of caregivers is likely to be prolonged. It is essential that they be able to continue in a role that is vital to the safety and well-being of the family member with AD. Caregivers should not expect to indefinitely perform all activities of care themselves. Very early in the caregiving journey it is important to consider what other community resources and personal supports are available. Knowing more about the purpose and availability of resources before they are needed will help caregivers adapt to a situation that changes dramatically.

Loved ones will change as will the relationship caregivers can have with them. Because of their intense involvement in the caregiving role, caregivers may no longer be able to participate in other important life activities. Alzheimer's caregiving has the potential to be extremely stressful on an ongoing basis. Successful caregiving will involve dealing not only with stress that comes and goes but also with chronic stress.

Caregivers bring their own skills and resources to the caregiving situation. These may be helpful, but Alzheimer's care is quite different from traditional family caregiving. Family caregiving addresses the time-limited needs of family members. Alzheimer's care is necessary from the time the disease is diagnosed until the death of the family member. It is dependent upon the resourcefulness and resiliency of the family member who assumes the primary caregiving role. The needs of the care recipient and the caregiver must be addressed.

Family caregivers are faced with difficult problems, and they must adapt to new and unfamiliar circumstances that are stressful. Managing the variable and multiple stressors of chronic care depends upon learning to cope with stress. Some caregivers are able to find meaning in their responsibilities and grow emotionally and spiritually as a part of the caregiving experience. Others find this difficult. Caregivers who feel hopeless and depressed also experience more health problems. Coping with stress distinguishes those caregivers who successfully negotiate the caregiving experience from the ones who do not, and, subsequently, suffer more detrimental effects to their mental and physical health. When caregiving has a negative impact on caregivers, it inevitably interferes with the successful completion of the task and may diminish their opportunities to resume a lifestyle that resembles the one they relinquished earlier in Alzheimer's care.

This chapter addresses coping. Stressors, stress, and different coping strategies are examined. Caregivers can examine how irrational beliefs create patterns of thought and behavior that heighten stress and make coping more difficult. These beliefs and the thoughts they foster can be major stressors. Reframing the situation is important.

Caregivers need to examine what they know about themselves. Here are some helpful questions:

- How have you coped with stressful situations in the past?
- How do you typically respond to stress?
- How does stress affect you?
- What are the emotional and physical effects you usually have when stressed?
- Do you believe you are capable of solving most problems?
- Do you believe you must do everything yourself?
- Can other people be helpful even though they cannot provide help like you?
- If you were having trouble managing a problem, who would you go to for help?
- Are you really helpful when you are feeling stressed?
- Who are the people you can trust and in whom can you confide?
- Alzheimer's disease affects the functioning of the other person in your relationship. What difference will that make?
- What part has that person played in handling the stressful demands of life that have affected both of you?
- How much confidence do you have in being able to cope without his or her involvement?
- Does it help to think about what that person would do in your situation?
- What do you think is the best way to handle things?

What is the best way for caregivers to handle things? This is an important question for caregivers to consider. It does not, however, have an easy answer. Caregivers must assimilate a great deal of knowledge and information to know the best way to personally handle their own unique caregiving situation. They need to consider the advice of family, friends, and professionals. Information available in books and from Alzheimer's Association chapters and support groups will be helpful. Guidance from their tradition of faith may provide strength. They must also look at what is healthy and possible for them. They may need to think in terms of all the resources available to them and not those limited by their own humanity. They should think of what kind of life they can have when caregiving is over and incorporate having a future in their plans for now. They need to remember what they know and identify what they need to learn. Finally, they need to decide the best way they can handle things.

Stressors, Stress, and Coping

Caregiver coping requires making a healthy adaptation to the stress associated with caregiving. It endorses the health of the caregiver as well as the care of the person with AD. Financial concerns can be an ongoing stressor. Caregivers have little time for themselves. They must deal with behavior problems while assisting with activities of daily living such as dressing and bathing. Other AD behaviors such as wandering, screaming, and destruction of property are highly stressful to caregivers. Agitation, hoarding, dangerous activities, and embarrassing activities add to caregivers' worries. Delusions and hallucinations may provoke agitation, uncooperativeness, and aggression in persons with AD. Repetitive questioning and clinging can be tiresome and annoying. It is particularly stressful to be the target of a loved one's paranoid beliefs.

Caregiver stress is not the result of one particular area of caregiving. Interrelated factors include socioeconomic status, culture and ethnic group, education, caregiving experience, family support, housing accommodations, and environment. The personal characteristics of caregivers have considerable influence on what is stressful and how they respond. One person's challenge is another person's stress.

Stressors are conditions or circumstances that have the potential to be stressful. Stress levels depend on how we appraise stressors and ascertain that a threat exists. Stress is the body's response to any demand made of it that disturbs or interferes with normal physiological equilibrium. Stress involves physical, emotional, or mental strain or tension. When stress occurs with such intensity that a person cannot manage it, pathological changes occur. A stressful situation is perceived as threatening when it is close to exceeding an individual's personal resources to manage it.

Several unique aspects of the caregiving situation contribute to the high degree of caregiver stress. The stress is chronic, which may be the most significant aspect, and it needs to be addressed by research. We already know that chronic stress is a major precipitating event for caregiver depression. Caregivers face increasing strain from the threat of exhaustion because of the continual need to assume more responsibilities as the functioning of the family member with Alzheimer's declines. They have minimal periods of relief, so continual adaptations and role changes are necessary. Their prolonged exposure to stressors results in wear and tear, which depletes their coping resources and increases their risk of becoming depressed.

Depression and other stress-related problems have more to do with the limits of human beings than the weaknesses of family caregivers. The nature of their human reserves limits the extent to which they can continue to cope with increasing demands. Caregivers with a high number of new demands or changes are more likely to suffer depression. The source of their stress is likely to develop out of new demands, not the situations with which they are more familiar. New behavioral problems and psychiatric symptoms are often the source of new demands.

The emotional and physiological arousal that stress produces is unpleasant. This state of arousal can become particularly distressing and harmful when it persists for long periods of time. Mental and physical health problems may develop under conditions of chronic stress. Hans Selye, one of the early researchers of the stress response, identified this relationship between stress and illness. Selye (1974) described three stages of the stress response, and caregivers experience all three.

The first stage is alarm. Alarm is a generalized state of arousal associated with the body's initial reaction to a stressor. A resistance stage follows. The body adapts to the stressor and is able to resist it, but functions at a high level of arousal. When stress persists for interminable periods, as occurs in Alzheimer's caregiving, the body is chronically overactive and less capable of adapting. Because it is unable to resist stress, the body moves into the exhaustion stage and is susceptible to disease. Death can even occur under extreme circumstances.

Many Alzheimer's caregivers are older and have age-related health problems. Their body is more vulnerable to stress. Hypertension, coronary artery disease, migraines, and irritable bowel syndrome have been linked to stress. Male caregivers have a high risk of heart attacks. Here is an example of a common stressful situation that sets the stage for chronic exhaustion and potential health problems.

After another long and tiring day, a caregiver finds a quiet, private moment. Suddenly a scream quickly followed by a crash at the back door breaks her peace and quiet. She is afraid. Her heart is racing. Her breathing is rapid. Her hands are moist. She doesn't know it, but her blood pressure is going up and her blood sugar level is climbing to give her body a quick source of energy to cope with the potential danger. Her senses, mind, and body are ready. She calls for her husband, but there is no answer. She goes to the back door. He isn't there, but the back door is ajar. He must be outside. She is about to step into the darkness of the backyard when the quiet is broken again, this time by the doorbell. She walks through the house to the front door. She turns on the porch light and peers through the small window in the door. No one is standing there. She's really afraid. Maybe her husband tried to get in. She opens the front door and steps out onto the porch. In the faint light of a streetlamp, she sees her husband walking toward the house next door. He is calling out her name like someone who is lost and scared. She calls out his name to slow him down. A moment later, she has caught up with him, turned him around, and is walking by his side. The stress is over—for the moment.

Unless she makes changes to secure her home, this incident might reoccur. Double locks on the doors, buzzers, and an identification bracelet for her husband. She has coped with other major stressors and daily hassles for a long time. She is wearing out and is worried that she cannot continue. She is closer to becoming a victim of the chronic stress of caregiving. Other factors contribute to this risk.

When we perceive something to be very threatening to us, our stress response will match this perception. Threatening situations may involve physical dangers, emotional hurt, or financial risks. Embarrassment, guilt, or shame may threaten a caregiver's self-esteem or identity. An innocuous situation can be viewed as a life-threatening catastrophe. Since we are responding to what we believe is a life-threatening event, our level of stress will reflect this. However, if we really appraised what was happening and determined there was nothing to worry about, we would not have any signs of stress.

Our thoughts are a source of stress and can either heighten the stress response or relieve it. The following example shows how a caregiver's worrisome thoughts about a future event create her present misery. For days she has dreaded taking her husband to his doctor appointment. She has even begun to feel resentful that her children have not offered to do it. Her dread develops into irritability and she is easily aggravated. Taking her husband to the doctor has developed into a major stress response. Her husband picks up on her irritable countenance and becomes agitated and uncooperative.

Another caregiver who was faced with almost the same situation responded quite differently. She kept her focus on how things were going in the present and didn't obsess about the appointment with the doctor. She was able to do this because she had learned to tell herself positive things. She thought to herself that she had handled this task before and could accomplish it again. Even if a problem developed, it was not the end of the world. She needed to maintain a calm countenance. On the day of the appointment, she and her husband went for a pleasant drive through some neighborhoods that were landscaped quite attractively. As they were enjoying the sights, she casually mentioned that they might as well drop by the doctor's office since they were already in the neighborhood. Her husband didn't object.

We are distressed by the view we have of events, not the events themselves. The belief that external events cause our stress promotes the idea that we have no control of things that happen to us when we really do. We determine our thoughts. Our perceptions of events and situations determine whether they are really stressors. We are the authors of our own stress. The venerable William Shakespeare knew this. He is credited with saying; "There is nothing either good or bad. Thinking makes it so."

Responding to Thoughts and Stressors

In Chapter 12 we learned to respond to behavior positively by viewing it as an expression of brain impairment rather than as an act intended to have a negative effect on caregivers. Our thinking changes our view of behavior, which helps us change our reactions to it. We are now ready to use this framework to look at how we respond to stressors. When we understand stressors differently, we can respond differently. We may discover there is no reason to be stressed.

Stressors.   What has happened, situations or events that are potential sources of caregiver stress.

Thoughts.   Interpretations and judgments; what we tell ourselves about the meaning and personal significance of what we perceive and know about the stressor.

Response.   The physical and emotional reaction to our thoughts about the stressor.

Using this framework to picture how people perceive, interpret, and respond to stressors will help caregivers appreciate the role of their thoughts in creating stress.

Stressor.   The husband loses mail, including bills, so they don't get paid.

Thoughts.   The caregiver believes her husband is possibly hiding the mail from her. At best she thinks he might be misplacing it. He denies these actions, so she thinks he is lying to her and acting as if he doesn't care about her.

Response.   Her thoughts create anger and suspicion. It hurts her feelings that her husband is unconcerned. She feels helpless. She has had more headaches and fatigue. At night she lies awake longer with alternating feelings of anger and sadness. Although she probably has several options, she is unaware of them. She tells herself this situation is terrible and there is nothing she can do. Her stress level builds. Her stress is caused by her appraisal of the stressor, not the stressor. She could have responded quite differently to this and other problems had she known he had Alzheimer's and understood how that affected his behavior. She could have changed their address to a post office box, gotten their bills, paid them, and let him keep going to the mailbox.

Caregivers are frequently faced with handling matters that a spouse or parent had previously managed. They need not burden themselves further with overwhelming feelings about the event or their ability to manage things themselves.

Caregivers may feel helpless watching the decline of memory and other cognitive functions. Care recipients may be unable to dress themselves appropriately and perform other activities of daily living. Caregivers cannot accept these problems as manifestations of the disease. They may try to do everything possible to keep loved ones functional. Thinking the problems are caused by care recipients' lack of effort or their intention that the caregivers do more for them, caregivers may push them harder. Because of their beliefs about what causes this behavior, caregivers feel angry, resentful, frustrated, and even unappreciated. It's not the behavior that causes these feelings. The caregiver's thoughts about the behaviors cause the stressful feelings.

Stressor.   *Richard's wife, Mary, does not dress herself appropriately or completely.*

Thoughts.   Richard believes that Mary is not paying enough attention to what she is doing and wants to depend on him to do more things for her that she could do for herself. He has enough to do.

Response.   Richard reacts to Mary with anger and frustration.

The importance of understanding dementia-related behavior is underscored by A and B below where different thoughts and response to the same stressor can produce more constructive interactions between Richard and Mary.

A: Thoughts.   Mary may not be dressing the way she used to but is doing the best she can. She really cannot take care of herself without some help. Richard needs to revise his expectations. Richard feels some sadness about this and tells himself he needs to learn to understand these changes in Mary's functioning. He upsets her when he pushes her to do things she is not always capable of doing, and then directs his frustration toward her.

A: Response.   He is kind as he assists with helping her dress.

B: Thoughts.   Mary becomes frustrated and embarrassed if Richard hurriedly dresses her instead of taking more time to patiently help her dress herself. He needs to remember she used to be so proud of her appearance. It will help her if he can compliment her on how nice she looks.

B: Response.   Richard has empathy for Mary and assists her with dressing step by step. He feels good telling her how nice she looks and even better when she smiles at him.

Many different responses can occur from different thoughts about the same stressor. Our appraisal of stressors has a lot of influence on how we will respond to something. We can learn to understand our own behavior and the behavior of care recipients if we listen to what we are thinking. Caregivers may not be able to change what loved ones do, but they can change the way they interpret and respond to the way loved ones act.

Stress and Self-Talk

We need to be able to understand how we view situations so that we can catch ourselves before we expend energy we need for something else. We must pay close attention to how we think about and interpret stressors. This is reflected in what we say to ourselves. We engage in self-talk every day. It reflects what we believe about what happens in our life. It gives us a glimpse of what we think about others and ourselves, and our view of why things happen to us. Self-talk guides our responses to stress. While it is a common part of our thinking processes, we are not always aware of how it influences our feelings and our thoughts. Unless we become more aware of what we are saying to ourselves and how it influences our reaction to stress, we will not be as successful in managing stress.

One caregiver trying to handle a behavior problem is very critical of how things work out. In his mind he hears himself repeatedly saying he is never able to get things right. It doesn't matter that he has unrealistic expectations because he doesn't see that these are the basis for the critical self-talk. Another caregiver has a more realistic view and tells himself that he will be able to get the hang of it. It may take a little time and effort, but things will be just fine. He'll be able to do it. Self-talk can encourage or discourage our coping efforts. We can beat ourselves up or pick ourselves up. We need to listen to what we are saying and to evaluate it. Our responses to stressful situations may be directed by self-talk arising from incorrect and irrational beliefs.

Rational self-talk reflects the caregiver's reality accurately and supports healthy functioning. Irrational self-talk increases distressful emotional and physical reactions to stressors. Irrational beliefs are built on an inaccurate perception. Caregivers may see things that loved ones think and do as irrational. They need to recognize their own irrational thoughts. Consider the following example.

Two caregivers with very similar situations both feel lonely. One caregiver tells herself that she will be able to learn to live with her loneliness. It is unpleasant but not the most awful thing in the world. Some of the feeling is probably related to her sense of loss. She has been able to make friends easily, and she has several important friends who help lessen this pain. Rational self-talk reduces stress and creates better opportunities for adaptation to life changes.

The other caregiver's self-talk sends an entirely different message. She tells herself she will never be able to make it alone. Her husband is her entire life. He made all of her decisions. She could not possibly make good decisions by herself. She could never find anyone like him. This woman doesn't doubt this questionable truth. She accepts it as reality. Her self-talk has constructed a frightening, hopeless future.

Two types of self-talk may be particularly troublesome to caregivers: statements that "awfulize" and "absolutize" events. Irrational self-statements that "awfulize" make catastrophes of events. This perspective predicts that what has or will happen is the worst possible thing. Because "awfulizing" is an overreaction to an event, it creates greater emotional reactions to stress, which reinforce the belief that the event is too much for the person to handle. We become overwhelmed by our "awfulizing" and are eventually paralyzed by it.

To recognize irrational self-talk that "absolutizes," caregivers should examine beliefs introduced with the words *never, always, should, have to, ought to,* and *must.* Self-talk that absolutizes has a tyrannical voice that is hard to question or disobey. Most of us will recognize it, since it has been with us since we were children. Our parents and other authority figures instilled these messages.

At first it is difficult to dispute these irrational beliefs because we feel guilty, ashamed, or unworthy if we fail to carry out what they direct us to do. Rigid responses result and demand that there is only one "right" way to do things. When we do not live up to this standard, we believe we are not good people. Absolutist statements are irrational and unreasonable. They take away all the other options people have to cope with stress. People are then inclined to believe that they—not their approaches to solving problems—are responsible for subsequent failures.

Irrational Beliefs Cause Stress

Albert Ellis is the founder of rational emotive therapy (Ellis, 1975), a type of cognitive therapy. Ellis determined that thinking and emotions are significantly interrelated. Distressing symptoms or consequences are caused by a person's beliefs about the activating experiences or events. For our purposes, this means a caregiver's stress is not caused by the occurrence of Alzheimer's. Trying to manage the care recipient's behavior problem is not the cause of stress. It is caused by the caregivers irrational beliefs about these situations. Ellis found that irrational and unrealistic beliefs cause unpleasant emotions. The goal of his approach is to identify and challenge the irrational beliefs that are the root of the emotional disturbances.

More specifically, emotional distress comes from unrealistic, negative appraisals of stressful situations. A caregiver, for example, looks at the lack of contact she has with her friends for the past month. The woman tells herself that nobody cares about her and her husband enough to stay in touch. She fears she won't see her friends anymore and tells herself her situation is terrible and hopeless.

Ellis identified 12 irrational beliefs that take the form of unrealistic, absolute, or overgeneralized expectations. These beliefs are often entangled in the things we say to ourselves and are very difficult to recognize as being unrealistic without facts to support them. Irrational beliefs are really the basis for our undesirable feelings and ineffective coping responses that we use to change these feelings, yet we strive to preserve these thought patterns because we do not see them as irrational. Irrational beliefs are embedded in and direct our self-talk.

Caregivers are particularly vulnerable to some of the beliefs that Ellis originally identified. Caregivers need to start monitoring their thoughts and self-talk for the appearance of these beliefs in some form. Then they must aggressively challenge them by finding rational, factual evidence to support them. Often, as in the example above, the evidence for what we believe is quite scarce. Caregivers may initially resist adopting another point of view. That's understandable, since the irrational beliefs have not been questioned for much of a lifetime. To cope and reduce their distress, it is vital that caregivers be open to seeing things differently. This makes it possible either to reappraise the stressor or look for other ways to cope.

1. *It is an absolute necessity for an adult to have love and approval from peers, family, and friends.*

   Caregivers who are isolated and overwhelmed find it easy to believe that no one cares about them anymore. They wonder if they are really loved. In fact, maybe people stay away from them because they are not lovable. It would be nice to have more frequent contact, but this is not a good measure for how people love us. Call them and ask them to come by.

2. *You must be unfailingly competent and almost perfect in all you undertake.*

Caregivers who try to adhere to such an unrealistic standard will suffer guilt, shame, depression, self-blame, and anger. Until they can acknowledge the inherent difficulties of Alzheimer's care and revise their expectations of themselves accordingly, they will not be able to enjoy relief from negative self-talk and the unpleasant thoughts and feelings it produces.

3. *It is horrible when people and things are not the way you would like them to be.*

This belief is a basis for "awfulizing." Caregivers will not get their way in many situations. Alzheimer's disease does not consider anyone. Caregiving burden and satisfaction coexist.

4. *External events cause most human misery—people simply react as events trigger their emotions.*

If caregivers believe what they feel is caused by external events, they are letting themselves be puppets on strings. Caregivers, not external events, control what they feel and their reactions to stress. They are the source of their misery. If we attribute the way we feel to external events, we fail to see that we make the choice to think, feel, and respond as we do.

5. *You should feel fear or anxiety about anything that is unknown, uncertain, or potentially dangerous.*

Caregivers who make mountains out of molehills will experience unnecessary anxiety and have less energy available to climb the real mountains. The unknown provokes anxious feelings in many people. Caregivers need to remind themselves of all the uncertain situations they never believed they could handle but were able to manage successfully.

6. *It is easier to avoid difficulties and responsibilities than to face them.*

Avoiding difficulties on a routine basis creates more difficulties to avoid. Then one day these difficulties surround you and there is nowhere left to go. Problem solving builds confidence in the ability to learn to deal with other difficulties.

7. *You need someone other or stronger than yourself on whom to rely.*

Those who adhere to this belief think they must rely on some higher authority, a person with more status, or one who knows more. Although caregivers need support and feedback from others, they are immobilized if they rely on someone else to direct every step.

8. *The past has a lot to do with determining the present.*

Sometimes the old ways are thought to be the best and only ways of dealing with problems. Caregivers need to be open to new methods and ideas.

Self-talk can be an ally in dealing with stressful situations. Here are some coping beliefs that give more flexibility for stress management:

- I can learn to accept mistakes.
- I may need some help.
- Some things I can put away.
- There is nothing wrong with that.
- Some things I need to act on now.
- I have more than one chance in most things.
- I cannot change some situations.
- I cannot always do my best, but I can live with it.
- I'll be able to make it through this.

Remember that it's not what happens to you that is critical but how you view what happens and then how you respond if necessary.

Coping Model

Coping with stress can be complicated. It is easier to understand in this model. The diagram on page 213 illustrates the process. In the diagram I have blocked "Caregiver Situations and Events" and linked it to the first step of active coping: "Potential Stressors." Certainly the potential for stress will exist in other areas of caregivers' lives. Consequently, managing stress will also involve dealing with stressors in these areas, for example, other family responsibilities or jobs. If recurring stressors do exist in other areas of life, caregivers might block these off as I did for caregiver situations and events. Then it will be possible to look at the process of coping for the stressors arising in other areas of life.

Stress occurring in other areas may have impact on caregiving, particularly if caregivers are not able to manage it. Even though it is external to the caregiving situation, stress that is not handled in one area increases the potential for stress in activities concerned with caregiving. A caregiver may in fact react to a specific caregiving situation as though it were causing her anger, tension, frustration when a stressor external to caregiving is really the source of her stress. If the real stressor originates in situations that are not directly related to caregiving, and caregiving situations and events only serve as the triggering event for something else, family caregivers will never be able to find ways to cope with the real stressor.

The connection between an observable behavior or event and stress is much easier to make than the connection between our thoughts and stress. Caregivers may need to pay more attention to what they are thinking just as they begin to sense early manifestations of stress. This may help them identify unresolved stressors triggered by some immediate demand on them. For example, imagine that you have an important appointment with your doctor. You begin to get ready and your husband begins to demand that you take him somewhere. You respond to your husband as though he asked you to do the impossible. Was the real stressor the husband's demand or the pressures you placed on yourself to keep the appointment?

Primary appraisal.   *The caregiver assesses what is happening to determine if the situation represents a threat or other stressful change.* The appraisal is an extremely important part of coping. However, it is quite common for people to react and feel stress without ever determining if there is a threat, or if what they are reacting to has actually happened. If caregivers determine that the situation exists, they can then decide if it poses a threat.

No threat, no stress.   *If the caregiver perceives no threat or significant change, no stress is experienced.* The perception of an event determines whether it is a threat. No matter what has happened or what thoughts we have, if we are not distressed or do not feel threatened, we do not experience stress.

Threat and stress present.   *The caregiver has perceived a threat or changes that are distressing and feels symptoms of stress such as tension, anxiety, anger, and a racing heart.*

Resources assessed.   *The caregiver determines if sufficient resources exist to deal with the stressor.* They include energy, problem-solving skills, psychological adaptability, social support, financial resources, and community services.

Coping strategy chosen.   *The caregiver may chose one or more coping strategies to manage the stress.*

Results of coping.   *The caregiver look at what has happened as a result of coping efforts.*

Secondary appraisal.   *The caregiver assesses if and how things have changed.* Is there still a threat? The secondary appraisal determines the effectiveness of coping efforts by reassessing the status of the stressor and manifestations of stress still observed in the caregiver. A secondary appraisal may become a stressor itself because the caregiver may be upset that coping efforts have failed. Caregivers can increase their stress by telling themselves they have failed, or concluding they are incapable of handling the situation.

Stress relieved.   *There is a return to the status of no threat—no stress.*

Stress remains.   *Coping has not been successful and stress is still present.* The process returns to assessing resources and choosing another coping strategy or the caregiver surrenders to the stress.

Recognizing a stressor seems simple, but it is difficult when there are multiple sources of stress affecting the caregiving situation and the caregiver is already suffering from prolonged stress. When we have been under stress for a long time, we often strongly react to innocuous events as though they were extremely threatening because they feel like the proverbial straw that broke the camel's back. Exhausted and overwhelmed, caregivers may react to benign events as catastrophes because there is one more thing to handle. They are, however, reacting to a stressor before they appraise how it will affect them. The first step in coping with another stressor is recognizing the event or circumstance that is the source of stress, then evaluating its consequence to the caregiver.

After identifying the specific source of distress, the caregiver can determine why it is stressful and develop alternative approaches to managing it. A list of possible ways to manage a stressor is a good idea. If these were kept in a journal, caregivers could keep track of them and the outcomes. As we discussed earlier, caregivers who learn to listen to their self-talk will find important leads to thoughts, beliefs, and values that trigger stressful reactions to different situations. Self-talk messages can be noted and tracked in a journal. As caregivers learn to identify what makes situations and events stressful, they can keep track of beliefs and other approaches to coping.

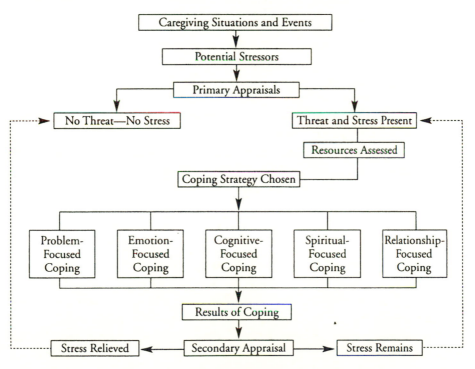

The Process of Coping with Caregiver Stress

Personality style, attitude, emotional and physical health status, and outlook on life guide how we perceive, interpret, and react to things that happen to us. Individual characteristics color how a stressor is perceived and interpreted, how the caregiver chooses to cope with it, and how long it will take the caregiver to successfully adapt. Caregivers who are optimistic, flexible, and resilient have more success coping with stress. They use diverse coping approaches. Caregivers who are meaningfully involved in what they are doing and have a sense of control over daily routines are also more resistant to stress. Greater stress is associated with a lack of knowledge about caregiving tasks, persistent behavior problems that caregivers cannot manage, rigidity, pessimism, limited endurance, provision of more direct care, and lack of resources to provide care. Family disharmony and limited support of the caregiver involve ongoing stressors.

Different Types of Stress

Chronic stress represents the greatest threat to a caregiver's well-being. The following stressors contribute to chronic caregiver stress:

1. Increased feelings of responsibility for another person
2. Guilt and frustration associated with unmet expectations
3. Increased pressures from decision making
4. Disruption of life and lifestyle
5. Isolation from family and friends
6. Alienation from friends, family, and coworkers

However, not all stress is chronic. Caregivers will find it helpful to make a distinction in the type of stressors they identify.

Chronic stress results from stressors that either continue indefinitely or reoccur. Marital and family conflicts are chronic stressors. The caregiver role and the overload that caregivers bear are chronic stressors. The declining memory of the person receiving care represents a chronic stressor until caregivers are able to accept that it is an irreversible symptom of the disease. This type of prolonged stress lasts for months or years and produces significant wear and tear. Caregiver depression is linked to chronic stress, as is breakdown in the body's immune system, which increases the caregiver's vulnerability to disease. Weakness, fatigue, and loss of interest are other consequences of chronic stress.

A major life event such as Alzheimer's disease triggers acute stress. The loss of a job, death of a loved one, financial loss, divorce, or natural or man-made disasters represent acute stressors, which set off long-term stress. When the intensity of the stress remains severe, it leads to decreased activity and withdrawal from social interaction and other activities.

All of us deal with daily hassles. These trials and tribulations can be unpleasant, boring, or irritating. At times, they seem like the dripping facet. They bother you until you do something about them. The routine caregiving activities, such as helping with bathing or dressing, can be hassles, but the stress ends with completion of the chore. If you keep thinking about problems related to these daily hassles, temporary stress may have a cumulative effect.

Manifestations of Stress

Reactions to stress are manifested as psychological and physical symptoms. Many reactions are minimal in intensity or of short duration, and they are forgotten when the stressor is no longer a threat. We become anxious or embarrassed, but once the source of these reactions has been addressed, these uncomfortable feelings dissipate. When persons function under conditions of chronic stress, however, the indications of stress and its harmful effects may be subtle and may develop insidiously over time. Signs of stress may resemble symptoms of other health problems; they might suggest decline in mental and physical health.

Thoughts.   Difficult to get thoughts together and express oneself, forgetful, difficult to concentrate and comprehend, hard to make decisions, more critical of self and others, self-focused, self-pitying, preoccupied with the future, fearful of failure, unorganized, irrational beliefs, worries and obsessions, hard to learn new information and skills, easily distracted, mental blocks, helplessness.

Behaviors.   Difficulty with self-expression, hesitant and overly cautious, stuttering speech, slowed or agitated motor movement, subordinate and dependent, withdrawn, pacing, immobilized, crying, impulsive, nervous laughter, teeth grinding, increased smoking and use of alcohol, increased use of tranquilizers, prone to accidents, changes in appetite, repetitive activities, increase in attention-seeking behaviors such as sobbing, trembling and somatic symptoms, insomnia, nightmares, frequent urination at night.

Emotions.   Anxiety, irritability, fear, resentment, anger, moodiness, guilt and shame, fidgety, frustrated, suspicious and paranoid, low self-esteem, lonely, embarrassed, sad, depressed.

Physical.   Chest and back pain, muscle tension, faintness, and dizziness, cold or sweaty hands, chronic fatigue, hot spells, dry mouth, difficulty breathing, rapid breathing, stomach distress, pounding heart, ringing in ears, constipation, diarrhea, nausea, acute illnesses, prolonged loss of sensation in limbs, sudden loss of auditory or visual acuity.

Many manifestations of stress suggest more serious psychiatric and physical health problems. Caregiving stress is chronic, and prolonged stress is associated with greater risks of physical and mental health problems. Caregivers need to have regular contact with their family doctor to monitor their health and adjustment to caregiving. If depression or other mental health disorders are suspected, caregivers should make arrangements to be evaluated by a mental health professional.

Coping Examples

In general, coping involves doing something to change what is stressful, or thinking differently about situations and events. Coping has important functions that support stress management (Pearlin et al., 1989), as discussed below.

Management of the Situation/Events Producing Stress
The following management tools are possibilities: behavior management; use of medications for behavior, psychiatric symptoms, and AD symptoms; prioritizing demands; emotional containment; telling half-truths to prevent agitation; modifying care environments; use of community resources; planning for legal and financial exigencies.

Management of the Meaning of the Situation/Event So That Its Threat Is Reduced
Search for ways to live with a situation that cannot be changed. Consider the following: positive comparisons that show you are better off than others; not contemplating the future but rather living day by day; not holding on to the past; accepting the person as he or she is and not the way you wish he or she could be; restructuring expectations to be more consistent with the behavior that is possible; using humor to dispel grimness; using prayer for divine intervention; being involved in organizations concerned with Alzheimer's.

Management of the Resulting Stress Symptoms
Avoid turning things that can cause long-term problems, for example, drinking alcohol, smoking, or excessive eating. Exercise and get plenty of rest. Find a relaxing hobby.

Problem-focused coping responses involve doing something that changes the situation or event that is stressful, thus diminishing or eliminating the stress. Changing a stressful situation may involve analyzing the problem and taking steps to deal directly with whatever is causing the stress. Not all stressful situations can be changed, however, so other types of coping responses must be used.

Coping Approaches for Different Stressors

Different stressors may call for different approaches. In this section, different approaches will be defined and caregiving examples will be provided. A caregiver may respond to a stressor with one or more of these coping strategies. A combination of coping approaches may be quite useful. In fact, we may use an assortment of approaches to solve the usual stressors that we face on a daily basis. Frequently, we respond to daily stress automatically without being conscious of how we are choosing coping approaches. Family members providing interminable care can face different and unpredictable situations. Stressors may be threatening because they are unfamiliar and a caregiver does not have the automatic, habitual coping response for that situation. Caregivers often face multiple stressors. Their usual patterns of handling stress may not apply to some of these. The nature and duration of caregiving stressors requires caregivers to be much more conscious of how they perceive stressors and how they choose to cope and evaluate if their coping response has effectively relieved their stress. Let's look at the following example.

As usual, a caregiver responds to thoughts about his mother's condition and needs with emotional distancing and avoidance to manage the painful awareness of how much his mother has changed over the past year and the fact that she needs more help than he can give. He has habitually used these approaches to manage stressors relating to her situation. He has done a few things to help her, which has helped him feel better about his involvement, but now he is hearing from her neighbors and friends. They are very concerned about her and her present living arrangements. His own suppressed fears and worries become too powerful to ignore now that others are also concerned. The distress becomes overwhelming. Over the next few days, he reappraises his mother's living situation and realizes that putting off the inevitable is hurting them both. After several hours of tearfulness and a heightened sense of loss, he concludes that he needs to act on his deepest fears. He needs to get his mother some help and company during the day when he is at work. He calls an information and assistance program affiliated with the Area Agency on Aging and begins to develop a list of potential resources. He learns that there are several ways to address her need for supervision, company, and meaningful activity during the day.

This man has used new approaches to cope with different stressors. He has also learned to view the stressors differently. He has acknowledged some facts about his mother's needs and himself. He has confronted some feelings he has tried hard to avoid. More effective coping has enabled him to identify things he can do to provide for the needs of his mother. The goal of successful coping is to utilize whatever responses are most helpful in managing the stressors perceived by caregivers.

Emotion-Focused Coping

When the stressful situation cannot be changed, caregivers might use an emotion-focused approach to coping. This approach helps us readjust our feelings about events that we cannot change so that the distress associated with the event is diminished for a period of time. On a short-term basis, it is important to use this approach to manage stress. We can decide to feel differently or choose not to have undesirable feelings about some unpleasant event. This allows people in a very stressful situation the chance to recoup energy and clear their minds about what to do next.

Managing stress in this way can be harmful when the real source of the stress has not been addressed and dealing with the problem is avoided indefinitely. Caregivers who wish the problem would go away or who avoid the problem have more symptoms of anxiety and depression. The use of emotion-focused strategies does have an important application in coping with the finality of such stressful events as a terminal illness and other interminable conditions. For example, acceptance of what is happening may be the most appropriate coping response to the cognitive decline associated with Alzheimer's disease. When the situation cannot be changed, caregivers may be able to change how they feel about what has already happened (Alzheimer's disease) or is happening (progressive decline of memory).

Examples of Emotion-Focused Coping

1. Denying the stressor for as long as necessary.
2. Using avoidance/escape, such as withdrawing from caregiving for short periods or not thinking about responsibilities and problems.
3. Using wishful thinking, such as wishing that the disease and caregiving pressures would go away.
4. Using distancing as suggested by the idea of not letting the stressor get to you, making light of the situation, or trying to look on the bright side.
5. Using humor, such as learning to play with problems or mistakes, teasing and joking with a relative, responding playfully to one's own behavior, intentionally finding humor in activities of the day.
6. Using stoicism and not letting others know how bad things really are.
7. Using medication and relaxation to acquire the desired emotional and mental states.
8. Using medications to change undesirable stress symptoms such as anxiety, depression, insomnia, fatigue, or tension; using other substances such as alcohol or nicotine.
9. Using social support to deal with a loved one's decline and one's own

emotional distress. Social support is a valuable form of emotional concern that reduces distressing feelings and the sense of being alone.

10. Being constantly vigilant or mentally preoccupied in order to ward off greater anxiety.

11. Using catharsis, which is the expression of feelings in order to reduce emotions such as sadness or anger.

12. Taking attention away from problems by putting one's mind on something else or engaging in other activities.

Cognitive-Focused Coping

Cognitive-focused coping offers another approach to managing caregiver stress. If we view something as a problem, then it has a certain meaning to us. If we can find other ways to think about the situation, the problem can be reframed and viewed differently. The problem is not what is happening but our view of it. Thoughts, belief, self-talk, and appraisals of potential stressors are examples of cognitive tools to prevent or decrease the impact of situations and events. These responses control the meaning of the stressful situation after it occurs but before stress develops.

Some caregiving stress can be reduced if family members view their role in other ways. For example, motivations for assuming the role can affect how caregivers view the activities they perform. For some, this will provide negative meaning to that role and thoughts that generate greater stress; for others, it will provide positive meaning, personal challenge, and a renewed sense of purpose.

Examples of Cognitive-Focused Coping

1. Making meaning occurs when caregivers remind themselves that a relative's behavior is disease related rather than the result of the kind of person he or she is. It is important to appreciate that some behaviors represent the care recipient's effort to cope and adapt.

2. Acceptance occurs when caregivers are able to understand that they are doing all that is possible and are making the most out of the situation, as well as finding meaning from their role.

3. Reframing approaches include taking one day at a time, treating caregiving as a job, making positive comparisons to see how one's own situation is better than another persons, learning to see a situation as humorous instead of sad, and accepting the situation.

4. Positive self-talk/affirmations can bring more positive meaning to the situation and create an ongoing sense of optimism to deal with problems.

5. With positive framing, caregivers focus on the positive aspects of situations and/or minimize the negative features (Gignac and Gottlieb, 1996).

6. With positive reappraisal, caregivers are able to look at their situations differently and find greater meaning because they conclude they have changed, grown as persons, accomplished things they had not believed they could, found new resolve and purpose in life, and gotten inspiration from their experiences.

7. Deeper awareness of the illness experience occurs when caregivers are able to make more sense of their experience through what they have been able to learn about themselves, their capabilities, and the impact others can have on their life.

8. Caregivers can be quite optimistic about their ability to manage caregiving responsibilities in the future.

9. Caregivers can be negative about their capabilities to manage future responsibilities, or fear a suffering fate like their loved one.

10. Finding positive purposes for what they are doing enhances caregivers' personal worth.

11. Reduced expectations help to be realistic. Adjustment to the disease can be viewed in terms of the obstacles loved ones presently face. Their behavior problems might represent attempt to cope with their own stressors.

Relationship-Focused Coping

Relationship-focused coping helps people relate more positively when they are not interacting well. One person boosts the other with empathy, encouragement, and other relationship enhancers. This decreases the negative reactions of the person with Alzheimer's to the caregiver, which in turn reduces the behavior problem that is experienced as stressful. Unfortunately, it is sometimes hard to recognize that our positive responses to loved ones can prevent some stressful situations from ever developing.

It may be easier to recognize how stress develops out of negative interactions. In relationships that have a history of negative interactions, the reaction of the person with Alzheimer's to what she perceives as stressful demands or comments can quickly trigger behaviors that are stressful to caregivers. Having positive alternatives to these reactive patterns in caregiver-care recipient relationships provides a constructive approach to coping with the present and relating in the future. Caregivers who frequently become argumentative or critical toward loved ones need not respond negatively when they appreciate that compromise and active listening serve as important relationship enhancers for care recipients. Relationship-focused coping acknowledges the value and personhood of the person with Alzheimer's who has very strong needs for a comforting connection to another person.

This approach to coping may demand more of the caregiver initially, but positive relating will help establish a positive pattern of interaction over the long term. Behaviors associated with the disease make it more difficult for care recipients to use this coping strategy, but at times they are capable of very meaningful, caring responses.

Let's look at situation that involves the person with AD not driving. Whenever they went somewhere in the car, the caregiver dreaded her husband's insistence that he drive and the problems that always seemed to occur when she tried to explain everything to him. Instead of attempting to explain all the good reasons he could not drive and be faced with anger, resentment, and uncooperativeness, she started responding to his questions about driving with warmth and concern about his feelings. Sympathetically she showed she understood what it must be like to lose the privilege to drive because of a disease. He was caught off guard by her response and accepted her interest in his feelings. A little later, it was possible for them to talk about something they could do together rather than all the reasons one of them could no longer drive. Relationship-focused coping should help reduce the frequency of interpersonal conflict and behavioral problems that increase the potential for stress.

Examples of Relationship-Focused Coping

1. Relationship enhancers include empathy, compromising, giving emotional and cognitive support; avoiding behaviors that are harmful to the relationship and individuals—that is, not confronting or criticizing people with Alzheimer's about errors in judgment or behavioral problems. When continually reminded of their deficits, some persons feel so discouraged that they withdraw further into themselves.

2. Communication skills that compensate for the patient's memory deficits and cognitive impairment such as the following:

   - Speak slowly.
   - Use simpler words and expressions.
   - Repeat and clarify content when the message is not understood.
   - Allow the care recipient to give opinions rather than facts. Facts are easy to forget.
   - Listen intentionally and give the individual enough time to respond.
   - Avoid corrections, which are disruptive. Instead, use a clarifying statement: "Do you mean . . . ? Are you saying . . . ? Do you believe . . . ?
   - Give the person encouraging and positive feedback when he or she is involved in tasks or other shared efforts. If rewarding him for the task or his assistance is not as meaningful, show appreciation for the person.

- Teach the care recipient ways to get you to allow him or her to communicate better; for instance, the person could say, "I need a little more time to find the right word"; "Can you remind me what we were talking about?"

Spiritual-Focused Coping

A person with Alzheimer's who is keeping a journal wrote, "How can I figure all this out when I'm losing the thing that I use to solve problems—my mind?" Spiritual-focused coping helps caregivers and people with Alzheimer's find meaning in their suffering. Spirituality offers a means of growth and a basis for support that may be more easily felt than remembered. It is a way to find acceptance of suffering, loss, and grief. Through spiritual support and relationships we are able to feel connected to life and rediscover what is really important.

Examples of Spiritual-Focused Coping

1. Religion: religious affiliations and related activities such as going to church and being part of that fellowship.
2. Spiritual support: prayers, concerns, and assistance offered as a part of personal contact from others, probably of one's faith.
3. Spiritual resources: Bible and other spiritually oriented books, music, videos, and television programs supportive of religious coping.
4. Pastoral care: guidance, support, counseling, and pastoral care from a pastor or another professional with spiritual and/or biblical orientation.
5. Personal prayer, meditation, and other spiritual practices: to be closer to God, practice one's faith, get in touch with oneself, find answers to suffering and loss that give meaning and comfort to one's own struggles and suffering.

Twelve Steps for Caregivers

Remember these twelve steps from Farran and Keane-Hagerty (1989):

1. I can control how the disease affects me and my relative.
2. I need to take care of myself.
3. I need to simplify my lifestyle.
4. I need to allow others to help me.
5. I need to take one day at a time.
6. I need to structure my day.
7. I need to have a sense of humor.

8. I need to remember that my relative's behavior and emotions are distorted by his or her illness.

9. I need to focus on and enjoy what my relative can still do.

10. I need to depend on other relationships for love and support.

11. I need to remind myself that I am doing the best I can at this very moment.

12. A higher Power is available to me.

15

Exploring Community Resources

Since the early 1980s, Alzheimer's disease has received considerable public attention. The media has given particular emphasis to the impact this illness has on both its victims and their families. Nonetheless, most communities do not have services and care facilities developed specifically for Alzheimer's patients. Nor do they provide the long-term needs of Alzheimer's patients. Nor do they provide support services for the family; for example, not all communities have sufficient day and respite programs which address the needs of both patient and caregiver. However, most communities do have agencies that provide for the various long-term care needs of the elderly, and these agencies often provide support and service to Alzheimer's patients and caregivers.

Drawing upon Community Resources
Reduces Strain on the Caregiver

This book stresses the importance of calling upon community resources. In this chapter, the creative and appropriate use of these resources is discussed in more detail. Such resources can allow the family to care for the person with Alzheimer's at home without a severely restrictive quality of life. The caregiver has been described as the hidden victim of this illness, and his needs cannot be ignored. But the physical and mental strain placed on the caregiver can be significantly reduced if both family and community resources are sufficiently utilized.

224

Before the Need Becomes Critical

Family members may feel at first that they prefer to manage alone. But community resources become more important as the primary caregiver grows more isolated and fatigued. Interest in exploring other resources naturally develops as the caregiver begins to wonder how much longer he can continue in the caregiver role. A need for outside help will also surface as the patient's deterioration produces greater difficulties in management and self-care. It is therefore advisable that families explore the resources available in their communities in the early stages of the disease so that they are prepared when the eventual need for more help arises. Families equipped with facts about what lies ahead find it easier to anticipate and plan for the future.

The first step in utilizing community resources is identifying what resources exist. The following are some good places to begin when searching for the resources in your community:

- *Health Professionals.*   Family physicians, psychiatrists, mental health professionals, social workers, and others already involved with the Alzheimer's patient are a natural starting point. Ask them for referrals and resource suggestions to address the needs and problems at hand.

- *Community Mental Health Centers.*   Mental health centers that have services for the elderly or offer more specialized Alzheimer's care can be a valuable information resource. These agencies can work with the person who has Alzheimer's and his or her family or spouse. After determining the types of resources needed, the agency can link families with the services that exist in the community.

- *Area Agencies on Aging.*   These agencies are involved in developing community resources supportive of the needs of the aging population. Persons with Alzheimer's represent a special part of this population, and area agencies on aging are likely to be knowledgeable about local resources that will support Alzheimer's care.

- *Medical Information and Referral Programs.*   These programs exist to aid persons seeking information about and help with medical conditions of all kinds. They may be attached to a governmental agency, a care facility, or a program for the elderly. To locate such a program in your community, contact a medical facility or the Agency on Aging.

- *Alzheimer's Resource and Information Centers.*   More recently, some communities have developed programs that specifically address the resource and informational needs of the Alzheimer's patient and family. Such programs may survey individual needs and help caregivers manage their situations.

They also may refer the family to other community social service or mental health programs developed for the aged or persons with Alzheimer's.

- *Alzheimer's Family Support Groups.* These groups provide important information about more formal local resources that support the care of the Alzheimer's patient. Such groups also may provide information about individuals who can be hired to stay with the person in the home and help with personal care and supervision.

Developing Goals for Caregiving

Once the family knows the full range of resources available, members can choose the ones most helpful in their situation. In determining how to use resources, the family may wish to reflect on the goals of caregiving. Often, the overall goal of caregiving is to keep the relative in the familiar surroundings of his home. However, refining this goal can provide caregivers with more definite guidelines for selecting community resources. They should draw upon those that can help them to:

1. *Maintain the patient's social and self-care abilities at the highest possible level.* Premature dependencies place an excessive strain on the family caregiver. To maintain the person's abilities, an appropriate degree of social activity and stimulation is needed, which the family cannot always provide.

2. *Support the patient's adjustment to the gradual losses and limitations associated with the illness.* Persons with Alzheimer's can benefit from supportive counseling, particularly in the disease's earlier stages, and they can appreciate emotional support for their adjustment throughout. Opportunities for the patient to continue in familiar activities with some degree of success are needed. These successes help support the patient's self-esteem and offset other losses that occur.

3. *Support the family's adjustment to the degenerative process of the disease and the stresses of care.* Family members may need supportive counseling to come to grips with the illness and to learn to work supportively with one another. The ongoing activity of caregiving must be supported to avoid the emotional and physical breakdown associated with stress.

4. *Maintain the safest and most supportive environment.* Basic needs must be provided for, and the person must be safe from danger, neglect, abuse, or exploitation. These concerns particularly apply to persons who live alone.

5. *Provide relief from the constant responsibility of caregiving.* Relief from constant supervision of the person, for example, may be possible when a nurse aide assists a few hours a day with personal care and housekeeping. Caregivers can use outside resources to care for their relative, providing opportunities to take care of their own needs.

Guidelines for Using Resources

Community resources are meant to support, not replace, family involvement. In relying on community services, family members should follow these guidelines:

- Ask questions to clarify their understanding of the situation.
- Express their own needs and concerns.
- Use contact with one community resource as an opportunity to learn about other resources that might be helpful.
- Seek information provided from community resources and professionals when making difficult decisions.

Some community resources that are helpful in caring for Alzheimer's are discussed in the following section. The Service/Resource Worksheet has been included in Appendix A for caregivers to use in comparing and selecting resources.

Community Resources for Alzheimer's Care

1. *Alzheimer's Family Support Groups.*   These groups provide caregivers with support in coping with the illness and in dealing with problems experienced in caregiving. Self-support groups also can be a source of information about the disease and community resources. Participants experience similar problems and assist each other in making decisions about care. The emotional adjustment of the family to the illness is promoted by such groups.

2. *Respite Care.*   This type of service provides family members with occasional relief from the pressures of continuous caregiving. Such relief can prevent premature institutionalization of the patient as a result of the caregiver's physical and emotional stress. Formal respite programs offer services ranging from several hours to several weeks' relief.

   Respite care also occurs when families hire persons to relieve them from duties in the home. Some families are able to take turns caregiving. In other situations, respite comes as a secondary benefit of medical or psychiatric hospitalizations.

3. *Shared Respite Care.*   A number of families with Alzheimer's relatives may join together to provide caregiving on a rotating basis. Typically, several family members watch over a group of patients to allow others to have some free time. Benefits are experienced as the Alzheimer's patient and spouse participate with other patients and their families in an activity setting outside the household. By caring for their loved one in company with

others, caregivers find that social isolation is reduced. The burden of providing activities becomes an opportunity that is shared by participants.

4. *Adult Day Care.*   Some day programs are designed specifically for persons with Alzheimer's. Others provide structured activities to a more heterogeneous group of impaired older persons or other age groups. Day care provides exercise, activities, recreation, support of daily living skills, counseling, and monitoring of the participant's general health. Such programs can help the person with Alzheimer's maintain some abilities that would otherwise deteriorate more quickly. Some provide more specialized social work, nursing, or physical and occupational therapy services. By utilizing adult day care, family members can remain employed, do errands, rest, and have a social life.

5. *Home Health Care.*   Home health programs usually can provide nursing and personal care services to patients in their homes. For persons with Alzheimer's disease, nursing care is usually not needed until the later stages of the illness, unless other coexisting medical problems exist. But supervision and personal care are very important needs of the Alzheimer's patient. Many home health programs have nurse aids, homemakers, or care providers that can assist with these needs. Self-employed persons also can be hired to provide supervision and assist with personal care needs. Persons with Alzheimer's will definitely need this type of care when they live alone and have no family who live nearby. Home health personnel can help with a broad array of supervisory and direct care needs such as meals and shopping, medications, cleaning and washing, transportation, appraisal of the person's condition, and companionship.

6. *Legal Services.*   Often family members must consider questions such as the person's ability to handle finances and make decisions for himself. Protection of the person and property must be considered, but not at the expense of his other rights and privileges. Alzheimer's disease does not automatically make a person incompetent. When some form of legal guardianship is being considered, the opinion of the treating physician, a psychiatrist, or other mental health professional should be solicited prior to legal consultation.

7. *Community Mental Health Centers.*   Some community mental health centers have specialized geriatric programs that can be very helpful in the management of the Alzheimer's client and supportive of the family caregiver. These programs can provide a wide range of services, including comprehensive assessment, psychiatric evaluations, individual, group, and family counseling. Additionally, case management services identify other com-

munity resources that can help with home maintenance. Referrals can be made and service linkages developed.

Some persons with Alzheimer's disease may present serious behavior management problems. Even when such problems are not apparent, however, the caregiver may find mental health centers helpful in planning care.

Mental health intervention may help in cases of an especially lengthy period of caregiving, a patient with difficult personality traits, a difficult living environment, or other large-scale problems. Among the specific behaviors that indicate a need for immediate attention are the following:

- Hallucinations and delusions that contribute to sleeping disturbances, agitated and combative behavior, or disruptive interactions with neighbors and community
- Severe confusion and disorientation
- Physically threatening behavior
- Harmful resistance to necessary care and management
- Potentially dangerous activities such as wandering, driving, and so forth that the family cannot stop
- Depressive symptoms early in the course of the illness
- Anxiety, agitation, or denial so extreme that they make care management difficult

Needs that can be addressed by a mental health center's case management services include:

- Severe lack of family support
- High level of caregiver stress
- An inadequate caregiving situation, such as that of a person who lives alone

8. *Psychiatric Hospitals.*   Private psychiatric hospitals offer assessment and behavior stabilization. They may be the best resort in cases of unmanageable behavior. The hospital staff can often assist the family with care planning and management.

Considerations for Nursing Home Care

Reevaluating Appropriateness of In-Home Care

Families can use other resources to maintain the loved one in the home. However, conditions may develop that require family members to reexamine the appropriateness of in-home care. Usually these conditions are beyond one's control. Professionals can assist families in deciding whether to place the person with Alzheimer's disease in a nursing home. The following questions should be considered:

1. Can the total needs of the loved one be adequately provided for on a 24-hour basis in the home?

2. Has the health status of the individual changed so that more nursing care and medical monitoring are necessary?

3. Is the stamina of the caregiver severely taxed by the care situation in the home?

4. If the person lives alone, is there adequate supervision and assistance available to provide for his needs on an ongoing basis?

5. Is it realistic to expect the family to deliver or purchase the services the relative now needs in the home?

6. Are the financial resources of the spouse becoming severely threatened?

7. Do health concerns for the caregiver begin to rival those for the Alzheimer's patient?

8. Has the caregiver's isolation become severe?

9. Is the in-home care contributing to the emotional/physical breakdown of the caregiver/spouse?

10. Is the nursing home placement as unacceptable as it first seemed?

11. Will the quality of contact with the person with Alzheimer's improve by placement in a nursing home?

12. Will the family be able to pull closer together around the nursing home placement?

13. Have physicians and other professionals recommended such a placement?

14. Have the caregiver's approaches to daily problems become ineffective?

Dementia Is Common in Nursing Homes.

Nursing homes are becoming more aware of the needs of the Alzheimer's patient and the family. Nursing homes have been dealing with this illness disguised by other names for a very long time, and a high percentage of the persons in nursing homes have some form of dementia or cognitive impairment.

Special Services

Some nursing homes have developed Alzheimer's units to more adequately address the total care needs of these individuals, and others are considering such approaches. Special Alzheimer's programs can provide a more meaningful role for family members. However, families must determine whether such units actually provide specialized services rather than just grouping the patients together.

When choosing a nursing home for a relative with Alzheimer's disease, families should consider these factors:

1. Is the staff physician familiar with Alzheimer's?
2. Are staff at all levels of the nursing home aware of the needs and problems associated with this disease (e.g., administrative, nursing, dietary, and activities staff)?
3. How do staff interact with residents who are similarly impaired?
4. What activities are provided for persons with Alzheimer's and other dementias?
5. Is the physical plan of the facility well organized, attractive, and designed to encourage either socialization or privacy as appropriate?
6. Does the facility encourage family involvement and support groups?
7. Is the atmosphere friendly?
8. What provisions are made to prevent wandering?
9. Is the building particularly noisy?
10. Is there a safe area for the person to walk outside?
11. How does the facility deal with residents who are noisy and hard to manage?
12. How are drugs and restraints used in behavior management?
13. Is the facility a reasonable distance from your home?
14. Do Alzheimer's units utilize a special approach to needs of these residents?

Some families may realize that a nursing home may be the most appropriate resource for the care of their relatives with Alzheimer's disease. Still, they may have built barriers to seeking the placement. Some concerns are practical, others psychological. The following example illustrates some psychological barriers that should be overcome.

Suzy was the middle-aged daughter of a 75-year-old man who had Alzheimer's disease. Suzy was the primary caregiver because her two brothers lived out of town. Her relationship with her father had not been particularly close. However, she shouldered the responsibility for his care, partly because she felt guilty about her past with her family. She had been divorced for 10 years, and during that time she had assumed a major role in caring for her parents. She still believed her brothers should help more, but their explanations for not being more involved were generally reasonable. They did help some-what with financial needs. Her mother had died a year before in a nursing home. Now her father was living with her.

The mother had a strong role in caring for Suzy's father until she had suffered a stroke, which eventually precipitated her placement in the nursing home. At that time, the father had objected to his wife's leaving. Suzy thought he had been angry with her since that time; certainly he was more agitated. Suzy had visited her mother in the nursing home, taking her father along. These visits had often upset her father. He would accuse her of trying to put him away.

Now the father required more care and supervision. Suzy still felt some guilt about the past, but she experienced new feelings of guilt about her mother's placement and how she thought it had affected her father. She was experiencing more guilt in caring for her father. It was painful to Suzy when he asked for his wife or called Suzy by his wife's name. One night he talked frequently about going home. Suzy did her best to assure him he was home, but in his state of agitation he would not listen. Later that night he wandered from the house.

Suzy's father was not found until the early morning hours by the police, who took him to a hospital emergency room. Suzy was awakened by a call after her name and number were found in his billfold. Her dad was so confused and agitated that he had to be placed in a psychiatric hospital for a few days.

The father responded well to that setting, yet it appeared to the hospital staff that he needed more care than Suzy could provide at home. Nursing home placement was recommended, but Suzy insisted that she must care for him at home. For a while, her position seemed unreasonable to staff until the past and current sources of guilt were uncovered. Suzy actually believed she could provide better care in her home, particularly now that her dad was more stable.

Hospital staff agreed to support this decision if Suzy would get help from some community services to help her manage her father and deal with her needs. Counseling eventually helped Suzy to accept her limitations in caring for her father. She finally reconciled her feelings of guilt to the extent that she was willing to look at some other nursing homes. She had gotten involved in an Alzheimer's family support group whose members helped her look at some facilities better equipped to care for Alzheimer's patients and to involve family members in constructive ways. Suzy also involved her brothers in the decision, so she did not have to feel it was her decision alone.

Three months later, the placement was made. After a month, Suzy was confident they had made the right decision when she saw her father doing a little better than he had at home. She became involved in some of the nursing home's activities and maintained a modified caregiving role with her father. She began to have a life of her own again.

Finances

Financial arrangements can be a practical barrier to nursing home placements even when families desire placement. Public assistance programs for nursing homes, such as Medicaid, have financial requirements that must be fulfilled before the cost is covered by a mixture of state and federal funding. Family members should investigate this resource long before their relative needs nursing home care. Too often, nursing home placement is sought in a crisis. A hospital may be about to discharge the person, or the caregiver may either have become too ill or too overwhelmed to continue to provide care himself.

In many states—Texas for one—there are two types of eligibility that must be met before nursing home placement can be covered by state and federal financial resources: financial and medical. This can be confusing to families. Not only are there two types of eligibility, but there are also two different state departments that approve the two types of eligibility. Since Alzheimer's disease is not yet uniformly considered a medical condition, there may be problems in getting medical eligibility established. The deficits in the person's functioning must be almost overemphasized for the person to qualify as having medical and nursing care needs. The treating physician may not be familiar with all aspects of daily functioning and mental status. (Forms in Appendix A should be helpful in establishing the degree of impairment.)

Families may need to elicit help from attorneys and other agencies in establishing financial and medical eligibility. Private pay does not require such planning, but many people with Alzheimer's disease cannot afford private pay at all. Contact with nursing homes may help families seeking nursing home placement if they start making their plans early. Agencies involved in establishing eligibility should be contacted to determine what information is required. Steps in that process should be fully understood by families. As a rule, if families are familiar with eligibility requirements and the process involved in nursing home care, the eventual placement will take place more smoothly. Early planning also enables family members, particularly the spouse who remains at home, a chance to plan for financial security.

Some patients with Alzheimer's disease may be eligible for other long-term care services, such as placement at a Veteran's Administration (VA) hospital or nursing home care unit. This too should be investigated so that family expectations can be based on facts and not assumptions. The placement may not be possible because the veteran does not meet eligibility requirements. Others who meet requirements may not stay in the VA system for long-term care. The VA also contracts with community nursing homes for placement.

Final Resource Considerations

Family members caring for a relative with Alzheimer's disease usually have more resources and services available to them than they utilize. Long-term care in the home is possible. In some cases, care can be provided in the home until the relative's death. Planning care will involve the need for strategic utilization of community resources, other family members, and friends. Services for Alzheimer's care vary from one community to the next. Rural areas and small towns usually have fewer services than urban areas.

Costs for services also vary. Some have state, federal, and local funding. Others are funded by foundations and other grant sources. Still others are private and require full payment unless other arrangements can be made. Insurance may cover some services, but at this point family members should not assume too much about insurance coverage. They should investigate what types of care and services insurance will cover and for how long. Some families face a difficult predicament when they assume insurance covers nursing home care. Although policies may cover some nursing home care, long-term care is not usually covered. Long-term care policies with more nursing home coverage are quite expensive and frequently do not cover Alzheimer's disease.

Few communities have sufficient and affordable resources for Alzheimer's care, particularly day care alternatives and respite care services. Other services may be unavailable or simply inadequate to meet the ongoing needs of in-home care. Many provider-type programs that supply in-home services such as cleaning and personal care cannot accept responsibility for supervision. The hours a week that such services can be provided are often limited. In-home supervision is, nevertheless, a major need. On a short-term basis, in-home respite care or a brief respite placement can be beneficial.

Persons living alone and suspected of having an Alzheimer's-type condition are quite difficult to help when family is absent or nonexistent. In these cases, some type of guardianship or protective services may be necessary to provide care. Mental health authorities may be able to help if these persons reach a point where they are a danger to themselves or others. Adult Protective Services may have to be contacted. However, there may be no long-range solutions.

Family caregivers are a source of ideas for what services are needed in their communities. In fact, families feel less helpless in these situations when they find a way to bring needs to the attention of agencies and others who develop program in the community. One of the better options is to contact an Area Agency on Aging, which is charged with the responsibility of identifying needs of the elderly, planning for those needs, implementing and monitoring programs funded under the Older Americans Act. (See the list of these agencies in Appendix B.) There may also be other community agencies active in planning and program development. The Area Agency on Aging may be able to direct caregivers to these other resources in the community.

Enigma

Isn't it strange . . .
That which we have long perceived
as a burden—
the care of a sick loved one—
the care that went on
and on and on—is over now?

It was tiring, and confining,
and discouraging and demeaning at times.
Yet—in a strange way—
I can feel no relief.

Perhaps, inadvertently,
he gave my life a purpose—
a purpose I hardly recognized
nor appreciated.

Now I need a new purpose
(and I am old for that).
That covenant has been kept
as best I knew how—
But my life goes on.

Help me to find a new purpose—
a new resolve—
and let it be a life that doesn't
just keep on living.

Maude S. Newton

PART II

Research and Treatment

In this part of the book, we deal with the more technical aspects of Alzheimer's disease, first describing the physiology of the brain and the changes that take place, then discussing treatment possibilities, keeping in mind that developments are happening daily. Finally, we describe medications typically used and possible side effects.

Survivors

For years I've watched
an old mesquite tree—
gnarled and bent and twisted—
buffeted by winds and droughts.

It starts to grow up
toward the sun and sky.
But the soil is so poor,
the water so scarce,
the heat so fierce,
so cold at times,
it was beat to the ground.

Each Winter you'd think,
—it's dead, for sure!
It's succumbed to the odds
stacked against it.

Yet wait 'til the Spring
and a miracle occurs,
New life springs up
from the gnarled old branches—
a tiny chartreuse sprout
heads straight for the sun!
It lives—overcoming
all that is hard,
telling all the world,
—I live, I will survive!

Sometimes I feel like that old mesquite tree
I feel battered by life's adversities,
I feel down—but not out!
When Spring rolls around,
I feel a fresh stirring of life.

I have things to do—
places I want to explore,
people I love!
I can hold my head high—
look the world in the eye—
and say,
—I live, I will survive!

Maude S. Newton

16

Abnormal Changes
in the Brain

For hundreds of years, the symptoms of what we now know as Alzheimer's disease were attributed to senility and old age, or perhaps in more recent times they were attributed to hardening of the arteries and psychosis. In the past, people feared that one day, just because they were old, they would "go crazy," lose their memory, and become completely helpless without ever knowing why. With the identification of Alzheimer's disease, however, it has become possible to properly diagnose persons suffering from this illness and to at least partially alleviate their suffering. The next step, at which medical researchers currently are at work, is to isolate the exact biological causes of the disease. Once these causes are known, we can begin to develop effective treatments for Alzheimer's and perhaps someday find a complete cure.

The next two chapters of this book offer a look at the research done to date on both the causes and treatment of Alzheimer's. This research has revealed physical and chemical changes present in brains affected by Alzheimer's, suggested possible causes of the disease, and included experiments with promising treatments.

Because the research leaves many questions unanswered, most of the material covered here must remain somewhat speculative. Although a great deal has been learned to date, no definitive answer to the mysteries posed by Alzheimer's disease has been found. The research findings are valuable, however, because they allow caregivers to understand more fully the changes occurring within the Alzheimer's patient. In addition, the very real progress gives hope that medical research will lead us to a clear-cut strategy for the disease's treatment and prevention.

The final chapter covers the use of current medications used in treating some of the psychiatric manifestations of Alzheimer's disease. Agitation, anxiety, delusions, and sleeping difficulties present behavior management problems to family caregivers. Careful use of psychiatric medications can make caregiving much easier.

Physical Changes in the Brain

Abnormality in the Brain

When a person is diagnosed as having Alzheimer's disease, the brain has already deteriorated to some degree. Almost without exception, physical abnormalities (such as neurofibrillary tangles, neuritic plaques, and others) are present in the cerebral cortex, the outer layer of the brain that governs such higher functions as memory, thinking, and reasoning.

Several of the abnormal characteristics of brains affected by Alzheimer's disease are associated with the most basic and important part of the brain, the neurons (also called nerve cells). The brain consists of many billions of neurons, which are its means of receiving and sending messages. Neurons can be viewed as the way different parts of the brain communicate with each other and the rest of the body. One neuron of the brain may communicate with as many as 1,000 other neurons, although these units of communication usually send messages to only a few neurons. Alzheimer's disease is somehow responsible for a loss of neurons. Some of the physical abnormalities, for example, neurofibrillary tangles, occur in the body of neurons. These changes might contribute to destruction of nerve cells or compromise their functioning.

Connection between Disease and Abnormalities

Because the tangles, plaques, and other physical abnormalities so consistently accompany the disease, researchers feel certain that some connection exists between these brain abnormalities and the mental and emotional changes that Alzheimer's patients experience. It is not well known whether these physical changes are directly related to the cause of Alzheimer's disease or whether other aspects of the disease itself cause the abnormalities. In the latter, the physical changes would be manifestations of the illness. These are questions future research will continue to address.

Connections between Abnormalities and Impairments

We do know that a direct correlation exists between the degree and the distribution of physical abnormalities and the severity of Alzheimer's-type dementia. We also know that the abnormalities discussed in this chapter tend to be concentrated in areas of the brain that control abilities most affected by Alzheimer's. These findings suggest that physical changes in the brain make some contribution to the disease's impairments.

Anatomy of the Brain

To understand how Alzheimer's affects the brain, we first must understand the basics of brain anatomy and the ways in which various areas of the brain are related to specific mental functions.

Brain's Cortex

The outer surface of the brain is known as the cerebral cortex (see Figure 1). Accounting for about 80 percent of total brain mass, the cortex is divided into two nearly symmetrical hemispheres: the left and the right. Each of these hemispheres is divided in turn into four lobes: the frontal, the parietal, the occipital, and the temporal.

Frontal Lobes

The frontal lobes mediate motor functions, govern emotional behavior, help organize sequential physical movements, determine some abilities of expressive speech, and influence personalities, inhibitions, and social behavior. As Alzheimer's disease affects this area of the brain, patients undergo a variety of personality changes, lose inhibitions, and become less able to organize behavior. With damage to the frontal lobes of the brain, persons do not recognize their errors.

Parietal Lobes

The parietal lobes are concerned with sensory functions such as physical sensations, touch, and spatial relationships. They also allow us to recognize patterns in our experience, perform intellectual tasks such as mathematics, and

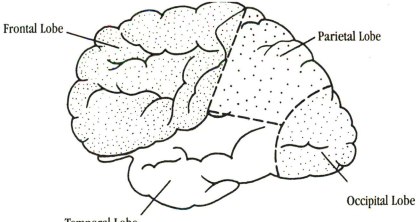

FIGURE 1. The Cerebral Cortex.   The lobes of the brain's cortex. The frontal lobe is at the front of the head. This is a side view of the left hemisphere. The right hemisphere is basically a mirror reflection of the left hemisphere.

maintain our physical orientation. Disorientation to places can result from damage to this brain area. When Alzheimer's strikes the parietal lobes, patients experience trouble with coordinated, purposeful movements, spatial perceptions, and recognition, among other functions.

Occipital Lobes

The occipital lobes are the brain's visual center, controlling very basic visual perceptions and bringing together the parts of visual information into a meaningful whole. Damage to this area can lead to loss of the visual field and problems in space perception.

Temporal Lobes

The temporal lobes are involved in a range of important functions, including hearing, memory, vision, and verbal comprehension. In conjunction with the brain's limbic system, these lobes also affect the experience and memory of emotions such as fear, jealousy, anger, or happiness. Our sense of time and individuality also seems to be located in these lobes (Restak, 1984). Of the four brain areas, the temporal lobes appear to be the area most severely affected by Alzheimer's disease. Memory problems, auditory perception, musical perception, difficulties in comprehension, and difficulties in execution of speech all appear to be connected with damage in this area. Problems in focused attention also can be attributed to damage in the temporal lobes.

The Limbic System of the Brain

Enveloped by the cortex are a number of other brain areas relevant to an understanding of Alzheimer's disease. Some of these are part of the limbic system, a group of brain structures that influence our emotions and behavior. The parts of the limbic system most involved in the damage associated with Alzheimer's disease include the amygdala, believed to affect emotion, and the hippocampus, believed to affect both short-term and long-term memory (see Figure 2).

The importance of the parts of the brain just described will become clear as we further explore the physical changes that Alzheimer's brings. The reader should note that the temporal, parietal, and frontal lobes of the cortex are more affected by physical changes. The hippocampus seems to be a prime target for physical abnormalities.

Neurofibrillary Tangles

Among the symptoms of the disease identified by Alois Alzheimer in his original diagnosis in the early 1900s was the presence in the brain of neurofibrillary tangles (see Figure 3). Simply put, neurofibrillary tangles are bundles of ordinary brain filaments that have become badly twisted. When such tangles

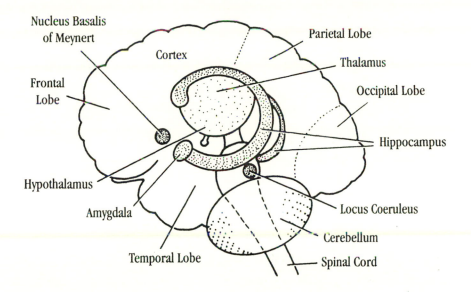

FIGURE 2. Brain Areas Affected by Alzheimer's Disease.   This picture of the brain shows areas impacted by Alzheimer's disease abnormalities. The location of the nucleus basalis of Meynert is an approximation. Other parts of the brain have been omitted because they are not relevant to our discussion. Some parts of the limbic system—the hippocampus, amydala, thalamus, and hypothalamus—are indicated.

are viewed under an electron microscope, little hairlike structures called filaments can be seen. When these filaments occur in pairs, they are wrapped around each other in a spiral fashion (Reisberg, 1981), somewhat like two pieces of yarn that have been twisted together and then stretched tightly. They are known as paired helical filaments, a term sometimes used to refer to neurofibrillary tangles. Filaments are normal; they become abnormal when their form is changed by twisting.

Interestingly, some degree of neurofibrillary tangle formation is found in virtually all examined brain tissue of persons over age 90 (Reisberg, 1981). Tangles also are found in specific brain areas of most normal middle-aged and older persons. When their brain tissue is examined microscopically, tangle formations are particularly evident in the hippocampus, the area that plays a role in both recent memory functions and the storage and retrieval of long-term memory (Beaumont, 1983). It has some involvement in learning. The hippocampus further seems to be involved in bringing together various forms of incoming sensory information (Bloom et al., 1985), the inhibition of responses, the organization of movement, and spatial organization (Kolb and Whishaw, 1980). Another area where concentrations of tangles are found is

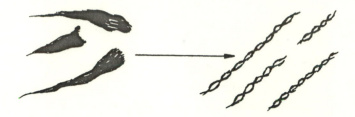

FIGURE 3. Neurofibrillary Tangles and Paired Helical Filaments. If the image of tangles to the left were enlarged, lines would take the appearance of the paired helical filaments to the right.

the amygdala, which has a role in fear reactions and aggressive behavior. It is also suspected of having some role in memory with the hippocampus. The reader will recall that both of these structures are part of the brain's limbic system, which has a major role in expression and experience of emotion (Kolb and Whishaw, 1980).

Since aging persons tend to exhibit a high incidence of tangles in brain areas associated with memory as well as memory problems, it seems possible that the development of slight short-term memory loss with age could be associated with subtle damage to the hippocampus. It further follows that the more severe memory disorders of Alzheimer's patients as well as related problems might be associated with more severe hippocampal damage. Similarly, the lack of emotional response to memory problems found early in Alzheimer's, sometimes called a blunted or flat effect, could be associated with damage to the amygdala, while damage to the overall limbic system could account for patients' loss of emotional control. Altogether, the damage caused by tangles to these parts of the brain could be responsible for some of the emotional disturbances and personality changes exhibited by persons with Alzheimer's.

Because tangles appear to occur naturally with age, the mere presence of tangles in the brain does not indicate disease. What is different about the brains of Alzheimer's patients, however, is the location and number of tangles. In these people, tangles tend to be significantly concentrated in the hippocampus and in far higher numbers than in the brains of normal aging persons. They also are concentrated in the cerebral cortex, particularly in the parietal-temporal region and the association cortex. The association areas of the cortex bring together information from the areas around which they are located. It is in these areas that the brain integrates immediate sensory information with memories and emotions, thus making it possible for us to think, decide, and plan behavior. Since such integrated thought typically becomes difficult for Alzheimer's patients, the damage observed in the association cortex seems particularly significant.

Other small but important areas of the brain are affected by neurofibrillary tangles. These small areas represent collections of nerve cells that serve as stimulation centers for neurons ascending into the brain's cortex. Neurons or brain cells of the brain comprise an intricate network through which information can be transmitted and received.

Groups of neurons within the brain's network are specifically adapted to communicate with their own chemical messenger, which is called a neurotransmitter. These special networks of neurotransmitters, specific nerve cells, each receive stimulation from their own collection of nerve cells deeper in the brain. For example, for the neurotransmitter acetylcholine, which is deficient in the Alzheimer's brain, the source of stimulation is called the nucleus basalis of Meynert (see Figure 2). This brain area has a significant concentration of tangles.

Tangles are also found in the localized areas of the brain that act as stimulation centers for neurons using the neurotransmitters norepinephrine, serotonin, and dopamine (Bondareff, 1986). Chemical changes in the brain are discussed later in this chapter.

The correlations discovered make it likely that tangles are directly linked to the impairment of brain function, though research has not yet uncovered precisely what that link might be. Some research suggests that tangles may have some role in neuronal deterioration and destruction. The loss of neurons may also be secondary to other unknown aspects of the disease process. Other research has shown that the larger the number of tangles found, along with another abnormality known as senile plaques, the higher is the degree of dementia observed in people with Alzheimer's.

Researchers have long thought that the composition of the tangles and paired helical filaments might reveal important information about what causes Alzheimer's and causes the loss of neurons. Recent findings indicate that the loss of neurons and the formation of tangles progress together. The twisted threads inside nerve cells that make up neurofibrillary tangles are comprised of a hyperphosphorylated form of a normal protein called *tau*. Normal *tau* proteins are important to the central nervous system because they help bind and stabilize microtubules, which are a part of the internal support structure of cells. Microtubules might be pictured as railroad tracks in healthy neurons that allow nutrients and molecules to pass from the cell body to the ends of its axon. An axon is a long, thin structure that extends out from the body of a cell to allow connections with other neurons. In Alzheimer's disease, normal *tau* is chemically changed, and this altered form can no longer hold together the track-like support structure of microtubules. As a result of this chemical alteration, microtubules collapse. This breakdown in the transport system of neurons may significantly disrupt communication between nerve cells and eventually lead to the death of the neurons.

Stabilization and support of the structure of microtubules may not be the only role that *tau* plays in brain function. For example, *tau* may be involved in cell growth. Much more research is required to completely understand this very complex protein and how it is regulated in the brain of persons with AD as well as in the normal brain.

Considerable research has focused on the role of amyloids. For example, a vaccine designed to counter the deposition of beta-amyloid and reduce that already present in the Alzheimer's brain has shown successful results in genetically engineered AD mice. Recently, reports show that the vaccine can have positive effects on behavior and cognitive function as well as brain chemistry. There is an area on chromosome 10 associated with amyloid plaques where researchers believe that a gene that may be associated with Alzheimer's disease is located. Although amyloid appears to have more backing than *tau* as having an instrumental role in the disease, research has not proven whether amyloid plaques are the cause of the disease or some by-product of the disease progression.

Tau appears to be the marker of the severity of the disease. The percentage of neurons with neurofibrillary tangles increases with the severity of the disease. Does this mean that they are more involved in causing the deterioration? Or are they an indication that *tau* is a by-product of the disease? With amyloid having a strong presence in the disease, one would expect it to increase in the same way as *tau*, but this is not the case. In fact, the amount of beta-amyloid in the Alzheimer's brain remains relatively constant over the disease course.

Other Dementing Illnesses

Neurofibrillary tangles also have been found in other types of dementing illnesses. Among these are dementia pugilistica (punch-drunkenness), a dementia observed in veteran boxers; the rare Parkinsonian dementia complex of Guam (Reisberg, 1981); postencephalitic Parkinson's disease (Bondareff, 1986); and other forms of infectious dementias. Another disorder in which tangles are very frequently present is Down's syndrome, the genetic abnormality that causes mental retardation. Persons with Down's syndrome who live past age 40 invariably develop tangles, plaques, and other pathological changes common to Alzheimer's disease (Katzman, 1986), and the tangles are similarly located in the brain (Reisberg, 1981).

Fronto-temporal dementia with Parkinsonism has been linked to *tau* gene mutations on chromosome 17. Numerous neurological diseases have prominent *tau* pathologies. The presence of *tau* within the cells may be enough to induce the onset, or progression, of Pick's disease, progressive supranuclear palsy, AD, and other neurodegenerative diseases found to have prominent *tau* pathology.

Senile or Neuritic Plaques

Significance of Plaques

Like neurofibrillary tangles, plaques were among the physical abnormalities noticed by Alois Alzheimer in his original diagnosis of the disease. As with tangles, plaques are found in the brains of normal aged persons; however, they appear in far more significant concentrations in the brains of persons with Alzheimer's, appear in those parts of the brain that are most affected by the disease, and are most prevalent in the most severely affected individuals. In fact, plaques appear to be an even better indicator of the degree of dementia than do neurofibrillary tangles.

Types of Plaques and Description

There are three types of plaques: primitive, classical, and amyloid. Classical and amyloid plaques both contain more amyloid. All types of plaques can be found in Alzheimer's disease. In classical plaques the amyloid is contained by the core; amyloid plaques consist almost entirely of this material (Wisniewski, 1983). The classical plaque is easier to picture (see Figure 4). There is the central core of amyloid that appears fuzzy and fibrous. This core is surrounded by a ring of degenerating fragments of cells that resemble a loosely arranged crown of thorns. The fragments are like the debris of brain cells and include axons, dendrites, and slender filaments. Paired helical filaments of neurofibrillary tangles can be found in the debris around the classical plaque's core. Neuritic or senile plaques are the more general terms used for the three types of plaques.

Plaques are found outside neurons, whereas neurofibrillary tangles are found in neurons. In Alzheimer's disease, plaques are abnormal, particularly

FIGURE 4. **Classical Neuritic Plaque.**   The primitive plaque consists mainly of the clustered debris outside the core of this plaque. Amyloid plaques consist of the core material of the plaque.

because they occur more frequently than in the brains of normal aged persons. Plaques also occur in other diseases of the brain.

Locations of Plaques

As with tangles, plaques tend to be more abundant in the cerebral cortex and are found in smaller numbers in other parts of the brain such as the thalamus. Rarely, they have been found in the cerebellum (Bondareff, 1986). The thalamus receives sensory information and has some control of our motor activity. It helps us be generally aware of touch, temperature, and pain. The cerebellum primarily coordinates muscular activity and receives information from other parts of the body such as skin, muscles, and joints.

Some indication of damage to the thalamus may be observed during the course of Alzheimer's disease. Damage associated with the cerebellum would be more difficult to observe until perhaps the later stages of the illness. Functions assigned to the hippocampus and cortex are more easily recognized and more severely disturbed. Memory impairment and disturbances in thinking, judgment, and speech are common features of Alzheimer's disease.

Amyloid and Plaques

With regard to this disease, the significance of plaques rests not only on their concentration in areas of the brain that are most impaired, but the presence of amyloid is also important. Amyloid is a part of the plaques, and research has shown enduring interest in amyloid because it is thought that understanding this abnormal protein might yield clues to Alzheimer's cause.

Amyloid and Disease

Amyloid has been associated with a variety of diseases that include tuberculosis, Hodgkin's disease, and cancer. Such severe neurological illnesses as Creutzfeldt-Jakob disease and kuru are associated with accumulations of amyloid. Both are caused by slow viruses.

Amyloid and the Immune System

Amyloid is known to be deposited in tissues that experience altered immunity (Thienhaus et al., 1985). For some reason, the body's immune system does not protect the body from disease effectively. The possibility is raised that Alzheimer's disease might result from breakdown in the body's immune system. Instead of protecting the brain, the immune system turns on the brain. This suggests an autoimmune response whereby the body produces antibodies that are directed against its own healthy tissue. The immune system cannot tell the difference between normal and foreign substances.

Amyloid and Prions

The understanding of amyloid has been advanced some by the work of Prusiner and his coworkers. Amyloid plaques were found in a slow virus disease (scrapie) in sheep and goats. This disease has been transmitted to a hamster brain. The brain tissue was found to contain very small rod-shaped particles called prions. Prions are protein-like infectious particles (Goldsmith, 1984) that are smaller than a virus. In a certain configuration prions have a remarkable resemblance to amyloid plaques, causing some researchers to hope that amyloid plaques may be found to be associated with prions. This would provide some evidence that a similar slow virus might cause Alzheimer's disease. However, the amyloid plaque in this disease could also be formed from proteins other than prions. The issue of what causes amyloid in plaques has not been settled.

Down's Syndrome

The significance of neuritic plaques has been examined from another perspective. The amyloid proteins found in Alzheimer's disease are thought to be the same amyloid present in Down's syndrome (Davies and Wolozin, 1987). In the Down's syndrome brain, neuritic plaques containing amyloid (as well as other abnormalities associated with Alzheimer's) typically appear in abundance and are distributed in much the same way as in Alzheimer's disease. Down's syndrome is characterized by extra copies of chromosome 21 and is a genetic disorder.

Chromosome 21 and Alzheimer's

In 1987, some significant findings occurred involving chromosome 21 and Alzheimer's disease. An abnormal gene on this chromosome shows a genetic defect that is thought to be responsible for a familial form of Alzheimer's disease, which indicates that some cases of Alzheimer's disease are under genetic control. This same chromosome contains a gene that is responsible for producing a major protein component of amyloid. The gene is now known as the amyloid precursor protein (APP). It is the parent protein of the smaller chain of amino acids that comprise the protein fragment beta-amyloid.

Amyloid in Down's Syndrome

The APP gene accounts for beta-amyloid in the Down's syndrome brain. Since there are extra copies of Chromosome 21 in this disorder, there would be more copies of the gene influencing the production of amyloid. This line of reasoning, however, cannot explain amyloid in Alzheimer's disease because there is no duplication of the amyloid gene.

Amyloid Mystery

Aging itself may be a factor. As we age, amyloid may be produced. This could explain why Alzheimer's disease increases in older persons. We know that amyloid is present in the walls of cerebral vessels of aged persons (Wisniewski, 1978). However, even with these deposits of amyloid, plaques do not necessarily occur.

It is not clear if vascular amyloid, which is fairly common in both Alzheimer's disease and old age, has the same origin and chemical composition as the amyloid in plaques. Amyloid's presence in plaques remains a puzzle.

Amyloid Near Cause of Alzheimer's

At present, we only know that amyloid plays a central role in Alzheimer's disease. We do not know how. It may very well be closely connected either with the cause of Alzheimer's disease or with other underlying conditions that will lead to the cause. Since it now appears that every person has a gene that plays a part in the production of amyloid, we must question why everyone does not get Alzheimer's disease. Researchers suspect that some other factor or factors must combine with the amyloid gene's role in order for Alzheimer's disease to develop. These factors might be a virus, some chemical extraneous to the brain or body, immune system breakdown, or factors that simply have not been identified.

Amyloid in plaques common in Alzheimer's disease raises many questions for research. Our understanding of amyloid is growing. It is associated with plaques, tangles, and cerebral vessels. We also know that the brain's loss of neurons corresponds with the distribution of plaques and tangles. Tangles and plaques particularly are indicators of the severity of dementia. The greater the concentration of plaques, the greater is the impairment of brain function. We cannot yet say that plaques cause the loss of brain cells.

Amyloid may act with other as yet unidentified factors in Alzheimer's disease that accelerate the production of amyloid. As a result, interaction in offensive proteins may be changed into harmful deposits of amyloids. Science may be able to discover ways to frustrate the genetic production of amyloid. Other factors must be identified that can explain why everyone who has an amyloid gene does not develop Alzheimer's disease.

Other Protein Abnormalities

Since cells are comprised of proteins, researchers have become interested in abnormal proteins. Other proteins act as conduits for chemical messengers. Two of these, tau protein and MAP (microtubule-associated protein), are found in increased amounts of abnormal forms in some persons with Alzheimer's disease (Mace and Rabins, 1991). According to the theory about these protein abnormalities, the body may not be able to break them down. As a result, abnormal proteins accumulate in the brain.

Granulovacuolar Degeneration

Description of GVD

A third type of brain abnormality, granulovacuolar degeneration (GVD), has an attraction to neurons in the hippocampus of the Alzheimer's patient's brain. GVD strikes the area of brain cells around their nucleus (see Figure 5), the area called cytoplasm. One or more fluid-filled spaces, vacuoles, form in the cell's cytoplasm with GVD. Within the vacuoles there is a dense, granular material (Ball, 1983) which under an electron microscope appears to have a crystalline structure (Conley, 1987). As these granulovacuoles develop, they cause a swelling of the cell's cytoplasm, which may eventually lead to degeneration or dysfunction of the brain cell itself.

GVD and Normal Aging

With normal aging, GVD also appears in the hippocampal area, but its concentration and severity are relatively low, and this degeneration occurs at a relatively slow rate with aging (Kemper, 1984). The rate of GVD is more rapid in Alzheimer's disease. Neurofibrillary tangles are also prevalent in the hippocampal area where high concentrations of GVD are found in Alzheimer's disease.

GVD and Memory Impairment Occur in Diminished Hippocampal Cells

The severity of impaired memory functions associated with the hippocampus in Alzheimer's disease can be more fully appreciated when one considers that GVD occurs within an already shrinking population of neurons. More than one-half of the original neurons of the hippocampus may have been lost, which is suspected to be up to five times more serious than cell loss in normal aging (Ball, 1983). Both GVD and tangles occur in this diminished cell population.

Role of Hippocampus

The hippocampus is commonly given a major role in memory functions. Cells in the rear portion of the hippocampus, an area thought to be more involved in remote memories, are especially vulnerable to GVD. It thus

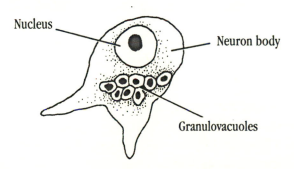

FIGURE 5. Granulovacuolar Degeneration in a Neuron.   Note that numerous granulovacuoles have formed in the body of this neuron around the nucleus.

appears that GVD may contribute to the disruption of more remote memories, a type of memory impairment that is most evident in later stages of Alzheimer's disease.

Future Research and GVD

Though much remains to be discovered about GVD, some researchers believe it may have an even stronger relationship with certain types of behavioral deterioration than plaques and tangles (Ball, 1983). This contention requires more investigation. Because GVD and tangles are closely matched in respect to their occurrence and location in the hippocampus, the possibility of related causes for both has been considered (Reisberg, 1983). GVD was first described as a characteristic of dementia in 1911, but investigation of this abnormality in Alzheimer's disease is relatively recent. For that reason it has not received the attention given to the classic brain abnormalities of Alzheimer's disease, the tangles and plaques.

Hirano Bodies

Description of Hirano bodies

A fourth abnormality of Alzheimer's disease, first described by Hirano in 1965, is known as the Hirano body. This is a discreet type of change primarily seen in the hippocampus. A microscopic spindle-shaped structure (Kemper, 1984), a Hirano body resembles a string of red blood cells (Davies and Wolozin, 1987). Under an electron microscope, Hirano bodies appear to have a crystalline structure (Brun, 1983). Hirano bodies invade the cell body of a neuron and also its processes (axons and dendrites). Neither the nature nor the importance of Hirano bodies has been clearly established, although these abnormal structures have been associated with actin (Davies and Wolozin, 1987), a major protein found in muscle fibers.

Age-Related Change

As with other abnormalities typical of Alzheimer's disease, the appearance of Hirano bodies in the brain is an age-related change. The bodies begin to appear in very small numbers during a person's teens, with a significant increase occurring only during and after the 60s. All persons over age 80 have Hirano bodies (Kemper, 1984).

Hirano Bodies and Memory Loss

Exactly how Hirano bodies affect the memory functions of the hippocampus is not known. However, some research suggests that Hirano bodies may trap ribosomes, rendering them dormant. Ribosomes are the agents that change RNA molecules—a basic unit of memory—into proteins, allowing the RNA to do its job of forming memories. If Hirano bodies are imprisoning the necessary ribosomes, then they may be preventing RNA from doing its job, so memories are not being formed. Further testing of this theory is needed.

Congophilic Angiopathy

Amyloid, the problematic protein found in senile plaques, also appears deposited abnormally in the walls of cerebral arteries, capillaries, and tiny veins. Because amyloid is a congophilic material (one that picks up a dye known as congo red, used to identify tissues), the presence of these abnormal deposits in blood vessels is called congophilic angiopathy, or simply amyloid angiopathy (angiopathy meaning a disorder of the blood vessels).

Somehow Related to Alzheimer's

The significance of congophilic angiopathy has not been clearly established, but there does appear to be some special connection between the deposits and Alzheimer's: while the condition appears in only 9 percent of neurologically normal individuals, it shows up in 92 percent of Alzheimer's patients. It also appears in all victims of Down's syndrome.

Angiopathy and Strokes

We further know that congophilic angiopathy sometimes leads to hemorrhaging and infarction—tissue death caused by the obstruction of blood vessels—in the Alzheimer's brain. Infarction and hemorrhaging in turn can cause strokes, and strokes can result in dementia. Indeed, multi-infarct dementia— a condition resulting from multiple large or small strokes—accounts for about 15 percent of all dementing brain disorders (Reisberg, 1981). A combination of multi-infarct dementia and Alzheimer's disease account for some 25 percent of all dementias in later life. Some researchers thus suspect that congophilic angiopathy is a contributing factor to stroke-induced dementia in Alzheimer's disease.

Possible Causes of Angiopathy

Other researchers theorize that congophilic angiopathy may signal an abnormality of the immune system of the brain or a deterioration of the blood-brain barrier, the special membrane that protects the brain from foreign substances. The deterioration of this barrier could cause both the angiopathy and the greater occurrence of infarcts and hemorrhage found in the Alzheimer's brain due to formation of amyloid deposits in the brain.

Major Points

Research has identified five physical abnormalities of the brain—neurofibrillary tangles, senile or neuritic plaques, granulovacuolar degeneration, Hirano bodies, and congophilic angiopathy—that are consistently present in the brains of Alzheimer's patients. All are present in those parts of the brain that control memory and behavior, particularly in the hippocampus. Some of these same abnormalities also are found in other neurological illnesses that cause dementia and in Down's syndrome, which causes mental retardation. The eventual appearance of all of these abnormalities in the brain is an age-related change, and normal aging brains generally show similar changes although in much lower quantities.

No definite facts are known about the link between these observed abnormalities and the cause of Alzheimer's disease. However, because these abnormalities tend to occur in those areas of the brain that control the functions most affected by the disease, and because they might somehow destroy or disable brain cells, researchers believe they may explain much of the mental impairment suffered by Alzheimer's patients. If the breakdown of nerve cells in Alzheimer's disease can be better understood, it might be possible to prevent the degree of cell destruction in this disease. The chemical treatments currently under investigation depend to a large degree on functional nerve cells that decrease as the disease progresses. Research must still determine if the physical abnormalities represent the debris of this disease process, or if they contribute in some way to the destruction of what had been a functional mind.

Chemical Changes in the Brain

Accompanying the physical abnormalities that appear in the Alzheimer's brain are chemical changes: lowered levels of crucial chemicals that the brain requires to record, process, and store information. These chemicals have been found most significantly lowered in the areas of the brain most affected by Alzheimer's, leading researchers to strongly suspect that chemical changes cause some of the disease's impairments.

More About Brain Anatomy

Neurons

At the cellular level, the brain is an intricate network of several billion interconnected cells, each equipped to perform a special task. Others included in this network are the billion or so nerve cells called neurons—the building blocks of a complex communication system that relays messages between the various areas of the brain and between the brain and the rest of the body. These messages travel along neuronal pathways. When plenty of healthy neurons are available to form the pathways, the whole communication system—and thus our thought processes themselves and other brain-related abilities—can function properly. However, when large numbers of neurons deteriorate or are destroyed, significant disruption of brain function occurs, severely limiting the ability to think, act, and remember.

Neurons Described

Neurons consist of a cell body and nucleus and protrusions called processes, which transmit electrochemical messages from one cell to another. Axons send a communication; dendrites receive communications from other neurons (see Figure 6). Each neuron usually has a number of dendrites (meaning tree with its branches). A remarkable feature of the brain's neurons is the fact that the axons, and dendrites link neurons together in circuits. One neuron could conceivably transmit messages to literally hundreds of other neurons. Usually neurons are linked with only a few other recipient neurons. The body of the cell may also have connections with adjoining neurons and receive that neuron's message.

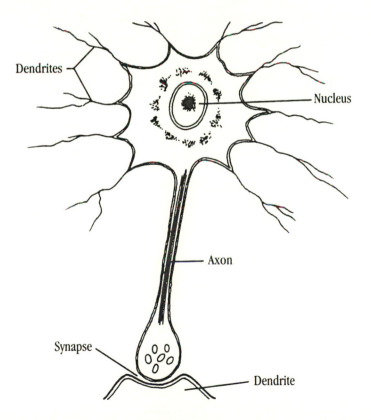

Dendrites

Nucleus

Axon

Synapse

Dendrite

FIGURE 6. Example of a Neuron from the Brain.   Note the axon, which carries the message a neuron sends to the synapse. Neurons have dendrites that receive messages from other neurons. (The synapse where the axon and dendrite communicate with a neurotransmitter is enlarged so that the reader can visualize this area.)

Synapse of a Neuron

The actual transmission from an axon to the receiving part of another cell (dendrites or cell body) takes place in the tiny gap between them, called a synapse (see Figure 7). Neurons do not communicate directly by touching each other; the synapse is important because of what happens there. For a message to be conveyed in the special gap (synapse), a chemical message must be transmitted.

Neurotransmitter

There is a specialized area at the end of a neuron's axon that secretes a chemical that combines with another chemical in that area of the synapse. The chemical process that occurs makes the neuron's special chemical messenger, a neurotransmitter. Without the neurotransmitter, neurons could not communicate; the information these chemical messengers carry would not be conveyed.

Neurons in Pathways Using Same Neurotransmitters

Many neurotransmitters exist in the brain. Different neurons in the brain's network use different neurotransmitters. Neurons utilizing the same neurotransmitter form pathways in the brain, often arising from areas deeper in the brain that serve as a source of stimulation for a pathway of neurons using a

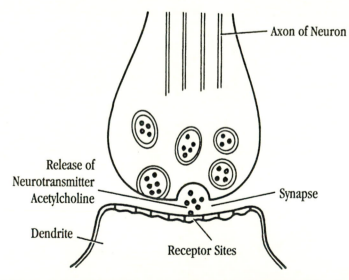

FIGURE 7. A Neuron's Axon Shown Communicating with a Dendrite of Another Neuron.
Neurotransmitter is released into the synapse and picked up at dendrite's receptor sites. The neurotransmitter is made when the enzyme CAT (choline acetyltransferase) combines with acetyl to make acetylcholine, the neurotransmitter of the cholinergic system.

common neurotransmitter to send messages. The neurotransmitter system thought to be involved in thought and memory is called the cholinergic system.

In Alzheimer's disease, problems develop in the brain's communication system. Disturbances or deficiencies in either the structural mechanisms (the neurons themselves) or the chemical messengers (the neurotransmitters) can lead to disturbances in behavior, thought, or emotion. In particular, Alzheimer's disables the brain's cholinergic system, which includes the neurotransmitter acetylcholine and its related network of neurons, known as the cholinergic neurons (Reisberg, 1981) or the cholinergic system.

To a lesser degree, the disease may also seem to affect the serotonergic system, which secretes the neurotransmitter serotonin; the noradrenergic system, which secretes the neurotransmitter noradrenaline (norephinephrine); and the system using the neurotransmitter somatostatin, which is also identified as a neuropeptide. We look at the changes wrought by Alzheimer's disease in each of these important chemical systems and at the subsequent disturbances in mental function and behavior that these changes appear to cause.

The Cholinergic System

Cholinergic neurons use the neurotransmitter acetylcholine. From a small area called the nucleus basalis of Meynert, these neurons and their processes reach up and out into the cortex of the brain. When these cholinergic pathways are not functioning, critical messages from one area of the brain to another cannot get through. Thus, a healthy cholinergic system—the neurons and their associated chemical messengers—may be essential to our memory, thoughts, judgment, personality, sensory perception, and other higher mental functions. Certainly it is involved in memory and in giving information meaning.

Cholinergic neurons communicate by means of a chemical chain reaction, and for the communication to work properly, all of the links in the chain must be in place. To start the process of transmitting information, a neuron secretes in its axon a chemical called acetyl (see Figure 8). The acetyl combines chemically with an enzyme known as choline acetyltransferase (CAT), and the CAT in turn creates the neurotransmitter, acetylcholine, which is released into the synapse. Acetylcholine, carrying its chemical message, is recognized by special sites (receptor sites) on the adjoining neuron. The message continues to be transmitted until another enzyme is activated. This enzyme is called acetylcholinesterase (AChE). Without the action of AChE on the acetylcholine, the neuron would be locked in to a message. Other messages could not be sent. Once the message is received by the adjoining cell and the acetylcholine is

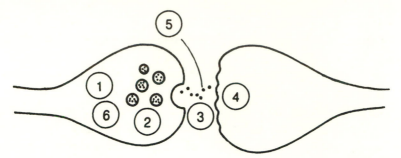

FIGURE 8. **Neurotransmission.**   (1) CAT combines with acetyl. (2) Acetylcholine results. (3) Neurotransmitter released into synapse. (4) Receptors on receiving neuron pick up acetylcholine. (5) Enzyme AChE breaks down acetylcholine. (6) New transmissions begin the process again.

broken down, the whole process can begin again. It is this simple chemical system that enables the brain's network of neurons to send hundreds of messages throughout the body each minute.

In Alzheimer's disease, however, this system breaks down. For unknown reasons, the cholinergic neurons begin to lose both their acetylcholine neurotransmitters and the two vital enzymes, CAT and AChE. Research has shown that the cholinergic system in particular is attacked by Alzheimer's disease, and cholinergic neurons are selectively destroyed; however, the cause for this destruction remains puzzling. Also in question is the precise role that the breakdown of this system plays in causing the impairments associated with Alzheimer's disease.

Loss of CAT and AChE Associated with Impairment

Some research has focused on the loss of the enzymes CAT and AChE, finding that deficiencies of these enzymes tend to accompany physical abnormalities such as plaques and tangles. Cholinergic dysfunction in the hippocampus and in the frontal/parietal areas of the cortex is quite pronounced. Such deficiencies also have been found to correlate with Alzheimer's patients' degree of cognitive impairment and severity of dementia. This suggests that a reduction in enzyme activity alone may impair the cognitive and memory abilities of the whole cholinergic system.

Deficiencies in the enzymes CAT and AChE mean that acetylcholine can neither be made adequately nor effectively broken down again. The cholinergic system's functioning depends heavily on these enzymes carrying out their role effectively.

Origin of Cholinergic System and Impact of Alzheimer's

Scientists consistently agree that there is a tremendous loss of neurons using acetylcholine in Alzheimer's disease. Now we know that the origin of this system, the nucleus basalis of Meynert, suffers a loss of from 44 to 75 percent of its neurons. This area of the brain is the major source of cholinergic stimulation (Davies and Wolozin, 1987; Tagliavini and Pilleri, 1983; Coyle et al., 1983). A network of axons from neurons in the nucleus basalis forms cholinergic pathways up to the cortex. The substantial loss of neurons in the origin of cholinergic stimulation will reduce the stimulation to the cortex and hippocampus. Researchers cannot explain why neurons in close proximity to this special nucleus, which do not depend upon acetylcholine, show no significant damage.

Other research has concentrated on the neurotransmitter acetylcholine. This chemical appears to play a unique role in our ability to perceive our environment in a detailed and meaningful way (Restak, 1984). It is connected with our ability to become intensely involved in the events around us and to remember what we experience—the appearance of a beautiful garden, perhaps, or the face of a new acquaintance. Conversely, when the amount of acetylcholine diminishes, Alzheimer's patients begin to lose their involvement with and enthusiasm for life. They become detached from the present and drift gradually into the past.

Memory Loss and Other Cognitive and Emotional Problems

Unfortunately, deficiencies in one or more of these associated chemicals may lead to the destruction of the cholinergic neurons themselves. Once large numbers of neurons are damaged, the crucial neuronal pathways leading to and from the frontal/parietal and temporal lobes, the hippocampus, and other brain areas begin to shut down. Damage to the cholinergic pathways in and out of the hippocampus, is particularly severe, leaving the hippocampus so isolated from the remainder of the brain that it might as well have been entirely removed (Hyman et al., 1984). This isolation most likely causes severe damage not only to memory functions but also to the patient's emotional health. It also may destroy necessary inhibitions, such as the fear of fire, that were learned through past emotional experience. In sum, damage to the cholinergic pathways linking the hippocampus with the cortex and the limbic structures, including the amygdala, as well as damage to other brain areas, seems to be responsible for much of the emotional and cognitive difficulty experienced by Alzheimer's patients.

The Serotonergic System

Serotonin

Believed to regulate both sleep and sensory perception, the serotonergic system also shows disturbance in Alzheimer's disease. This system relies upon the neurotransmitter serotonin, which is also the chemical thought to induce sleep in the brain. Just as acetylcholine is deficient in the cholinergic system, serotonin is significantly reduced in a variety of brain areas when Alzheimer's disease is present (Volicer et al., 1985; Carlsson, 1983). Also deficient is serotonin's metabolite (5-HIAA), which is a product of chemical changes related to metabolism. Some research suggests that deficiencies of these two chemicals are related to the sleep disturbances, mood changes, and overly aggressive behavior typical of some Alzheimer's patients (Volicer et al., 1985).

Link with Alzheimer's Uncertain

Numerous studies have found the neurotransmitter, serotonin, deficient in Alzheimer's disease. It is reduced from 50 to 70 percent (Cummings et al., 1998). Changes in the serotonergic system are not strongly correlated with cognitive changes, but noncognitive symptoms such as aggressive behavior and depression are believed to be associated with the loss of serotonin (DeKosky, 1996). Persons with Alzheimer's whose depression is characterized by more agitation and aggressiveness may respond favorably to antidepressants called serotonin reuptake inhibitors (SSRIs) such as sertraline (Zoloft) and peroxetine (Paxil). Changes in serotonin and norepinephrine levels are often involved in persons whose disease onset occurs before age 65. These persons face major changes in their lives and psychosocial losses are common. The development of depression would not be an unreasonable reaction to their circumstances. However, changes in the levels of serotonin and norepinephrine may be more involved in the etiology of these depressive disorders. With a psychological and chemical basis for depression, these persons would benefit from a treatment approach that combines therapy with medications.

The Noradrenergic System

Changes in Alzheimer's Disease

This system appears to counter the serotonergic system by triggering wakefulness and arousal. Too much of the operative neurotransmitter, noradrenaline, may produce severe stress reactions; too little may cause depression and excessive sleeping. One study reports that noradrenaline is reduced in the Alzheimer's brain by 57 to 74 percent (Gottfries, 1985); another indicates that about half of all Alzheimer's patients suffer deficits of noradrenaline in the cortex, with a severe loss in only about 20 percent of that group (Davies and Wolozin, 1987). The hippocampus and the hypothalamus also show deficiencies of noradrenaline, of from 49 to 73 percent (Winblad et al., 1982).

Noradrenaline

Given the interplay of this system and the serotonergic system, disturbances in either or both neurotransmitters could cause the sleep disturbances found in Alzheimer's disease. Deficits of these chemicals could also explain why some patients become unusually heavily sedated by tranquilizers. In contrast, a deficit of noradrenaline could also trigger emotional arousal. Loss of this neurotransmitter has some correlation with symptoms of depression, but no correlation with the cognitive loss in AD.

Somatostatin

Role in the Brain and Alzheimer's Disease

Among the other neurotransmitter chemicals suspected of playing a role in Alzheimer's are the neuropeptides: somatostatin, substance P, neurotensin, and cholecystokin (Perry and Perry, 1985). Neuropeptides are peptides made from amino acids that are now known to function as neurotransmitters in the brain.

In particular, a lack of somatostatin appears to accompany the disease and contribute to its impairments. Although research on this chemical is still in the early stages, somatostatin has been shown to be significantly reduced in several brain areas, including the parietal lobe, a region thought by many to be affected first and most profoundly in Alzheimer's disease (Tamminga et al., 1987). Other findings suggest that a loss of somatostatin neurons may be directly related to Alzheimer's dementia (Tamminga et al., 1987).

There is continued evidence that memory can be enhanced with somatostatin (Craft et al., 1999). The therapeutic role for this neurotransmitter in supporting memory and neuronal communication is recognized. More research is need to increase our understanding of the role of somatostatin in AD in conjunction with deficits known to exist in other neurotransmitter systems. Researchers currently believe that a combination of drugs or compounds with multiple functions might provide additional therapeutic value. Levels of somatostatin, serotonin, noradrenaline are lower than normal in some persons with AD and may contribute to sensory disturbances, aggressive behavior, and neuron death. These lower levels appear to have a role in cognitive and behavioral deficits. The cholinergic deficit in Alzheimer's disease needs to be studied further.

The Glutaminergic System

Glutamate is a form of glutamic acid, which is a nonessential amino acid in proteins. Glutamate is the major excitatory neurotransmitter in the brain. About 70 percent of excitatory synapses in the central nervous system utilize this neurotransmitter. Under conditions of overexcitation, glutamate can cause neurotoxicity; this situation is called excitotoxicity. Dysfunction of the neurotransmission of glutamate is one mechanism of degeneration thought to be involved in Alzheimer's disease.

Neurons need an adequate supply of oxygen and glucose to survive. A sustained deprivation of glucose, as occurs in strokes and asphyxiation, has devastating consequences: Glutamate, which otherwise is essential and harmless, is changed into a potent neuron killer under conditions of chronic glucose insufficiency.

Glutamate is an excitatory amino acid that is essential for the development and normal functioning of cells—in appropriate amounts. In excessive amounts this neurotransmitter becomes toxic to the exact same neuron it normally stimulates in the appropriate way (Khachaturian and Radebaugh, 1996). Neurotoxicity occurs when too much glutamate is present at a synapse. It also happens when glutamate excites a glucose-starved neuron. The excitatory effect of chronically released glutamate causes the degeneration of cortical and subcortical cells, thus leading to the development of dementia symptoms.

Glutamate toxicity is mediated when calcium normally flows into the cell. However, breakdown in this normal chemical process results in an excessive internal concentration of calcium that eventually kills the cell.

The effects of glutamate are normally mediated through three classes of receptors named according to the agonist associated with each. An agonist is a drug that is chemically attracted to, and stimulates activity at, cell receptors normally stimulated by naturally occurring substances. One of these receptors is called NMDA, and the Alzheimer's brain has an extensive loss of the NMDA receptor sites (Shihabuddin and Davis, 1996).

Altering the activity of glutamate is an approach to treating Alzheimer's that is gaining support. It is, however, one that must take into account the fact that glutamate can enhance learning and memory as well as produce neurotoxicity. A way must be found to reduce toxicity without causing cognitive impairment. One medication that seems to do this, Memantine, will be described in Chapter 17.

Treating Neurotransmitter Deficiencies

Drug Interventions

Some drug treatments already exist for treating deficits in the cholinergic system, although to date they have not proven particularly effective. It may be that this system needs to be treated in conjunction with other affected systems. As research into the disease and its effects on the brain continue, it is highly likely that other neurotransmitters and chemical systems that have a bearing on Alzheimer's disease will be discovered as well. Because the disease's symptoms can vary widely from one individual to the next, it may be that a number of different neurochemical deficiencies are involved. A given individual's symptoms could hold the clue to treatment: a patient suffering from early dementia, pronounced visual-spatial deficits, and lesser intellectual and memory impairment, for example, might be more responsive to cholinergic drug treatment alone.

Other Drug Treatments for Other Chemical Systems

As we learn more about the full range of neurotransmitter and other chemical deficiencies associated with Alzheimer's disease, it seems likely that drug treatments will become available that can at least partially compensate for these deficits and the problems they cause.

Summary

The levels of certain neurotransmitters and related chemicals crucial to the brain's information communication process are lowered by Alzheimer's disease. The absence of these chemicals may cause the destruction of neurons, particularly the cholinergic neurons, that form the pathways to the hippocampus, the frontal/parietal lobes, and other areas of the brain's cortex. By cutting off effective communication between these areas, chemical disturbances in the brain may be responsible for many of the emotional, cognitive, memory, and behavioral changes suffered by Alzheimer's disease patients. Most Alzheimer's disease treatment-oriented research has sought ways to correct chemical abnormalities.

17

Treatment Possibilities

Role of Drugs in Alzheimer's Treatment

As medical researchers gradually come to understand the physical and chemical changes that occur in the Alzheimer's brain, they can use their knowledge to develop treatments that effectively prevent or reverse these changes. Many experimental studies using drug therapies on Alzheimer's patients already have been tried, with varying degrees of success. While no "wonder" drug for Alzheimer's disease—or even a clear and consistent treatment approach—has yet emerged, research has shown that some drugs help some of the people some of the time. Unfortunately, the studies completed thus far often show puzzling inconsistencies in response from one patient to the next. To achieve more consistent results, we no doubt need to learn more about the nature of the illness and its causes.

Cholinergic Deficits Target of Treatment

To date, several major groups of drugs have been investigated. Many of the drug interactions in research have attempted to correct the deficiencies in the brain's cholinergic system. Since the neurotransmitter acetylcholine is deficient in the Alzheimer's brain and these deficiencies have been associated with Alzheimer's-related impairments, it has been thought that finding ways to increase this chemical messenger might hold promise in treating the disease.

Basis for Drug Research

Additionally, lecithin and choline, which increase the availability of acetylcholine, have received some research attention. Drugs such as physostigmine and THA (tetrahydroacridine) which make acetylcholine available longer in the brain by blocking its destruction, have seemed promising in developing an effective treatment of Alzheimer's disease. Drugs that directly increase the amount of acetylcholine and those that prevent its chemical destruction are called cholinergic agents.

In 1993, the Federal Drug Administration (FDA) approved the use of THA under the name Cognex. In 1996, a similar medication, Aricept (donepezil), was approved by the FDA, and Exelon (rivastigmine) was approved in April 2000. These drugs are known as cholinesterase inhibitors because they slow the breakdown of the neurotransmitter acetylcholine and enhance its availability at the synapse so that information transmission is more likely to occur. They depend upon a fairly intact system of neurons, their processes, and synaptic connections. Originally they were approved for people with mild to moderate dementia. There is evidence that this type of medication may also be helpful to people with more advanced Alzheimer's.

An approach supporting the survival and protection of nerve cells was needed. Drugs preventing damage to nerve cells resulting from the deleterious effects of oxidation and inflammation would support the survival of nerve cell highways and their neurochemical transmission. As the result of epidemiological research, two kinds of drugs that can prevent or slow the development of Alzheimer's disease have been identified: estrogen and anti-inflammatory agents. The use of antioxidants, also promises to aid in the survival of neurons by the prevention or inhibition of oxidation. Free radicals generated through oxidative mechanisms are thought to play a role in Alzheimer's disease. A fine balance exists between oxygen-free radical formation and antioxidant defense. When the balance is tipped in favor of the reactive free radical, oxidative stress results, thus making neurons especially vulnerable to free radical attack (Markesbery, 1996). The accumulation of damage resulting from oxidation then causes nerve cells to degenerate.

In this chapter, we examine different groups of drugs and their effects singularly and in combination with others. We consider possible explanations for the inconsistent results of drug studies to date, including the possibility that Alzheimer's disease has different subtypes that respond to different treatments. Other novel treatments are being considered. For example, neuronal transplants may be possible. Studies began recently to determine if a vaccine that worked in mice with extensive plaque formation will be safe and effective in humans. Alzheimer's research is developing possibilities for preventing, delaying, or slowing AD at a more rapid pace. Medications are being developed and becoming more readily available. While many of these are still cholinesterase inhibitors similar to Aricept, they have slightly different characteristics. Before we look more closely at medications, we need to cover issues relevant for participating in drug research studies.

Should You Participate in Drug-Research Study?

Consider Risks, Costs, and Motivation

In order for Alzheimer's treatments to be adequately developed and tested, it is necessary to conduct research using human subjects who have Alzheimer's disease. Subjects who volunteer for such studies do a great service both for medical research and for their fellow Alzheimer's sufferers. However, it is important that persons who elect to participate in a research study clearly understand the study's potential risks, results, and requirements, as well as their personal motivation for participating.

Families and subjects must not hold unrealistic expectations of significant improvement. Generally, persons with severe impairment have little chance of benefitting from drug treatment, while those in earlier stages of the disease may experience substantial, little, or no improvement. The drugs might even cause a worsening of the patient's condition. Also, families and subjects sometimes cannot be told whether the subject will in fact be receiving the treatment medication or a placebo used for the control group.

Issues to Consider

Other issues that must be carefully considered include:

- Purpose and rationale of the study
- How the study will be conducted
- Size and safety of the dosage given
- Method of administering the drug
- Potential side effects
- Responsibilities of the family
- Consent of the subject
- All expenses connected with participation (including travel, lodging, etc.)
- Researchers' attitude toward study participants (including family members)
- Researchers' credentials

Inconsistencies in Drug Studies

Unknown or Uncontrolled Variables

Many uncontrolled variables exist in drug studies that may account for the frustrating inconsistencies found in Alzheimer's research. The many individual factors that may vary from one subject to the next, affecting or masking a drug's effects in a study, include:

- Degree of the subject's dementia
- Severity of the loss of cholinergic neurons
- Incorrect diagnosis of Alzheimer's
- Coexisting disabilities (i.e., stroke)
- Other coexisting conditions (i.e., infection)
- Unrelated fluctuations in behavior and mood
- Age at onset of dementia

Unknown Variables May Be Significant

For example, a severe presenile dementia (onset before age 65) may be intrinsically different in terms of brain pathology than a severe senile dementia (onset after age 65), and thus it may respond very differently to a certain drug treatment. Any of the variables listed above may or may not prove to be an important indicator for Alzheimer's drug research.

Other variables that must be controlled relate to the study itself. These include:

- Dosage amounts
- Length of treatment and study
- Method of administration (oral, intravenous, etc.)
- Ways of measuring improvement
- Assumptions about the drug and effects expected
- Choice of symptoms to be measured

Distinct Subtypes that Respond Differently to Treatment

Another possible explanation for the inconsistencies found is that Alzheimer's disease may have distinct subtypes, each associated with slightly different manifestations of symptoms and rate of progression. Different subtypes may respond differently to the same drug treatment. One researcher posits that two subtypes of Alzheimer's disease exist: AD-1 and AD-2 (Bondareff, 1983). As defined, AD-1 begins in old age and follows a slow, subtle progression; AD-2 begins in middle age and shows a more rapid course and greater impairment. Other neurochemical and anatomical differences established between the two groups would seem to support this distinction. For example, AD-2 might develop under more genetically controlled influence.

Another researcher has suggested four distinct subtypes of the disease: extrapyramidal, myclonic, benign, and typical (Mayeux et al., 1985). As compared to the typical group, the extrapyramidal and myclonic groups each show certain accentuated features, while the benign group shows underexpressed features. The groups also differ as to severity of impairment in cognitive and memory functions.

Attention to Subtypes May Produce Better Treatment Strategies

Other researchers now are looking into the validity and significance of the subtypes, and overall, the concept of subtypes may prove rewarding to research treatments. It may be that attention to these subtypes, and to other distinguishing indicators such as age of onset and severity of dementia, will lead to the creation of better drug treatment strategies with more predictable and reliable results.

Despite the many variables to be controlled and the inconsistencies found in studies to date, it has been shown definitively that drug therapies can produce improvements in Alzheimer's symptoms. The challenge now is to identify some clear pattern that will show us which drugs can be expected to help which patients, in what ways, and for how long.

Cholinergic Agents

As seen in the Chapter 16 discussion of chemical changes, Alzheimer's disease is accompanied by a lowered level of the neurotransmitter acetylcholine in the brain. Insufficient acetylcholine causes dysfunction of the brain's cholinergic system, which may lead to impairment of memory and cognitive abilities.

Among the first treatments for Alzheimer's to be explored, then, are drugs that can increase the level of acetylcholine in the brain. The drugs tried include two substances that are precursors of acetylcholine: choline and lecithin. These substances increase the availability of acetylcholine. We also consider physostigmine and THA, which prevent the breakdown of this neurotransmitter. In this role, these two drugs prolong the availability of the acetylcholine. Finally, we consider drugs that make the receptors for acetylcholine more sensitive, essentially heightening the potency of the available acetylcholine.

Choline

A component of various foods and of commercially available lecithin, choline can increase the availability of acetylcholine in the brain and enhance its synthesis and release in synapses between the neurons. Because of these potential effects, it first was approached with a great deal of hope. In the numerous studies completed, however, choline therapy has been associated with only extremely modest improvements in Alzheimer's patients or no improvements at all.

In some cases, a modest increase in alertness and awareness has been reported, although the increase has been accompanied by mild irritability; in a few others, a reduction in confusion has been noted (Fovall et al., 1983). But all of these improvements have been so mild that they could have been simply ordinary behavioral fluctuations unrelated to the choline therapy. Those patients who have appeared to improve were in the earlier stages of the illness; no effect from choline therapy seems possible in more advanced cases. Some research findings suggest that choline might prove more beneficial when used in combination with other drugs.

Side effects from choline include nausea, abdominal pain, diarrhea, incontinence, and fishy odor in the sweat. This last side effect has been avoided by substituting phosphatidylcholine, a more complex form of the drug of which choline is a component. The availability of choline and lecithin encourage their use.

Lecithin

Lecithin is a naturally occurring dietary substance found in many foods, including egg yolks, meat, fish, and soybean products. The dosages of lecithin used in treating Alzheimer's disease, however, are much higher than those obtainable through a healthy diet. Like choline, lecithin increases the availability of acetylcholine; it also raises the body's blood choline level and maintains that level longer than does straight choline (Etienne, 1983). It has been shown to produce small improvements in some patients.

The most important finding is that lecithin could be capable of slowing deterioration in a few patients. This may mean that long-term lecithin therapy can be used to slow down the disease's progress (Dysken, 1987). Supporting this theory is the finding in the Dysken study that patients who discontinued use of lecithin showed more rapid deterioration. However, this very limited evidence must be replicated in other studies before stronger conclusions can be drawn.

At present, lecithin treatment requires further exploration. No compelling evidence suggests that it alone can produce significant or consistent improvement, though it may prove an effective supplement to other drug therapies. Furthermore, there is no scientific evidence in support of the idea that lecithin can prevent Alzheimer's. Lecithin therapy has shown some very modest improvements in some patients some of the time. The idea behind lecithin and choline, increasing the amount of acetylcholine, remains a promising direction for future research.

Side effects of lecithin can include nausea, diarrhea, irritability, and dry mouth. These are more likely to occur in older persons. Lecithin is not otherwise harmful. It can be purchased in health food stores, but this form is usually 20 percent lecithin (Henig, 1981). It would be impossible to take enough of this form of lecithin to be of any benefit with Alzheimer's disease.

Physostigmine

This drug works by slowing down the chemical destruction of acetylcholine in the brain's synapses. By keeping the existing acetylcholine available longer, it increases cholinergic activity at active synapses, although it cannot help synapses that have been damaged or destroyed by the disease. Since physostigmine is thought to effectively cross the blood-brain barrier (Smith et al., 1979), it will be more effective in blocking the breakdown of acetylcholine by the enzyme acetylcholinesterase.

A danger of physostigmine is its narrow dose range: only a slight difference exists between a safe dose and one that is toxic. Additionally, it does not stay in the body very long; thus, it must be given more frequently. Despite the disadvantages, more positive results have been achieved with physostigmine than with either choline or lecithin. The improvements noted are modest: in mid-sized dose, it improves verbal recognition memory; in larger doses, it improves nonverbal recognition memory (Dysken, 1987). Overall, it seems to have positive effects on visual memory, that is, memory of information that is presented in a visual form (e.g., recognizing pictures).

Physostigmine also seems to improve certain types of learning measured by psychological tests, and the improvement is the greatest in patients with only mild symptoms. It will not be as effective when other neurotransmitter systems are impaired in addition to the cholinergic system—a condition that seems to be more frequent with early-onset dementia (Mohs et al., 1982).

Overall, the studies with physostigmine are encouraging. Because they have shown such widely varying kinds and degrees of improvement—including no improvement in many patients—further research is needed to pinpoint the best uses for this drug: the most effective doses, the types of functions improved by various doses, and the kinds of patients who respond best. It is now available to researchers in oral form. The potential for toxicity can be monitored, although it remains a risk factor for physostigmine. Although this drug has not produced dramatic improvements and its effects on the progression of Alzheimer's disease have not been determined, physostigmine shows promise for further research.

Available Cholinesterase Inhibitors

Tacrine

Tacrine, or THA (tetrahydroacridine) as it was known in earlier studies, was the first drug to become available for usage outside of research settings. Multicenter clinical trials were conducted, and in September 1993, it was approved by the U.S. Food and Drug Administration under the name Cognex (tacrine) for treatment of Alzheimer's disease despite concerns about its effectiveness. It has the same chemical action as physostigmine: it slows the chemical breakdown of acetylcholine in the brain's synapses and allows the small amounts of neurotransmitter released to remain longer than usual at the synaptic junction. Presumably, this action would more effectively support the transmission of information at the synapse. Keeping the neurotransmitter at the synapse longer might make up for the deficiency that has already been identified in the cholinergic system of the Alzheimer's brain. Tacrine is known as a cholinesterase inhibitor because it inhibits cholinesterase, the enzyme that breaks down acetylcholine.

Study of tacrine began in 1981. In that study, 75 percent of the subjects showed subjectively measured improvement from treatment with tacrine alone (Summers et al., 1981). Another study by Summers in 1986 also indicated improvement (Summers et al., 1986). Studies reported by others have investigated tacrine with and without lethicin. Lethicin is not essential and does not contribute much to the therapeutic effect (Stearn and Davis, 1996). Tacrine may slow cognitive deterioration by 6 to 12 months. This time can be meaningful to patients and their caregivers.

The patient response to tacrine is heterogeneous and benefits vary. Significant benefits were experienced by 10 percent of patients. More modest benefits were demonstrated by 20 percent, and 20 percent showed smaller but significant improvement in clinical status or performance. Remaining patients exhibited no short-term benefits (Stearn and Davis, 1996).

Side effects from tacrine include nausea, belching, and diarrhea. Because of the potential for liver toxicity, people taking tacrine must have regular blood tests to monitor liver function. Rash, anorexia, and rhinitis are other fairly common adverse effects. Tacrine use has declined with the introduction of donepezil because dosing is easier and there is no need to monitor liver function.

Aricept

Aricept (donepezil) is more selective for the cholinesterase in the central nervous system; it has fewer of the peripheral cholinergic effects such as nausea, vomiting, and diarrhea. Dosage is easy: 5 or 10 milligrams can be given at bedtime. It is indicated for persons with mild to moderate dementia of the Alzheimer's type. Adverse effects reportedly are mild and transient, and they are resolved during treatment with the medication. This type of symptomatic treatment may slow or delay disease progression for 6 months or more. The cholinergic deficit is much greater in more advanced stages of the disease. The use of donepezil is now being considered for people with more advanced AD.

Exelon

Exelon (rivastigmine) works a little differently from Aricept. It prevents the breakdown of acetylcholine by inhibiting two cholinesterase enzymes: acetylcholinesterases and butrylcholinesterases. The presence or activity of butrylcholinesterases may be higher in the Alzheimer's brain, so inhibiting this enzyme may be beneficial in treating AD.

People involved in large clinical trials with Exelon have demonstrated benefits in several key areas of functioning: activities of daily living like eating and dressing, global functioning, and cognition. Exelon's impact on preserving activities of daily living appears to be most significant in moderate-stage dementia. Improvement in social interaction and participation in hobbies have also been observed. Exelon is given twice a day. It is usually initiated at 1.5 milligrams twice a day and gradually increased to a maximum dose of 6 milligrams daily (an oral solution may eventually be available). Most people with dementia are older and take multiple medications. Exelon has a low potential for negative interactions with other prescribed medications. Like other cholinesterase inhibitors, the medication has gastrointestinal side effects such as nausea and vomiting, and it is best tolerated when taken with food. Side effects have been reported as mild and transient, and they subside with continued treatment. This medication may be beneficial for people with moderately severe to advanced AD. Its drawbacks are multiple daily doses, slow titration, and gastrointestinal side effects.

Switching from one cholinesterase inhibitor to another without some functional deterioration is tricky. When people on Cognex were switched to Aricept, a washout of the Cognex was necessary; thus, for 2 weeks Cognex was discontinued before treatment with Aricept was initiated. Deterioration was noted in people during this transition period. By the time the therapeutic dose of Aricept was reached, the functional status present before the switch could not be restored.

For this reason, it seems most appropriate for Exelon to be a consideration for people who have not responded to Aricept or Cognex, or who have not yet been started on any cholinesterase inhibitor. Treatment of people with more advanced Alzheimer's, who have not been seen as appropriate candidates for this kind of treatment should be reconsidered and given a trial on Exelon. Questions about switching from another similar medication to Exelon should be answered by a physician.

Metrifonate

Many of the antidementia drugs being developed are cholinesterase inhibitors. One, galantamine, received FDA approval in February 2001. It will be marketed by Jannssen under the brand name Reminyl. The development of another, metrifonate, has been stopped.

Galantamine

Galantamine has been used in Europe to treat several neuromuscular diseases. It is extracted from the bulb of a species of daffodils and is well tolerated.

Galantamine is unique among cholinesterase inhibitors. It binds to acetylcholine receptors and stimulates the function of cells. Galantamine modulates specialized acetylcholine receptors on neurons called nicotinic receptors, which are activated by nicotine and various other substances. Galantamine is one of the substances capable of activating these receptors. This is important because nicotinic receptors play an important role in learning and memory. Stimulation of nicotinic receptors may also be associated with inhibiting the buildup of beta amyloid and the resulting damage to brain cells.

Studies are promising. Galantamine appears to help preserve memory and function in people with AD. Benefits have lasted 12 months. People with mild to moderate AD were able to maintain memory function and the ability to learn. They were able to perform activities of daily living at the same level or better than the level seen before the drug was started. Galantamine has gastrointestinal side effects, particularly at higher doses, including nausea, diarrhea, dizziness, and headaches.

The deficiency of the neurotransmitter acetylcholine is only one of a cascade of biochemical events occurring in Alzheimer's disease. Treatments based solely on reversing the cholinergic deficiency cannot be expected to be completely successful. Exploration of potential treatments for Alzheimer's disease have expanded significantly.

Cholinergic Receptor Agonists

Other drugs that seem to help the brain's cholinergic system are cholinergic receptor agonists. These drugs work by stimulating the receptors that receive acetylcholine. Two such drugs, arecoline and RS-86, have been tried in studies on Alzheimer's patients, but unfortunately they produced little or no significant improvement (Bruno et al., 1986). Another drug, benthanechol chloride, did produce improvements such as decreased confusion, increased initiative, and greater productive activity in a four-subject study (Dysken, 1987).

One interesting aspect of the benthanechol study was the pioneering drug-administration technique used. A drug infusing pump was implanted into the subject's abdominal wall and connected to an intracranial catheter (Dysken, 1987). The pump allowed the drug to reach the brain directly and to cross the blood-brain barrier; it also allowed direct measurement of the amount of drug in the brain, something impossible with other administration techniques. The pump's improved measurement abilities, together with the steady, guaranteed dosage it provides, may make it a more desirable administration technique for all studies of brain-altering chemicals, allowing more precise findings. These benefits, however, must be weighed against the undesirable physical intrusiveness of the pump and catheter.

Naxolone and Naltrexone

Treatment with these drugs represents a very sophisticated investigation of the role of more fundamental biological systems of the brain affected by dementing illnesses. Although they have been tried on Alzheimer's patients in several studies, they have failed to produce any real, consistent improvement. Only one study with Naloxone has shown significant benefits from the drug (Reisberg et al., 1983). Several others have found the drug to exacerbate undesirable symptoms. At present, there is little evidence to suggest that these drugs hold promise for future treatment.

Vasodilators and Nootropic Agents

Vasodilators are a group of drugs that improve blood flow to the brain by expanding narrowed blood vessels. In a brain stricken by Alzheimer's disease, a rapid and diffuse reduction in cerebral blood flow occurs after the onset of symptoms; vasodilators can help offset this reduction. In fact, vasodilators are more effective in raising cerebral blood flow in Alzheimer's patients than in normal persons of the same age (Reisberg, 1981) or in persons with arteriosclerotic brain changes often referred to as "hardening of the arteries."

Two types of vasodilators exist: primary and secondary. Primary vasodilators—such as nylidrin, the only one drug shown to improve dementia—act directly on vascular deficiencies. Secondary vasodilators, such as piracetam, increase blood flow indirectly by stimulating cerebral metabolism. Metabolism is a chemical process necessary for the body and brain to maintain and regenerate themselves. Energy is a product of metabolism.

Piracetam

Piracetam is also one of the nootropic agents—a group of compounds that seems to improve functioning in mild to moderate senile dementia (Jenike, 1985). Piracetam increases the response of neurons in the hippocampus (Cooper, 1984) and appears to stimulate cerebral glucose metabolism (Jenike et al., 1986) and enhance release of acetylcholine in the hippocampus (Rosenberg et al., 1983).

Cerebral blood flow has a strong relationship with metabolic activity. Disturbances in metabolism seem tied to reductions in cerebral blood flow found in Alzheimer's disease. For instance, persons with Alzheimer's have significantly lower levels of oxygen and glucose utilization in the frontal, temporal, and parietal areas of the brain. Secondary vasodilators stimulate the brain's metabolism to increase cerebral blood flow.

In animal studies, piracetam has increased brain energy reserves, increased learning, and protected against learning impairment. The same studies indi-

cate that piracetam does not have side effects or toxic effects at normal therapeutic doses (Schneck, 1983). Preliminary evidence suggests that a combination of piracetam and choline given for one week improved memory storage,
recall, and delayed recall (Schneck, 1983). It may be that piracetam is most
effective when combined with drugs that increase the availability of acetylcholine. As with other drug treatments, more mildly impaired patients—
those whose cholinergic systems are least damaged and thus most
responsive—seem to show the greatest benefit.

At this time, neither nylidrin nor piracetam are commercially available in
the United States. In Canada, nylidrin is sold under the brand names of
Arlidin, Arlidin Forte, and PMS Nylidrin, and is used to treat problems due
to poor circulation. Piracetam is marketed under many different names and
can be purchased over the counter in Mexico. Outside the United States, it is
used to improve impaired cognition due to hypoxia (lack of oxygen) and as a
treatment for stroke, alcoholism, and vertigo.

Neuropeptides

Neuropeptides are short chains of amino acids that have strong effects on the
nervous system. Certain types of neuropeptides act as hormones in the body
and have roles as neurotransmitters in the brain; they also assist in the communication between body cells, tissues, and organs (Reisberg, 1981). Research into
possible uses for neuropeptides in treating Alzheimer's is still in the early stages.

In animal studies, neuropeptides have produced reversal of memory
impairment. They also have been shown to boost human cognitive abilities
and to play a role in neurotransmission and in memory and learning. However, drug research with Alzheimer's patients to date has not had particularly
encouraging results. Neuropeptides have been shown to produce mood
improvements such as reduced depression, increased energy, and increased
attention and concentration (Ferris, 1983), and they may prove to have a role
as geriatric antidepressants.

Vasopressin

Both a neuropeptide and a secondary vasodilator, vasopressin has improved
memory and learning in animal studies. In one particularly interesting study
with rats, vasopressin helped the animals remember things they had previously
forgotten. In a study with Alzheimer's patients who suffered memory disturbances, use of a vasopressin nasal spray helped memories appear more quickly.
Normal adult men have shown improved attention, concentration, and recall
in response to vasopressin (Reisberg et al.,1982).

Vasopressin analogs—such as LVP, ODAVP, and DGAVP—also have been
tried on Alzheimer's patients, with mixed results. One study has shown small

but statistically significant improvements in memory, retrieval, and reaction time when an analog was administered (Ferris, 1983). Possibly the more potent, longer-acting analogs will prove to have the greatest effects. Further research is needed to determine how vasopressin and its analogs work: by genuinely improving memory, by stimulating enhanced concentration, or by acting as an antidepressant.

Because of the role they seem to play in memory, learning, and communications between neurons, neuropeptides represent a promising frontier for further research. At the very least, they may prove helpful as antidepressant agents.

Psychostimulants

This group of drugs stimulated the central nervous system, increasing motor activity and reducing fatigue. Although psychostimulants do not improve cognitive or memory abilities, they can benefit other symptoms of Alzheimer's disease. Research has focused on treating three clusters of symptoms: (1) apathetic and withdrawn behavior, (2) mild depression, and (3) impaired short-term memory (Prien, 1983).

Of the psychostimulants tried, a number of drugs, such as Ritalin, have generally proven unhelpful. These drugs may exacerbate behavior that is already agitated. Metrazol has received mixed reviews, but it has seemed to help with apathy, withdrawal, drive, and self-care (Prien, 1983). However, it has a number of very undesirable side effects. Procaine hydrochloride, the primary active ingredient in a drug called Gerovital-H3, seems to have potential only for the treatment of geriatric depression (Prien, 1983).

To date, then, psychostimulants have not proven particularly helpful, although they may have some use in treating specific subtypes of Alzheimer's. The side effects associated with these drugs require that they be carefully monitored, however, and may limit their usefulness.

Glutaminergic Agents

The cholinergic deficit in Alzheimer's disease has driven much of the research on antidementia drugs. Medications addressing this deficit have been moderately successful in managing symptom maintaining activities of daily living, reducing some behavior problems, and slowing down the progress of the disease. Research needs to be broadened to consider other treatment approaches.

Memantine is a glutaminergic agent and acts on glutaminergic neurotransmission and the loss of specific glutamate receptors. One of these, the NMDA receptor, is implicated in the deterioration found in Alzheimer's disease. Memantine is an agonist of the NMDA receptor. Studies of the brains of persons with Alzheimer's have found extensive loss of the NMDA receptor sites. Memantine protects the neuronal system from the neurotoxicity that leads to cell death. It preserves, or restores, appropriate levels of activation necessary for the appropriate functioning of glutaminergic neurotransmission. Since glutamate is thought to be one mechanism involved in AD neurodegeneration, a receptor agonist such as Memantine should slow down the disease progression.

Memantine, developed by Merz and Co. of Frankfurt, Germany, has been approved for the treatment of dementias in Germany for 10 years. Recently, research trials using this drug have occurred in the United States. Forrest Labs of New York and Merz have entered into a partnership. Efforts are under way to seek FDA approval in order to market the drug in the United States.

Reports suggest that Memantine slowed the progression of symptoms in persons with moderately severe to severe Alzheimer's disease. It was well tolerated and caused few, if any, side effects. Compared to placebo, persons taking this substance manifested improvements in clinical global, cognitive, and behavioral functions (Reisberg, 2000). Fewer declines were noted in the progression of the disease. Memantine has both neuroprotective and symptomatic treatment effects. While this study involved persons with more advanced AD, Memantine has been used for treatment of persons with earlier stages of the disease. It may be an important edition to the short list of anti-dementia drugs in the United States, especially for persons with more advanced dementia.

Combination Drug Studies

Lecithin and THA Work Well Together

Often two or more drugs are given in combination so that each can help the other do its job. As we saw in the 1986 Summers study, for example, THA and lecithin were successfully combined to produce different but complementary actions. The lecithin increased the availability of acetylcholine in the synapses between neurons, while the THA inhibited the activity of the enzyme that breaks acetylcholine down in the receiving neuron. Together they produced the desired effect: more usable acetylcholine in the brain. In another study, lecithin and THA were given together to a group of Alzheimer's subjects with relatively high education and an average age of 61.5 years; some improvement in learning was noted, particularly among the more mildly impaired (Sitaram et al., 1983).

Lecithin Combined with Choline and Physostigmine

Lecithin has also been paired in studies with physostigmine. One study noted some improvements in long-term memory when lecithin and physostigmine were given together (Peters and Levin, 1982). Another study of the same drug pairing produced even more impressive results. Eight out of the 12 subjects showed clear improvements in recall from long-term memory and a decrease in intrusions—memories seemingly forgotten but later interjected into another context (Thal and Fuld, 1983). The results were repeated in a subsequent trial. Somewhat surprisingly, other studies of this drug combination have shown a greater degree of improvement in more severely impaired subjects.

Combination drug treatments, like single drug treatments, generally have not shown the kind of consistent results for which one might hope. Subjects who share similar characteristics—such as degree of dementia, early or late onset of dementia (before or after age 65), and so forth—do not seem to respond similarly to the drugs. This makes it very difficult to predict subject response or identify any pattern in the study results.

Estrogen, Anti-Inflammatory Agents, and Antioxidants

Several disease-related processes produce cell death. This process also involves apoptosis—programmed cell death. It is a genetically determined process thought to exist and be activated by some stimulus, which causes the orderly breakdown and elimination of cells that are no longer needed. If there were a way to stop this process—to protect and preserve nerve cells along with their synapses and connections—then it might be possible to prevent Alzheimer's disease or at least delay its onset or severity. Scientists are looking at ways to do this. Estrogen may play a role.

Estrogen is a hormone that is thought to have important roles in the brain and other parts of the body in addition to its role in the female reproductive system. Like the antioxidants and anti-inflammatory drugs, estrogen may help nerve cells survive by preventing damage from inflammation and oxidation. There is growing evidence that estrogens serve a normal maintenance role in the same area of the brain most affected by Alzheimer's (Simpkins et al., 1994). Estrogen appears to promote the growth of cholinergic neurons and may interact with apolipoprotein E (Tang et al., 1996). Acting as a neurotropic factor, estrogen stimulates neurite growth and synapse formation in responsive neurons (Henderson et al., 1994). It also seems to work as an antioxidant by stopping the harmful action of oxygen molecules on cells, and is thought to promote cell metabolism.

One study suggest that the increased incidence of Alzheimer's in older women may be due to estrogen deficiency. Estrogen replacement therapy may be useful for preventing or delaying the onset of Alzheimer's disease (Paganini-Hill and Henderson, 1994). Earlier studies showed that women who had taken estrogen after menopause had lower rates of Alzheimer's than those who had not. Estrogen use has even been associated with better cognitive performance in women with Alzheimer's compared to others with the disease who did not use it (Henderson et al., 1994). More recent studies are supportive of the protective role of estrogen but less supportive of it being a helpful treatment for women with AD.

Although a significant role for estrogen may develop in Alzheimer's prevention, estrogen replacement therapy following menopause is not recommended for all women. This factor, and how men might benefit from the protective role of estrogen need further investigation. Cholinergic neurons of the brain have numerous estrogen receptors, which occur on the same neurons that have receptors for nerve growth factor. Does this mean that estrogen and nerve growth factor share a common role in preventing the degeneration of cholinergic neurons? This issue is being addressed by research.

Preventing damage associated with brain inflammation and oxidation helps nerve cells in the brain survive. Studies have shown that persons who take anti-inflammatory drugs or suffer anti-inflammatory diseases such as rheumatoid arthritis have a reduced risk of developing Alzheimer's disease. Another study shows that Japanese leprosy patients who have continuously taken a medication that has anti-inflammatory activity have a low incidence of Alzheimer's. One study identifying the protective role of anti-inflammatories notes that the role may be greater in persons over 70. Anti-inflammatory treatment was also more effective in persons without the apoE4 allele (Breitner, 1996). Anti-inflammatory agents include steroidal medications such as prednisone and nonsteroidal anti-flammatory drugs (NSAIDs). The latter includes over-the-counter drugs such as aspirin and ibuprofen. Indomethacin and naproxen are NSAIDs that require a prescription.

A recently released study indicates that persons taking NSAIDs had half the risk of developing the disease than people who did not use the drugs. Researchers also established for the first time that longer use of these drugs decreases the risk of Alzheimer's disease. Shorter-term use might also reduce the risk. The most commonly used anti-inflammatory drug was ibuprofen. Aspirin and acetaminophen, which is not an NSAID, had little or no effect on reducing risk. The aspirin dosages may have been too low to affect the central nervous system (Stewart, 1997), so aspirin may have an effect at higher doses.

A 6-month study of indomethacin in patients who had Alzheimer's compared to Alzheimer's patients who did not take the drug indicated that those taking the drug had stable cognition. Function declined in patients without the drug. Adverse effects must be carefully monitored and might limit its use (Aisen and Davis, 1994).

The reader is reminded that these findings are still preliminary, and potentially serious side effects are associated with the chronic use of anti-inflammatory drugs, for instance, gastric irritation and bleeding, peptic ulcer disease, and even impaired renal and kidney function. A physician should supervise ongoing use.

Aging and Alzheimer's disease are associated with increased free radical formation. Oxidative stress results when antioxidant defenses are overwhelmed by free radical formation. The beta-amyloid protein glutamate or other toxic factors can also cause free radicals. Antioxidants protect neurons from oxidative damage and could have beneficial effects in Alzheimer's by reducing the free radical formation and preventing the associated cell injury and loss.

Selegiline, or deprenyl, is used in the treatment of Parkinson's disease. It is also an antioxidant. Selegiline and vitamin E (alpha-tocopherol) are both presumed to reduce oxidative stress and to have neuroprotective functions. Vitamin E traps free radicals and interrupts the chain reaction that damages cells. It also prevents cell death caused by glutamate and beta-amyloid protein. Selegiline is thought to act as a scavenger of free radicals (Shihabuddin and Davis, 1996). It may improve cognitive deficits.

The results of a long-anticipated study involving selegiline and vitamin E, given separately and in combination to patients with Alzheimer's, have been published (Sano et al., 1997). The authors chose to focus on functional losses instead of cognitive deterioration. Both drugs were reported to delay functional deterioration as indicated by the decreased need for institutionalization. There were no differences reported in the results of the group receiving the combined treatment and either of the groups receiving individual treatment. Falls and syncope were noted to be more frequent in treatment groups. Treatment with either selegiline or vitamin E slows the progression of the disease in patients with moderately severe AD and is recommended for persons with moderate dementia.

More study of these drugs must be carried out to determine their value in long-term management of Alzheimer's. Vitamin E is available without prescription, but can cause nausea and cramping at high doses. The risk of bleeding in people taking blood thinners, or who have coagulation abnormalities, may increase. A prescription is needed for selegiline.

Statins

Statins are cholesterol-lowering drugs widely used to prevent heart disease and stroke. Higher cholesterol has been implicated as another risk factor for Alzheimer's disease. Scientists have suspected that cardiovascular disease and cholesterol levels were related to dementia. Finding that the cholesterol transport protein apolipoprotein E4 (apoE4) increases the risk for Alzheimer's disease provided one explanation for this relationship. Even more important is the discovery that older people who take statins have a significantly reduced risk of developing Alzheimer's disease and other dementias. These drugs were not specifically designed for treatment or prevention of dementia, but subsequent research will hopefully substantiate the role statins appear to have in the delay and possible prevention of Alzheimer's disease.

Researchers are not certain how statins reduce the risk for Alzheimer's, but evidence is mounting that they reduce the production of the beta-amyloid protein. Beta-amyloid accumulates around brain cells, becomes toxic to these cells, and promotes cell death. It may be the cause of AD.

The fact that a relationship has been found between beta amyloid and cholesterol is very important to research. In animal models of Alzheimer's disease a diet high in cholesterol and fat increases the amount of beta-amyloid in the brain; brains of people with lower cholesterol levels have less brain amyloid. Both beta-amyloid and cholesterol may stimulate an inflammatory response in blood vessels and cause them to constrict, so statin drugs may modulate immune responses by decreasing inflammation. More research must be done, but statins may be capable of delaying the onset or progression of Alzheimer's disease, and may even play a role in prevention of the disease. Statins are currently available by prescription.

We now have several pharmacological approaches for Alzheimer's disease. Prevention and delay of the disease are possible. We do not have a cure, but research is rapidly advancing.

Neuronal Transplants

In the future, it may be possible to graft healthy neuronal tissue onto impaired areas of the Alzheimer's brain, thus stimulating the regeneration of neuron networks and improving certain brain functions. This transplant technique could offer an important alternative for more severely impaired persons, since drug therapies rarely seem to help those with extensive neuron damage.

Neuronal transplants already have been tried on subjects suffering from Parkinson's disease. One such study reported a slowing of degeneration (Moore, 1987), while another reported an improvement in motor functioning (Madrazo et al., 1987). Animal research with neuronal transplants has shown that the technique can achieve desired results for specific behavioral and cognitive impairments (Gash et al., 1985; Merz, 1987; Fine, 1986; Gage et al., 1984).

The use of neuronal transplantation as a treatment for Alzheimer's disease is a growing possibility emerging from nearly two decades of research, particularly with Parkinson's disease. This treatment holds promise for other degenerative brain disorders such as strokes. Implanting cells directly into the brain can restore lost functions. This is accomplished by replacing dead neurons with healthy neurons. For Parkinson's disease, embryonic tissue rich in dopaminergic nerve cells has been injected into the brain. Results of a recent study involving 17 persons who were injected with the dopaminergic neurons taken from embryonic tissue have been quite encouraging (Melton, 2000) in terms of improvement and safety. The success of this approach forces us to look for other sources of neuronal cells.

Major ethical issues are raised when one considers how much fetal tissue would be needed to treat the number of people with Parkinson's disease, Alzheimer's disease, and other degenerative brain disorders. Practical barriers arise as well and become insurmountable when one considers that up to six human fetuses were needed to provide enough tissue to treat one person with Parkinson's disease.

Scientists need to find other sources of healthy cells for implantation. Several new approaches are being investigated. Growing cultures of human cell lines in the laboratory is one alternative. Another is supported by recent findings about stem cells: Stem cells have the ability to divide for indefinite periods in culture and give rise to specialized cells. Embryonic stem cells are derived from the earliest developmental stages of an embryo and can spawn almost any type of cell in the body. These stem cells could be used to repair damage caused by neurological conditions such as Alzheimer's. There may be ways to activate adult stem cells in the brain to replace cells that die or are damaged by the disease. It seems possible that other sources of cells can be developed for neuronal cell transplantation.

Nerve cells outside the body's central nervous system have the capacity to be regenerated after being damaged. The nerve cells of the brain were not thought to have this ability. These cells and others in the body do develop in specific patterns under the direction of special chemicals called nerve growth factors. Scientists are now investigating these chemicals to determine if they might be used to regrow or regenerate deteriorating nerve cells in the brain (Mace and Rabins, 1991). If this process were better understood, it might be possible to stimulate the replacement or regrowth of damaged brain cells. This, in turn, could allow treatment with medications to be better utilized. Some restoration of the pathway necessary for the brain's chemical messengers might be possible.

18

Psychiatric Medications and Dementia

Psychiatric medications can be effective in managing some symptoms of Alzheimer's disease. An overview of these various medications is helpful to caregivers. Since side effects, some quite adverse, can develop, these medications require close monitoring by physicians and family members. Individual responses to psychiatric medications can vary considerably, from clear benefits, to no change, to even worse symptoms. The elderly generally have a lower tolerance for these medications than younger persons, and brain impairments often interfere with the effectiveness of a medication.

A good rule of thumb with psychiatric medications is to start persons at low dosages, increasing dosages slowly. This approach may be frustrating to family members who are seeking rapid relief from some symptoms. It is a safer approach, however, and allows physicians to monitor an individual's response to a medication. Side effects are more likely to occur at higher dosages. If the person is going to experience adverse side effects, these probably will occur in a milder form at a lower dose. Additionally, it is critical to determine over a period of time whether a person can tolerate a specific psychiatric medication; lower doses allow the body to gradually adjust to the medication.

Only a Physician Should Change Prescribed Dosages

Only physicians should change dosages. Family members should consult the physician if side effects develop or if the medication is simply not working. Families should have realistic expectations about changes they can expect; generally medications can produce moderate changes. Target symptoms should be discussed with the prescribing physician, who must be informed of any other medications the patient is currently taking. Family must not change the dosage even if behaviors such as agitation or angry outbursts are still occurring. In fact, more of the medication could create more severe symptoms, which is especially true with major tranquilizers. Administering more medication than prescribed can also create more side effects, which can be dangerous, especially for the person with Alzheimer's disease. The following example illustrates some problems associated with increasing the dosage of a major tranquilizer without the advice of a physician.

Case Example of Harmful Effect of High Dose of Major Tranquilizer

Emma Day, an elderly woman, had been prescribed a 150 mg total daily dosage of a major tranquilizer. This particular medication (Mellaril) had high sedative effects. The dosage had been increased over a month to reduce symptoms of agitation, sleeping difficulties, and delusional beliefs about her husband. These symptoms were reduced but still occurred occasionally. Jim, the husband, had diabetes and severe arthritis. The diabetes was not well controlled, thus causing periods of depression.

On this particular day, Jim was somewhat agitated himself due to fatigue and worry over caregiving and financial problems. He was abrupt and aggravated with Emma's slowness in bathing. He saw her behavior as resistant and uncooperative. As he became more forceful, Emma became more upset. The more he pushed, the more hostile she became. Later she calmed down, but Jim decided on his own to increase her medication. That night he doubled the dosage.

The next morning Emma was a little more confused and sedated; Jim doubled the dosage again. Later that morning she was still in bed, and Jim wanted her to get up. He got her out of bed with some difficulty, pointed her toward the bathroom, and left for another part of the house. On his way he heard her fall. She was not seriously injured, but her shoulder and elbow were badly bruised. For several weeks, Jim had to help her more with dressing and bathing. Emma's fall and Jim's increased workload were direct results of too much tranquilizer given without a doctor's order.

Major Tranquilizers Should Not Be Used as Chemical Restraint

Except in extraordinary circumstances, the use of major tranquilizers as a chemical restraint is inappropriate. This should never be done at home by family members. Two other points are made in the example above: (1) caregivers, particularly those who are older, often have health problems that can interfere with caregiving and their response to daily stressors, and (2) it is to the benefit of the caregiver and patient to use problem-solving and coping skills, rather than to increase medication.

In this chapter, we cover three groups of medications used in treating symptoms associated with dementia or other coexisting psychiatric conditions, such as depression. Side effects are discussed and listed by groups of medications that may produce them. The reasons these medications are prescribed, as well as their generic and brand names, are noted.

Side Effects

Major tranquilizers are the most frequently prescribed medications for symptoms associated with dementia. One potential side effect that must be monitored is *hypotension*. This results in a lowering of blood pressure, which can increase the risk of falls caused by dizziness and loss of balance.

Another type of side effect is called *extrapyramidal reactions,* which causes decreased or slowed movements, muscle rigidity, resting hand tremor, shuffling gait, drooling, and a mask-like face. Some of these symptoms can accompany dementia, particularly if true Parkinson's disease coexists with Alzheimer's disease. The drug-induced or "pseudoparkinsonism" is likely to appear sometime between the first week and two months after beginning treatment with a major tranquilizer. These symptoms can be reduced with careful additions of other medications, which in turn may be discontinued later if the symptoms fade.

When major tranquilizers are given to reduce agitation and restlessness but instead produce these symptoms, the person is having a paradoxical reaction to the medication. The patient cannot sit still, may be constantly pacing, and feels anxious and agitated. In addition, the person may find it difficult to sleep; no position is comfortable. A change in medication, reducing the dosage, or use of an anti-Parkinson-type medication might help some people with this side effect.

If persons with Alzheimer's disease have taken major tranquilizers for a long time, they run the risk of another type of extrapyramidal reaction called tardive dyskinesia. Advancing age can also be a risk factor. This type of side effect is characterized by involuntary lip and tongue motions and writhing movements of the arms and legs. In more severe tardive dyskinesia, speech, eating, walking, and even breathing can be impaired. Reducing the dosage or adding an anti-Parkinson medication does not consistently help reduce this side effect. The best treatment is preventive; that is, avoid the use of major tranquilizers whenever possible or use low dosages.

Another possible side effect is a delirium or reversible dementia that is related to an anticholinergic effect that some major tranquilizers can have. The more common features involve dry mouth, blurred vision, dilated pupils, constipation, urinary retention, nasal congestion, and increased heart rate. A few major tranquilizers can inhibit ejaculation. The cholinergic system of the brain, which is vital to memory functions, is already impaired in Alzheimer's disease. Major tranquilizers and some classes of antidepressants block the function of acetylcholine, the chemical messenger intrinsic to the cholinergic neurons of the brain.

In addition, a syndrome can develop that appears as an acute toxic confusional state. This state is characterized by disorientation, visual hallucinations, irritability, and impaired attention. The syndrome can be treated by discontinuing the drug(s) with anticholinergic effects. Symptoms should clear in 2 to 3 days. The medication can then be changed to one with less anticholinergic properties or resumed if the syndrome developed from a toxic buildup.

Several other side effects can occur with some major tranquilizers. One that applies particularly to elderly persons is greater sensitivity to heat and cold. Weight gain can also occur when taking major tranquilizers. Cardiac side effects, while rare with some of the major tranquilizers, are possible and must be taken into consideration for those patients with heart conditions.

Other side effects can occur but are quite rare. A physician should monitor the Alzheimer's patient carefully, as should family members.

Three groups of psychiatric medications, major tranquilizers, minor tranquilizers, and antidepressants, are described next.

Major Tranquilizers (Neuroleptics or Antipsychotics)

Purpose
Manage symptoms of agitation/anxiety, suspiciousness, hostility, delusions, hallucinations, preoccupations, poor self-care resulting from psychotic state, social withdrawal, uncooperativeness, belligerent and hostile behavior.

Drugs have a tranquilizing or sedating effect. There is an antipsychotic effect or normalizing effect on mood, thought, and behavior.

Side Effects

Drowsiness	Sensitivity to light	Decreased sweating
Dry mouth	Shakiness	Difficulty urinating
Constipation	Muscle spasms in neck/back	Restlessness
Blurred vision	Dizziness/light-headedness	Hypotension
Stiffness	Stuffy nose	Fast heartbeat
Drooling	Decreased sexual ability	Shuffling gait

Any side effects of concern should be brought to the attention of the physician prescribing the medication. The newer atypical antipsychotic medications—risperidone (Risperdal), quetiapine (Seroquel), and olanzapine (Zyprexa)—are associated with more favorable side effect profiles and are being used to treat the behavioral and psychological symptoms of dementia that do not respond to other approaches. Lower doses are often successful. More severe agitation, aggressiveness, delusions, and hallucination may require higher doses.

The mood stabilizers valproic acid (Depakote) and carbamazepine (Tegretol) have been effective in treating these problems when major tranquilizers have not been successful. These medications can be used alone and with antipsychotics and antidepressants to control AD-related noncognitive problems. The following table notes some common major tranquilizers and side effects.

Major Tranquilizers

TRADE NAME	GENERIC NAME	SEDATIVE	ANTI-CHOLINERGIC	EXTRA-PYRAMIDAL
High Potency				
Haldol	Haloperidol	Low	Low	High
Navane	Thiothixene	Low	Low	High
Prolixin	Fluphenazine HCL	Low	Low	High
Stelazine	Trifluoperazine HCL	Moderate	Low	Moderate
Moderate Potency				
Trilafon	Perphenazine	Moderate	Moderate	Moderate
Loxitane	Loxapine Succinate	Moderate	Moderate	Moderate
Moban	Molindone HCL	Moderate	Moderate	Moderate
Low Potency				
Thorazine	Chlorpromazine	High	High	Low
Mellaril	Thioridazine	High	High	Low

Minor Tranquilizers

Minor tranquilizers are used to treat some symptoms that accompany Alzheimer's disease. They may be more appropriate for controlling anxiety/agitation when psychotic features are not evident. These medications can build up in the body over time, thus those medications with a shorter half-life should be used to prevent this buildup. The longer the half-life of a medication, the longer it stays in the body. We note the half-life below and each drug's action rate (rate of onset). In some cases, it may be more appropriate to dispense this medication as needed rather than regularly. We only note the antianxiety agents.

Purpose
Reduce symptoms of anxiety/agitation and related insomnia.

Minor Tranquilizers

GENERIC NAME	BRAND NAME	RATE OF ONSET	HALF-LIFE (HOURS)	DOSE RANGE MG/DAY FOR ELDERLY
Diazepam	Valium	Fastest	26–53	2–10
Clorazepate dipotassium	Tranxene	Fast	30–200	7.5–15
Triazolam	Halcion	Fast	2–5	0.25–0.5
Lorazepam	Ativan	Intermediate	20–200	0.5–4
Chordiazepoxide HCl	Librium	Intermediate	8–28	5–30
Alprazolam	Xanax	Intermediate	6–15	0.125–0.5
Oxazepam	Serax	Intermediate to slow	5–15	10–30
Temazepam	Restoril	Intermediate to slow	12–24	15–30
Prazepam	Centrax	Slow	30-300	10–15

Side Effects

Oversedation	Dizziness	Fatigue
Drowsiness	Light-headedness	Depression
Unusual excitement	Headache	Blurred vision
Nervousness	Irritability (paradoxical)	Breathing problems

As with other medications, use of minor tranquilizers may not be appropriate with other medical conditions. The physician will consider this factor. Withdrawal from this type medication should be supervised by a physician, since there can be problems if the person has taken the medication for a long time.

Antidepressants

While there is some question about how often Alzheimer's patients are depressed, there is no question that depression can precede or coexist with Alzheimer's disease. Some depression can be treated successfully, and the person's mental status will improve. However, side effects are a major concern with antidepressants. Anticholinergic effects can occur with antidepressant medications. While all side effects can be significant, those that produce more confusion and delirium must be prevented. In dementia, these effects compound existing memory and cognitive deficits. Careful use of the appropriate antidepressants can sometimes avoid these side effects. (See Chapter 3 for more detailed information about depression with Alzheimer's.)

Antidepressants

Trade Name	Generic Name	Sedation	Anti- cholinergic	Orthostatic Hypotension
Elavil	Amitriptyline	High	High	High
Asendin	Amoxapine	Moderate	Low	Moderate
Wellbutrin	Bupropion	Low	Low	Low
Annafranil	Clomipramine	High	High	High
Norpramin	Desipramine	Low	Low	Low
Sinnequan/ Adapin	Doxepin	High	Moderate-High	High
Prozac	Fluoxetine	Low	Low	Low
Tofranil	Imipramine	Moderate	Moderate	Moderate
Ludiomil	Maprotiline	High	Low	Low
Pamelor/ Aventyl	Nortriptyline	Low	Low	Low
Paxil	Paroxetine	Low	Low	Low
Zoloft	Sertraline	Low	Low	Low
Desyrel	Trazadone	High	Low	Moderate

The selective serotonin reuptake inhibitors (SSRIs) and other types of new antidepressants are showing promise in treating depression with Alzheimer's and have side effect profiles that are better tolerated than those of tricyclic antidepressants such as amitriptyline and imipramine. New generation antidepressants that are not listed in the table are nefazodone (Serzone), venlafaxine (Effexor), fluvoxamine (Luvox), citalopram (Celexa), and mirtazapine (Remeron).

Purpose
Decrease aspects of depressed mood, improve appetite and sleeping habits, improve social functioning, increase level of energy.

Side Effects

Drowsiness	Increase in heart rate	Hypotension
Dry mouth	Blurred vision	Arrythmias
Urinary retention	Constipation	Weight gain
Nasal congestion	Dizziness/fainting	Stomach upset
Delirium	Tremors	Nausea
Increased appetite for sweets	Slow pulse	

There is some interest in another type of antidepressant medication, the monoamine oxidase inhibitors (MAOs or MAOIs). This antidepressant may be considered when others do not work. However, special care must be taken regarding dietary restrictions and combining MAOIs with other medications. This type of medication also has side effects that must be carefully considered.

Most antidepressant medications take several weeks to a month to reach a therapeutic level. Families must take this into account and be patient. With the elderly, a lower dosage is often initiated to determine how well the antidepressant will be tolerated.

Summary

Psychiatric medications—when carefully prescribed and monitored—can be helpful in the management of psychiatric symptoms associated with Alzheimer's disease. Family must understand why these medications are prescribed and what side effects can be expected. Many times a simple explanation will encourage Alzheimer's patients to take their medications. All psychiatric medications can help with relaxation, and sleep. Families must be responsible for monitoring side effects and reporting these to the prescribing physician. Family members must avoid the temptation to exaggerate or over-report disturbing symptoms in order to increase prescribed dosages. Finally, the help of a professional should be sought to learn more appropriate ways to handle behavior problems and caregiver stress. Depending solely on psychiatric medications will not be sufficient.

An Afterword

When I was about 17, I found an old German drinking mug hidden among the rubble heaped along a creek near my grandparents' home in an isolated rural area near Waco, Texas. The creek, one of my favorite places, was exciting to explore, partly because I could hide in the sea cane and splash through the water, but also because I always hoped I would find something ancient and valuable there. My eyes alert for old coins and arrowheads, I would find instead rusty cans and buckles from old mule harnesses—until the day I spotted the old mug. The handle was broken, but as with many decorative mugs of its type, there were inscriptions on it in old German. Surely, I thought, there was some great truth revealed there, if only I could find someone to translate it.

My family had long since stopped speaking German and had largely forgotten the language, but I searched for someone to help me understand what the words meant. Finally, a high school German teacher found someone to translate the ancient German saying:

> God protect you.
> Things have happened
> Differently than I imagined

and

> God protect you.
> It would have been nice.

In my adolescent frame of mind, I thought at the time the inscription must have related to a long ago youth who had lost his first love. Later when I began working with the elderly and their families, however, that saying deepened in meaning with an application to losses of a very different nature. It is hard to accept lost dreams, unfulfilled at the end of a brief romance. It is quite another thing to see plans and dreams made over decades slowly but unrelentingly ripped apart by an illness that seems to go on forever before it ends.

The ancient saying takes on new meaning when I look at it today, applying those words to the people I work with daily—people with Alzheimer's and their families, engaged in a long goodbye filled with the acceptance of something that is not over, at least not yet.

I remember how the mug had been chipped in a number of places, the porcelain finish cracked from the ravages of time and weather. As a teenager, I imagined how beautiful the mug must have been long ago. I thought of all the history it could have shared with me if it could have talked. Many times, I tried to find ways to restore the mug to its original condition. The chips were filled in, but that did not help much. It could not be restored.

Finally, I accepted the mug for what it was. It was still special, and the message it carried became more meaningful as time passed. I could not put the mug back into its original shape. Its personal value to me cannot be fully appreciated by others. Its original function and purpose has been lost, but it still occupies an honorable place on a bookshelf in my home, and its message serves to remind me that life is full of losses and disappointments, but it is also full of hopes.

It is common to look back on what has happened, the good and the bad, when we have lost someone. In the case of Alzheimer's, your caregiving made a difference to the one you loved. You need to hear that now, to accept it, and to let it make a difference to you.

Any one of us could say that things have worked out differently than we imagined. If we are thinking of only what could have been, we are probably pondering how nice it could have been. We might ponder instead what was and still is—the experiences, the memories, and the accomplishments of one's whole life. And they are nice, too, aren't they?

Behut dich Gott,
(God Protect You)

Howard Gruetzner
Waco, Texas

Worksheets

Use of the Behavior Profile

The Behavior Profile can be helpful to the family caregiver and professional. We will briefly discuss its contents and uses.

Behavioral areas: There are 58 behaviors listed in five categories. These behaviors occur with Alzheimer's disease, although some may not occur as frequently in all persons. Certainly on an infrequent basis some occur with almost everyone. The behavior problem can occur with other conditions, particularly psychiatric disorders.

How often it occurs: Many problems are not significant unless they occur frequently. This is certainly the case with symptoms and their manifestations in Alzheimer's disease. More supervision may be indicated if a behavior occurs frequently, such as not eating or bathing; others need attention even if a behavior occurs infrequently, such as wandering or leaving the stove turned on. The caregiver can use the frequency of a behavior to plan the necessary degree of assistance and supervision. Some behaviors will require more intervention than others. Potential consequences of a behavior will influence the type of intervention and how quickly an intervention must be made. For instance, if a person begins to get lost driving, action must be taken to stop his driving. Denial of problems may occur. This will be bothersome but does not pose a problem unless the person insists on doing things anyway that could have harmful consequences.

How much it bothers you: This will help point out behaviors that need more understanding and attention. For instance, if toileting accidents are extremely bothersome to the caregiver, this area should be addressed to reduce the number of accidents. If the person has delusional ideas, these will probably be accompanied by agitation. These behaviors usually bother caregivers a great deal initially. Psychiatric medication will probably be needed. As caregivers are trying to adjust to the symptoms of Alzheimer's disease, they may be bothered more by a larger number of symptoms.

Completing the profile: For each behavior, check the most appropriate box under the two categories: *How often it occurs* and *How much it bothers you.* If the behavior is no longer a concern because you have taken over that area, scratch through the behavior and the row of boxes to the right. For example, if you pay bills for the person now, scratch through "forgets to pay bills" and the boxes to the right.

Use of the profile: Both caregivers and professionals can use the profile. Caregivers can complete the profile and refer to it to see how behaviors change and how their perception of problems change. The more seriously impaired person will have more behaviors occurring more frequently. This, however, usually occurs over time. If the frequency of numerous behaviors increases abruptly, an underlying medical condition may have developed. Medications might need to be reviewed.

If the person has not been diagnosed, the completed profile will provide information to the physician about the individual's functioning and the caregiver's concerns. The profile is not intended to be a diagnostic tool, but when a person is not testable, a reliable family informant can provide a more complete picture of functioning by completing the profile.

For counseling purposes the profile can indicate behaviors that need more problem-solving work and understanding. It also more quickly identifies behavior areas that are of great concern to the caregiver and thus require additional support and/or intervention.

Behavior Profile

NAME: _____ CAREGIVER: _____

DATE: _____ LENGTH OF CAREGIVING: _____

Check the appropriate category for each behavior.

BEHAVIORAL AREAS

Orientation

	How Often It Occurs				How Much It Bothers You				
	Always	Usually	Sometimes	Never	Extremely	Very much	Moderately	A little	Not at all
1. Fails to recognize friends									
2. Fails to recognize family									
3. Forgets year									
4. Forgets month									
5. Forgets day of week									
6. Unable to name place (town, etc.)									
7. Fails to recognize familiar places									
8. Gets lost in neighborhood (walking)									
9. Gets lost driving									
10. Gets lost in own home									
11. More confused at night									
12. More confused in new places									
13. Wanders and gets lost									

Memory

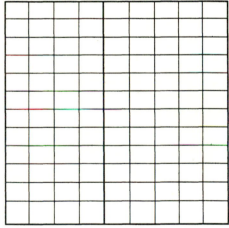

14. Loses/misplaces small items
15. Loses/misplaces valuable things
16. Forgets to pay bills
17. Forgets to eat
18. Unable to recall what was read
19. Forgets to turn things off
20. Forgets what conversation is about
21. Unable to follow what's on TV
22. Forgets to bathe
23. Forgets major events of the day
24. Forgets major events of the week
25. Forgets major events from distant past

Language

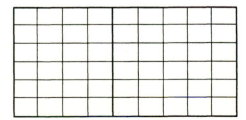

26. Unable to initiate conversation
27. Misunderstands what others say
28. Unable to respond to questions
29. Has trouble finding right words
30. Just speaks in phrases
31. Avoids questions

295

	How Often It Occurs				How Much It Bothers You				
	Always	Usually	Sometimes	Never	Extremely	Very much	Moderately	A little	Not at all
32. Unable to verbalize needs									
33. Repeatedly says same things									
34. What is said makes little sense									

Ambulation/Movement

	Always	Usually	Sometimes	Never	Extremely	Very much	Moderately	A little	Not at all
35. Walks short, shuffling gait									
36. Gait slow and labored									
37. Tires easily when walking									
38. Unable to get up from chair alone									
39. Unable to use stairs									
40. Unable to use eating utensils									
41. Unable to write name									
42. Hands/arms shake									

Behavior Problems

	Always	Usually	Sometimes	Never	Extremely	Very much	Moderately	A little	Not at all
43. Has problems sleeping									
44. Has toileting accidents									
45. Talks excessively about past									
46. Denies problems									
47. Gets upset easily									
48. Becomes physically violent									
49. Shows poor judgment									
50. Has trouble taking medication									
51. Drives unsafely									
52. Very withdrawn, refuses to leave house									
53. Very nervous and restless									
54. Walks and paces constantly									
55. Very suspicious/paranoid									
56. Has delusional ideas									
57. Has hallucinations									
58. Sexually inappropriate									

Other

	Always	Usually	Sometimes	Never	Extremely	Very much	Moderately	A little	Not at all
59.									
60.									
61.									
62.									
63.									

Using the Personal/Social Support Resources

Family members often become isolated in caregiving; however, this is not inevitable. Contact with the outside world can be maintained. As stress and pressures of caregiving build, it is difficult to think of who can help. Thus, it is a good idea to identify persons to call on for assistance before you become overwhelmed by too many demands and have no time to think.

First, it is helpful to evaluate the supports within the family and neighborhood. As independent people, many caregivers like to think they can always take care of themselves, but constant caregiving can change things. They may need much more support and help. Caregivers can turn to family, friends, neighbors, church members, or professionals for help.

We have found in our work that it is often difficult initially for caregivers to complete this form. Too often, only one person is the support for all areas covered by the questions. It is important for others to be considered as backup resources and for the caregiver to begin to rely on at least one or two people to cover some of the areas. Family support groups can be important resources.

Some of the questions point to a need for a more immediate source of security. For example, when the caregiver is frightened, he or she needs to talk to someone quickly. If the behavior of the relative is threatening, the caregiver may want to call the doctor or mental health professional. If the caregiver suspects a burglar is in the house, he or she must call the police.

Different resources may be more appropriate for different questions. Caregivers are encouraged to use this form to examine closely their total support network. A confidant is a valuable resource, but other personal resources may need to be developed.

Personal/Social Support Resources

NAME: _____ DATE: _____

Using your own situation, check the most appropriate Personal/ Social Supports to the right of each question. Try to check at least 3.

	Yourself	Spouse	Children	Other Family	Friends	Neighbors	Church	Pastor/Priest	Doctor	Other Professional	Support Group	Agency Staff	Other
1. Who can you count on for transportation?													
2. Who can you count on for financial help/decisions?													
3. Who helps most with household chores?													
4. Who can you count on to get to appointments?													
5. Who do you enjoy doing things with during the week?													
6. Who can you count on in time of crisis?													
7. Who can you count on when you're physically sick?													
8. Who can you count on to console you when you're very upset?													
9. Who would you seek out when you're frightened?													
10. Who would you talk to when you're lonely?													
11. When you need to talk, who can you count on to listen?													
12. With whom can you really be yourself?													
13. Who do you trust completely?													
14. Who do you feel really appreciates you as a person?													
15. With whom do you have the most frequent contact?													
16. Whose advice are you most likely to accept?													
17. Who supports your independence the most?													

Using your own situation, check the most appropriate Personal/Social Supports to the right of each question. Try to check at least 3.

	Yourself	Spouse	Children	Other Family	Friends	Neighbors	Church	Pastor/Priest	Doctor	Other Professional	Support Group	Agency Staff	Other
18. Who seems to understand you best?													
19. Who helps you to be honest with yourself?													
20. Who helps you keep a positive outlook?													
21. Who do you enjoy being with the most?													
22. Who best understands your current situation?													
23. Who helps you work out your problems most?													
24. Who could temporarily take your place in caregiving?													
25. Who do you trust regarding legal matters?													
26. Who can you talk to about family problems?													

In-Home Care List

This form may be used by family members to determine how much assistance their relatives actually need to perform activities of daily living. Realistic expectations can develop, and this information can be communicated to other persons who help with caregiving. Alzheimer's patients should be encouraged to do what they can for themselves; family members must avoid doing things for them unnecessarily.

Some persons with Alzheimer's disease still live alone. In these cases, the In-Home Care List will help family members to determine how much assistance the person needs.

Nursing homes can use this form to get a better idea of how much assistance the resident will require in daily living activities, socialization, and leisure/recreational activities. This scale is a planning, communication, and monitoring tool. Other professionals may use it to help families secure appropriate community resources.

For each behavior check the category that best describes how it occurs. For example, for the behavior to occur appropriately or as one desires, verbal assistance, physical assistance, or complete supervision may be necessary. On the other hand, there may be no need for assistance of any kind for the behavior to occur as desired on a regular basis. In some cases the behavior may not be carried out as desired or appropriately even with complete supervision. In that case, check that the behavior does not occur appropriately. Put NA for "not applicable" when that behavior does not apply.

Definitions

Without assistance: The behavior occurs appropriately with no assistance or corrective devices (e.g., glasses, hearing aid, walker, etc.).

With verbal assistance: The behavior occurs appropriately or as desired with *only* verbal cues, reminders, instructions, directions, and so forth.

With physical assistance: Verbal assistance is not enough; physical assistance is required for the behavior to occur appropriately; the caregiver physically assists or does for the person; glasses and other adaptive devices represent physical assistance.

With total supervision: The behavior occurs only if totally supervised. Both verbal and physical assistance may be necessary as part of the supervision.

Behavior does not occur appropriately: The behavior does not occur as desired even with assistance and supervision.

In-Home Care List

NAME: _____ DATE: _____

I. Activities of Daily Living

Basic

	Behavior Occurs Appropriately:				Behavior Does Not Occur Appropriately
	Without Assistance	W/Verbal Assistance	W/Physical Assistance	W/Total Supervision	
A. Dresses self					
B. Bathes regularly					
C. Eats regular meals					
D. Takes prescribed medication					
E. Takes over-the-counter medications					
F. Uses bathroom as necessary					
G. Grooms self regularly					
H. Wears clean clothing					

Advanced

A. Prepares meals					
B. Does food shopping					
C. Pays bills					
D. Uses telephone					
E. Uses stove safely					
F. Follows medical advice					
G. Handles money					
H. Washes clothes					
I. Keeps house clean					

J. Follows daily routines
K. Wears suitable clothing for weather
L. Seeks help when needed
M. Drives car
N. Has regular contact with doctor

II. Socialization

A. Leaves house for social activities
B. Good interaction with friends, neighbors
C. Good interaction with spouse
D. Good interaction with other family
E. Expresses self
F. Understands what others say
G. Recognizes familiar people
H. Generally gets along with people

III. Leisure Activities

A. Follows specific instructions
B. Walks in yard
C. Walks in neighborhood
D. Reads newspaper
E. Watches TV
F. Plays games
G. Looks at magazines
H. Enjoys gardening
I. Listens to music
J. Enjoys arts and crafts
K. Does exercise
OTHER:

303

Care Management Stress

This form can be useful for the family caregiver and professionals involved with the caregiver and the Alzheimer's patient. It is another approach to problem solving and making changes in the caregiver situation. Some changes must occur as a result of psychological adjustment, but family support and outside resources can help. For example, when it is hard to accept the diagnosis of Alzheimer's, the caregiver needs time to adjust and plenty of information in order to understand what lies ahead for both patient and caregiver. For a caregiver who experiences frequent financial problems, family meetings to discuss possibilities and an investigation of community resources may prove helpful.

When a caregiver often feels isolated and abandoned, other people showing their care and concern can help. Other statements reflect the caregiver's response to frequent stress. Another cluster of statements may suggest depression or other adjustment problems that may require professional treatment. For example, being overly upset or fatigued, sleeping poorly, or feeling nervous, all suggest the need for more support, counseling, and perhaps treatment for the caregiver.

Family problems or feelings of estrangement may be evident if statements concerning family are rated frequently. These kinds of problems may require counseling or other approaches to bring the family back together or to develop ways to accept dissenting family views.

This stress scale can assist caregivers in assessing how they are coping over the duration of the caregiving experience.

Care Management Stress

CAREGIVER: _____ DATE: _____ AGE: _____

CLIENT: _____ AGE: _____ DURATION OF CAREGIVING: _____

Please check a response for each.

	Never	Rarely	Sometimes	Frequently	Nearly Always
1. I'm uncomfortable leaving my relative alone.					
2. Worries bother me a lot.					
3. I get tired and worn out doing everything.					
4. Family fail to understand what I'm experiencing.					
5. Everyone fails to appreciate what is happening.					
6. Family members could help a lot more.					
7. I'd like to see friends more.					
8. My relative's behavior frightens me.					
9. It's hard now to accept this diagnosis.					
10. It's hard for my family to accept this diagnosis.					
11. I'm feeling more tense and nervous.					
12. I have a lot of financial concerns.					
13. My relative asks too much of me.					
14. I feel abandoned by doctors/professionals.					
15. I feel my health is suffering because of this.					
16. Decisions are hard for me to make.					
17. I feel I need more rest and sleep.					
18. Family members think I should do more.					
19. I feel I need more privacy.					
20. I'm unable to get out to do what I need to.					
21. I'm embarrassed by my relative's behavior.					
22. I get easily upset with my relative.					
23. I feel I need more help.					
24. I feel I'm getting isolated.					
25. I'm afraid of what the future will be.					

Staff Stress Measure

This form is designed for use in nursing homes and day programs that care for Alzheimer's patients. For persons in supervisory and staff development positions, it can be useful in developing training programs and in working individually with employees. Direct care staff have the most contact with the Alzheimer's patient; therefore, they need a better understanding of the illness, how to deal with the behavior, and how to cope with this behavior emotionally. They need skills and sensitivity.

These staff in an open and supportive learning environment can be open and honest about their frustration and fears. They can also be receptive to suggestions when they begin to understand that the behavior of brain-impaired individuals can be more predictable and manageable.

Staff Stress Measure
Dementia Care

All statements below reflect feelings and beliefs that apply to work with residents who have Alzheimer's disease or a similar degenerative dementia. For each statement, check how often you are affected in such a way.

	Never	Rarely	Sometimes	Frequently	Nearly Always
1. Their forgetfulness really gets on my nerves.					
2. I believe these residents should do more for themselves.					
3. I'm afraid these residents will get violent and hurt someone.					
4. I get tired of repeating things to them so much.					
5. Their families just don't appreciate what we do for these people.					
6. Their babbling and rambling speech gets on my nerves.					
7. It's very hard for me to communicate with these people.					
8. I get mad when they deny problems and blame others for things.					
9. I really get tired working with these residents.					
10. It's hard to accept what is happening to these residents.					
11. I get frustrated and angry working with these people.					
12. I think more medication would make it easier to help them.					
13. I have trouble talking to their families.					
14. I take my work with them home with me.					
15. I feel these residents should appreciate our help more.					
16. It worries me these people will wander off.					
17. I feel it takes too long to do things for them.					
18. It bothers me how helpless these residents become.					
19. I believe we should have more training to work with them.					
20. It's difficult to explain their behavior to other residents or families.					

SERVICE/RESOURCE WORKSHEET
Example

Name of agency: ___Home Health Care___

Type of service/resource needed: ___Supervision of Alzheimer's patient in the home and assistance with basic personal care (bathing)___

What the service/resource will accomplish: ___give caregiver time to get away, and do necessary errands, visit, shop___

Agency/individual providing service—contact person: ___Home Health Care: Jodie Smith___

Eligibility requirements (income, age, geographic): ___none for this type of service___

Fees/cost of service: ___$5.00 an hour for 10 hours___

Projected cost of service over time: ___about $200.00 a month times 12 months___

Sliding scale for fee structure: ___none—different hourly rates for total monthly hours___

Insurance coverage—how much, how long: ___none, unless nursing care needed___

In-home and/or office services: ___All services provided in the home___

Benefit of service to family: ___gives caregiver a break, time to do other things___

Other services provided by this agency: ___Agency also has medical equipment, nursing services; occupational, physical, and speech therapists___

Providers recommended by professionals and/or friends: ___This agency and Home Help Health Care (which is $8.00 an hour regardless)___

Self-Help Groups and Organizations That Can Help

Alzheimer's Association

A network of self-support groups exists through the Alzheimer's Association. Groups that have just become affiliated may not be listed here. There are also local support groups in some areas that are not affiliated with the Alzheimer's Association. These groups may be helpful to the caregiver. To find out about a support group in your area, contact the Area Agency on Aging or the Information and Referral Program. The Alzheimer's Association will have information about affiliated groups, and information about the disease and caregiving.

National Office—Alzheimer's Association, 919 N. Michigan Ave., Suite 1000, Chicago, IL 60611-1676; 312-335-8700

The Alzheimer's Association has an Information and Referral Service Line. Through it you can locate the support group nearest you. Call: 800-272-3900.

Alzheimer's Disease Education and Referral Center, P.O. Box 8250, Silver Spring, Maryland 20907-8250; 800-438-4380

American Health Assistance Foundation

The American Health Assistance Foundation (AHAF) is devoted to funding scientific research on Alzheimer's disease as well as other age-related and degenerative diseases. AHAF's Alzheimer's Family Relief Program provides direct emergency financial assistance to persons with Alzheimer's disease and caregivers when no other means are available. The foundation also offers free educational materials on Alzheimer's disease upon request.

The American Health Assistance Foundation, 15825 Shady Grove Road, Suite 140, Rockville, MD 20850; 301-948-3244 or 800-437-2423

Area Agencies on Aging

Area Agencies on Aging carry out implementations of programs for older persons that are indicated by the Older American's Act. The Administration on

Aging has this responsibility at the federal level. Area Agencies on Aging are a local extension of the federal agency. Usually there is a state Department on Aging that governs Area Agencies on Aging for each state. The reader may call the State Department to determine what Area Agency on Aging covers his particular location. State Departments or Area Agencies on Aging can also provide information concerning Nursing Home Ombudsman Programs.

Administration on Aging
330 Independence Avenue
Washington, DC 20201
General Information: 202-472-7257

Alabama—Region IV
Melissa M. Galvin, Executive Director; **Alabama Commission on Aging**, RSA Plaza, Suite 470, 770 Washington Avenue, Montgomery, AL 36130-1851; 334-242-5743; fax: 334-242 5594

Alaska—Region X
Jane Demmert, Director; **Alaska Commission on Aging**, Division of Senior Services, Department of Administration, Juneau, AK 99811-0209; 907-465-3250; fax: 907-465-4716

Arizona—Region IX
Henry Blanco, Program Director; **Aging and Adult Administration**, Department of Economic Security, 1789 West Jefferson Street, #950A, Phoenix, AZ 85007; 602-542-4446; fax: 602-542-6575

Arkansas—Region VI
Herb Sanderson, Director; **Division of Aging and Adult Services**, Arkansas Department of Human Services, P.O. Box 1437, Slot 1412, 1417 Donaghey Plaza South, Little Rock, AR 72203-1437; 501-682-2441; fax: 501-682-8155

California—Region IX
Lynda Terry, Director; **California Department of Aging**, 1600 K Street, Sacramento, CA 95814; 916-322-5290; fax: 916-324-1903

Colorado—Region VIII
Rita Barreras, Director; **Aging and Adult Services**, Department of Social Services, 110 16th Street, Suite 200, Denver, CO 80202-4147; 303-620-4147; fax: 303-620-4191

Connecticut—Region I
Christine M. Lewis, Director of Community Services; **Division of Elderly Services**, 25 Sigourney Street, 10th Floor, Hartford, CT 06106-5033; 860-424-5277; fax: 860-424-4966

Delaware—Region III
Eleanor Cain, Director; **Delaware Division of Services for Aging and Adults with Physical Disabilities**, Department of Health and Social Services, 1901 North DuPont Highway, New Castle, DE 19720; 302-577-4791; fax: 302-577-4793

District of Columbia—Region III
E. Veronica Pace, Director; **District of Columbia Office on Aging**, One Judiciary Square, 9th Floor, 441 Fourth Street, N.W., Washington, DC 20001; 202-724-5622; fax: 202-724-4979

Florida—Region IV
Gema G. Hernandez, Secretary; **Department of Elder Affairs**, Building B, Suite 152, 4040 Esplanade Way, Tallahassee, FL 32399-7000; 904-414-2000; fax: 904-414-2004

Georgia—Region IV
Jeff Minor, Acting Director; **Division of Aging Services, Department of Human Resources**, 2 Peachtree Street N.E., 36th Floor, Atlanta, GA 30303-3176; 404-657-5258; fax: 404-657-5285

Guam—Region IX
Arthur U. San Augstin, Administrator; **Division of Senior Citizens, Department of Public Health and Social Services**, P.O. Box 2816, Agana, Guam 96910; 011-671-475-0263; fax: 671-477-2930

Hawaii—Region IX
Marilyn Seely, Director; **Hawaii Executive Office on Aging**, 250 South Hotel Street, Suite 109, Honolulu, HI 96813-2831; 808-586-0100; fax: 808-586-0185

Idaho—Region X
Lupe Wissel, Director; **Idaho Commission on Aging**, P.O. Box 83720, Boise, ID 83720-0007; 208-334-3833; fax: 208-334-3033

Illinois—Region V
Margo E. Schreiber, Director; **Illinois Department on Aging**, 421 East Capitol Avenue, Suite 100, Springfield, IL 62701-1789; 217-785-2870; Chicago Office: 312-814-2916; fax: 217-785-4477

Indiana—Region V
Geneva Shedd, Director; **Bureau of Aging and In-Home Services, Division of Disability, Aging and Rehabilitative Services**, Family and Social Services Administration, 402 W. Washington Street, #W454, P.O. Box 7083, Indianapolis, IN 46207-7083; 317-232-7020; fax: 317-232-7867

Iowa—Region VII
Dr. Judy Conlint, Executive Director; **Iowa Department of Elder Affairs**, Clemens Building, 3rd Floor, 200 10th Street, Des Moines, IA 50309-3609; 515-281-4646; fax: 515-281-4036

Kansas—Region VII
Connie L. Hubbell, Secretary; **Department on Aging**, New England Building, 503 S. Kansas Avenue, Topeka, KS 66603-3404; 785-296-4986; fax: 785-296-0256

Kentucky—Region IV
Jerry Whitley, Director; **Office of Aging Services**, Cabinet for Families and Children, Commonwealth of Kentucky, 275 East Main Street, Frankfort, KY 40621; 502-564-6930; fax: 502-564-4595

Louisiana—Region VI
Paul "Pete" F. Arcineaux, Jr., Director; **Governor's Office of Elderly Affairs**, P.O. Box 80374, Baton Rouge, LA 70898-0374; 504-342-7100; fax: 504-342-7133

Maine—Region I
Christine Gianopoulos, Director; **Bureau of Elder and Adult Services**, Department of Human Services, 35 Anthony Avenue, State House—Station #11, Augusta, ME 04333; 207-624-5335; fax: 207-624-5361

Maryland—Region III
Sue Fryer Ward, Secretary; **Maryland Department of Aging,** State Office Building, Room 1007, 301 West Preston Street, Baltimore, MD 21201-2374; 410-767-1100; fax: 410-333-7943; E-mail: sfw@mail.ooa.state.md.us

Massachusetts—Region I
Lillian Glickman, Secretary; **Massachusetts Executive Office of Elder Affairs,** One Ashburton Place, 5th Floor, Boston, MA 02108; 617-727-7750; fax: 617-727-9368

Michigan—Region V
Lynn Alexander, Director; **Michigan Office of Services to the Aging,** 611 W. Ottawa, North Ottawa Tower, 3rd Floor, P.O. Box 30676, Lansing, MI 48909; 517-373-8230; fax: 517-373-4092

Minnesota—Region V
James G. Varpness, Executive Secretary; **Minnesota Board on Aging,** 444 Lafayette Road, St. Paul, MN 55155-3843; 612-297-7855; fax: 612-296-7855

Mississippi—Region IV
Eddie Anderson, Director; **Division of Aging and Adult Services,** 750 North State Street, Jackson, MS 39202; 601-359-4925; fax: 601-359-4370; E-mail: ELANDERSON@msdh.state.ms.us

Missouri—Region VII
Andrea Routh, Director; **Division on Aging,** Department of Social Services, P.O. Box 1337, 615 Howerton Court, Jefferson City, MO 65102-1337; 573-751-3082; fax: 573-751-8687

Montana—Region VIII
Charles Rehbein, State Aging Coordinator; **Senior and Long Term Care Division,** Department of Public Health and Human Services, P.O. Box 4210, 111 Sanders, Room 211, Helena, MT 59620; 406-444-7788; fax: 406-444-7743

Nebraska—Region VII
Mark Intermill, Administrator; **Division on Aging,** Department of Health and Human Services, P.O. Box 95044, 1343 M Street, Lincoln, NE 68509-5044; 402-471-2307; fax: 402-471-4619

Nevada—Region IX
Mary Liveratti Administrator; **Nevada Division for Aging Services,** Department of Human Resources, State Mail Room Complex, 3416 Goni Road, Building D, Carson City, NV 89706; 775-687-4210; fax: 775-687-4264

New Hampshire—Region I
Catherine A. Keane, Director; **Division of Elderly and Adult Services,** State Office Park South, 129 Pleasant Street, Brown Building #1, Concord, NH 03301; 603-271-4680; fax: 603-271-4643

New Jersey—Region II
Eileen Bonilla O'Connor, Acting Assistant Commissioner; **New Jersey Division of Senior Affairs,** Department of Health and Senior Services, P.O Box 807, Trenton, NJ 08625-0807; 609-588-3141 or 800-792-8820; fax: 609-588-3601

New Mexico—Region VI
Michelle Lujan Grisham, Director; **State Agency on Aging,** La Villa Rivera Building, 228 East Palace Avenue, Ground Floor, Santa Fe, NM 87501; 505-827-7640; fax: 505-827-7649

New York—Region II
Walter G. Hoefer, Executive Director; **New York State Office for the Aging,** 2 Empire State Plaza, Albany, NY 12223-1251; 518-474-5731 or 800-342-9871; fax: 518-474-0608

North Carolina—Region IV
Karen E. Gottovi, Director; **Division of Aging,** Department of Health and Human Services, 2101 Mail Service Center, Raleigh, NC 27699-2101; 919-733-3983; fax: 919-733-0443

North Dakota—Region VIII
Linda Wright, Director; **Aging Services Division,** Department of Human Services, 600 South 2nd Street, Suite 1C, Bismarck, ND 58504; 701-328-8910; fax: 701-328-8989

North Mariana Islands—Region IX
Ana DLG Flores, Administrator, Director; **CNMI Office on Aging,** P.O. Box 2178, Commonwealth of the Northern Mariana Islands, Saipan, MP 96950; 670-233-1320/1321; fax: 670-233-1327/0369

Ohio—Region V
Joan W. Lawrence, Director; **Ohio Department of Aging,** 50 West Broad Street, 9th Floor, Columbus, OH 43215-5928; 614-466-5500; fax: 614-466-5741

Oklahoma—Region VI
Roy R. Keen, Division Administrator; **Aging Services Division,** Department of Human Services, P.O. Box 25352, 312 N.E. 28th Street, Oklahoma City, OK 73125; 405-521-2281/2327; fax: 405-521-2086

Oregon—Region X
Roger Auerbach, Administrator; **Senior and Disabled Services Division,** 500 Summer Street, N.E., 2nd Floor, Salem, OR 97310-1015; 503-945-5811; fax: 503-373-7823

Palau—Region X
Lillian Nakamura, Director; **State Agency on Aging,** Republic of Palau, Koror, PW 96940; 9-10-288-011-680-488-2736; fax: 9-10-288-680-488-1662 or 1597

Pennsylvania—Region III
Richard Browdie, Secretary; **Pennsylvania Department of Aging,** Commonwealth of Pennsylvania, 555 Walnut Street, 5th Floor, Harrisburg, PA 17101-1919; 717-783-1550; fax: 717-772-3382

Puerto Rico—Region II
Ruby Rodriguez Ramirez, M.H.S.A.. Executive Director; Commonwealth of Puerto Rico, **Governor's Office of Elderly Affairs,** Call Box 50063, Old San Juan Station, PR 00902; 787-721-5710, 721-4560, 721-6121; fax: 787-721-6510; E-mail: ruby-rodz@prtc.net

Rhode Island—Region I
Barbara A. Raynor, Director; **Department of Elderly Affairs,** 160 Pine Street, Providence, RI 02903-3708; 401-277-2858; fax: 401-277-2130

American Samoa—Region IX
Lualemaga E. Faoa, Director; **Territorial Administration on Aging,** Government of American Samoa, Pago Pago, American Samoa 96799; 011-684-633-2207; fax: 011-864-633-2533/7723

South Carolina—Region IV
Elizabeth Fuller, Deputy Director; **Office of Senior and Long-Term Care Services,** Department of Health and Human Services, P.O. Box 8206, Columbia, SC 29202-8206; 803-898-2501; fax: 803-898-4515; E-mail: FullerB@DHHS.State.sc.us

South Dakota—Region VIII
Gail Ferris, Administrator; **Office of Adult Services and Aging,** Richard F. Kneip Building, 700 Governors Drive, Pierre, SD 57501-2291; 605-773-3656; fax: 605-773-6834

Tennessee—Region IV
James S. Whaley, Executive Director; **Commission on Aging,** Andrew Jackson Building, 9th floor, 500 Deaderick Street, Nashville, TN 37243-0860; 615-741-2056; fax: 615-741-3309

Texas—Region VI
Mary Sapp, Executive Director; **Texas Department on Aging,** 4900 North Lamar, 4th Floor, Austin, TX 78751-2316; 512-424-6840, fax: 512-424-6890

Utah—Region VIII
Helen Goddard, Director; **Division of Aging and Adult Services,** Box 45500, 120 North 200 West, Salt Lake City, UT 84145-0500; 801-538-3910; fax: 801-538-4395

Vermont—Region I
David Yavocone, Commissioner; **Vermont Department of Aging and Disabilities,** Waterbury Complex, 103 South Main Street, Waterbury, VT 05671-2301; 802-241-2400; fax: 802-241-2325; E-mail: dyaco@dad.state.vt.us

Virginia—Region III
Dr. Ann Magee, Commissioner; **Virginia Department for the Aging,** 1600 Forest Avenue, Suite 102, Richmond, VA 23229; 804-662-9333; fax: 804-662-9354

Virgin Islands—Region II
Ms. Sedonie Halbert, Commissioner; **Senior Citizen Affairs,** Virgin Islands Department of Human Services, Knud Hansen Complex, Building A, 1303 Hospital Ground, Charlotte Amalie, VI 00802; 340-774-0930; fax: 340-774-3466

Washington—Region X
Ralph W. Smith, Assistant Secretary; **Aging and Adult Services Administration,** Department of Social and Health Services, P.O. Box 45050, Olympia, WA 98504-5050; 360-493-2500; fax: 360-438-8633

West Virginia—Region III
Gaylene A. Miller, Commissioner; **West Virginia Bureau of Senior Services,** Holly Grove, Building 10, 1900 Kanawha Boulevard East, Charleston, WV 25305; 304-558-3317; fax: 304-558-0004

Wisconsin—Region V
Donna McDowell, Director; **Bureau of Aging and Long-Term Care Resources,** Department of Health and Family Services, P.O. Box 7851, Madison, WI 53707; 608-266-2536; fax: 608-267-3203

Wyoming—Region VIII
Wayne Milton, Administrator; **Office on Aging,** Department of Health, 117 Hathaway Building, Room 139, Cheyenne, WY 82002-0710; 307-777-7986; fax: 307-777-5340

Internet and World Wide Web Resources

The Internet and World Wide Web are important resources for caregivers. I have listed several helpful Web sites for Alzheimer's disease and for caregiving. The reader can find many more by using a Web browser to search the Internet for the word "Alzheimer's" or "caregiver." Many sites include chat rooms and e-mail for caregivers to share their problems and solutions and recognize that others appreciate their experiences. Addresses change, but usually you are redirected to the new Web site.

For Alzheimer's disease:

Alzheimer's Association of Australia
http://www.alzheimers.org.au/

Alzheimer's.Com
http://www.alzheimers.com/

Alzheimer's Disease Education and Referral (ADEAR), The National Institute on Aging
http://www.alzheimers.org/

Alzheimer's Disease International
http://www.alz.co.uk/

Alzheimer's Disease Society
http://www.alzheimers.org.uk/

Alzheimer's Disease Society, London, England
http://www.alzheimers.org.uk/alzheimers/

Alzheimer's Europe (most languages)
http://www.alzheimer-europe.org/

Alzheimer Research Forum
http://www.alzforum.org/

Alzheimer's Society of Canada
http://www.alzheimer.ca/

Alzheimer Italia (Italy)
http://www.alzheimer.it/

Asociacion Mexicana de Alzheimer y Enfermedades Similares
http://www.spin.commx/alzheimer/

Association of Family Caring for Demented Elderly (Japan)
http://www2f.meshnet.or.jp/~boke/boke2

Doctor's Guide to Alzheimer's Disease Information and Resources
http://www.pslgroup.com

John Hopkins Health Information
http://www.intelihealth.com.

National Alzheimer's Association
http://www.alz.org/

Mayo Health Oasis Alzheimer's Resource Center
http://www.mayohealth.org/

For Caregiving:

AARP
http://www.aarp.org/

Administration on Aging
http://www.aoadhhs.gov/

Caregiving Online
http://www.caregiving.com/

Family Caregiver Alliance
http://www.caregiver.org/

Family Caregivers Association
http://www.nfcares.org/

Mediconsult.com: Senior Health and Caregiving-
http://www.mediconsult.com/

National Alliance for Caregiving
http://www.caregiving.org/

Senior-Directions.Com
http://www.senior-directions.com./

Bibliography

Agbayewa, O. M. "Earlier Psychiatric Morbidity in Patients with Alzheimer's Disease." *Journal of the American Geriatric Society,* 34 (1986):561–564.

Aisen, P., and Davis, K. "Inflammatory Mechanisms in Alzheimer's Disease: Implications for Therapy." *American Journal of Psychiatry,* 151(1994):1105–1113.

American Psychiatric Association. *Diagnostic and Statistical Manual of Mental Disorders,* 4th ed. Washington, DC, 1994.

Aneshensel, C. S., et al. *Profiles in Caregiving: The Unexpected Career.* San Diego: Academic Press, 1995.

Backman, L., et al. "Episodic Remembering in a Population-Based Sample of Nonagenarians: Does Major Depression Exacerbate the Memory Deficits Seen in Alzheimer's Disease?" *Psychology and Aging,* 11(1996):649–657.

Ball, M. J. "Granulovacuolar Degeneration." In *Alzheimer's Disease—The Standard Reference,* Reisberg, B., ed., pp. 62–68. New York: The Free Press, 1983.

Ball, M. J., et al. "A New Definition of Alzheimer's Disease: A Hippocampal Dementia." *The Lancet* (January 5, 1985):14–16.

Bartus, R. T., et al. "The Cholinergic Hypothesis of Geriatric Memory Dysfunction." *Science,* 217(1982):408–417.

Beaumont, J. G. *Introduction to Neuropsychology.* New York: Guilford Press, 1983.

Blacker, D., et al. "Alpha-2 Macroglobulin Is Genetically Associated with Alzheimer's Disease." *Nature Genetics,* 19(1998):357–360.

Blass, J. P., et al. "To the Editor." *New England Journal of Medicine* (1983): 309.

Blazer, D. "Evaluating the Family of the Elderly Patient." In *A Family Approach to Health Care of the Elderly,* D.Blazer and I. Siegler, eds., pp. 13–32. Menlo Park, CA: Addison-Wesley, 1984.

Blenkner, M. "Social Work and Family Relationships in Later Life, with Some Thoughts on Filial Maturity" In *Social Structure and the Family: Generational Relations,* E. Shanas and F. G. Streib, eds. Englewood Cliffs, NJ: Prentice-Hall, 1965.

Bloom. T. E., et al. *Brain, Mind, Behavior.* New York: W. H. Freeman and Company, 1985.

Bodnar, J. C., and Kiecolt-Glaser, J. K. "Caregiver Depression After Bereavement: Chronic Stress Isn't Over When It's Over." *Psychology and Aging,* 9 (1994):372–380.

Bondareff, W. "Age and Alzheimer's Disease." *The Lancet* (June 25, 1983):1447.

Bondareff, W. "Biomedical Perspective of Alzheimer's Disease and Dementia in the Elderly." In *The Dementias: Policy and Management,* M. L. M. Gilhooly et al., eds., pp. 13–37. Englewood Cliffs, NJ: Prentice-Hall, 1986.

Breitner, J. "Inflammatory Processes and Anti-Inflammatory Drugs in Alzheimer's Disease: A Current Appraisal." *Neurobiology of Aging,* 17(1996):789–794.

Breitner, J. C. S., and Folstein, M. F. "Familial Alzheimer Dementia: A Prevalent Disorder with Specific Clinical Features." *Psychiatric Medicine*, 14(1984):63–80.

Breitner, J., and Gau, B. "Inverse Association of Anti-Inflammatory Treatments and Alzheimer's Disease: Initial Results of a Co-Twin Study." *Neurology*, 44(1994): 227–232.

Brookmeyer, R., et al. "Projections of Alzheimer's Disease in the United States and the Public Health Impact of Delaying Disease Onset." *American Journal of Public Health*, 88(1998):1337–1342.

Brun, A. "An Overview of Light and Electron Microscopic Changes." In *Alzheimer's Disease: The Standard Reference*, B. Reisberg, ed., pp. 37–48. New York: The Free Press, 1983.

Brun, A. "The Structural Development of Alzheimer's Disease." *DMB, Gerontology*, 1(1985):25–27.

Bruno, G., et al. "Muscarinic Agonist Therapy of Alzheimer's Disease." *Archives of Neurology*, 43(1986):459–661.

Callahan, D. "Families as Caregivers: The Limits of Morality." *Archives of Physical Medicine and Rehabilitation*, 69(1988):323–328.

Carlsson, A. "Changes in Neurotransmitter Systems in the Aging Brain and in Alzheimer's Disease." In *Alzheimer's Disease: The Standard Reference*, B. Reisberg, ed., pp. 100–106. New York: The Free Press, 1983.

Carlsson, A. "Neurotransmitter Changes in the Aging Brain." *DMB, Gerontology*, 1(1985):4043.

Chui, H. C., et al. "Clinical Subtypes of Dementia of the Alzheimer's Type." *Neurology*, 35(1985):1544–1550.

Clyburn, L. D., et al. "Predicting Caregiver Burden and Depression in Alzheimer's Disease." *Journal of Gerontology: Social Sciences*, 55B(January 2000):S2–S13.

Cohen, D. "The Subjective Experience of Alzheimer's Disease: The Anatomy of an Illness as Perceived by Patient and Families." *The American Journal of Alzheimer's Care and Related Disorders and Research*, (May/June 1991):6–11.

Cohen, D., and Eisdorfer, C. *The Loss of Self—A Family Resource for the Care of Alzheimer's Disease and Related Disorders*. New York: W. W. Norton and Company, 1986.

Cohen, S., and Whiteford, W. *Caregiving with Grace*. Video Production. Baltimore Life Care, Inc. 1987.

Conley, Charles, M.D. Personal communication with author, July 1987.

Cooper, S. J. "Drug Treatments, Neurochemical Change and Human Memory Impairment." In *Clinical Management of Memory Problems*, Barbara Wilson and Nick Moffat, eds., pp. 132–147. London: Aspen Publication, 1984.

Corder, E., et al. "Gene Dose of Apolipoprotein E Type 4 Allele and the Risk of Alzheimer's Disease in Late-Onset Families." *Science*, 261(1993):921–923.

Coyle, J. T., et al. "Alzheimer's Disease: A Disorder of Cortical Cholinergic Innervation." *Science*, 219(1983):1184–1189.

Craft, S., et al. "Enhancement of Memory in Alzheimer's Disease with Insulin and Somatostatin, But Not Glucose." *Archives of General Psychiatry*, 56(1999):1135–1140.

Cummings, J. L., and Benson, D. F. *Dementia: A Clinical Approach*. Boston: Butterworths, 1983, pp. 35–167.

Cummings, J. L., et al. "Alzheimer's Disease: Etiologies, Pathophysiology, Cognitive Reserve and Treatment Opportunities." *Neurology*, 51S(1998):2–17.

Davies, P. "The Genetics of Alzheimer's Disease: A Review and a Discussion of the Implications." *Aging*, 7(1986):459–466.

Davies, P., and Wolozin, B. L. "Recent Advances in the Neurochemistry of Alzheimer's Disease." *Journal of Clinical Psychiatry*, 48(1987):23–30.

DeKosky, S. "Advances in the Biology of Alzheimer's Disease." In *The Dementias: Diagnosis, Management and Research*, M. Weiner, ed., pp. 313–330. Washington, D. C. : American Psychiatric Press, Inc., 1996.

Devanand, D. P. "The Interrelations Between Psychosis, Behavioral Disturbance, and Depression in Alzheimer's Disease." *Alzheimer's Disease and Related Disorders,* 13(November 1999):S33–S38.

Doody, Rachelle S. "Therapeutic Standards in Alzheimer's Disease." *Alzheimer's Disease and Associated Disorders,* 13(November 1999):S20–S26.

Dunn, A., and Brody, S. *Functional Chemistry of the Brain.* New York: Spectrum Publications, 1974.

Dura, J. R., et al. "Spousal Caregiver's of Persons with Alzheimer's and Parkinson's Disease Dementia: A Preliminary Comparison." *The Gerontologist,* 30(1990):332–336.

Dysken, M. W. "A Review of Recent Clinical Trials in the Treatment of Alzheimer's Dementia." *Psychiatric Annals,* 17(1987):178–191.

Ellis, Albert. *A New Guide to Rational Living.* North Hollywood, CA: Wilshire Books, 1975.

Etienne, P. "Treatment of Alzheimer's Disease with Lecithin." In *Alzheimer's Disease: The Standard Reference,* B. Reisberg, ed., pp. 353–354. New York: The Free Press, 1983.

Evans, D. A. "Estimated Prevalence of Alzheimer's Disease in the United States." *The Milbank Quarterly,* 68(1990):267–289.

Eyde, D., and Rich, J. *Psychological Distress in Aging: A Family Management Model.* Rockville, MD: Aspen Publications, 1983.

Farran, C.J., and Keane-Hagerty, E. "Twelve Steps for Caregivers." *American Journal of Alzheimer's Care and Related Disorders and Research,* 4(Nov/Dec 1989):38–41.

Ferris, S. H. "Neuropeptides in the Treatment of Alzheimer's Disease." In *Alzheimer s Disease: The Standard Reference,* B. Reisberg, ed., pp. 369–373. New York: The Free Press, 1983.

Fine, A. "Transplantation in the Central Nervous System." *Scientific American,* 255(1986): 52–59.

Folstein, M. F., et al. "The Meaning of Cognitive Impairment in the Elderly." *Journal of the American Geriatric Society,* 33(1985):228–235.

Fovall, P., Dysken, M. W., and Davis, J. M. "Treatment of Alzheimer's Disease with Choline Salts." In *Alzheimer's Disease: The Standard Reference,* B. Reisberg, ed., pp. 346–353. New York: The Free Press, 1983.

Gage, F. H., et al. "Intrahippocampal Septal Grafts Ameliorate Learning Impairments in Aged Rats." *Science,* 225(1984):533–536.

Gallagher, D., Rose, J., Rivera, P., Lovett, S., and Thompson, L. "Prevalence of Depression in Family Caregivers." *Gerontologist,* 29(1989):449–456.

Garity, J. "Stress, Learning Style, Resilience Factors, and Ways of Coping in Alzheimer's Family Caregivers." *American Journal of Alzheimer's Disease,* 12(July/August 1997): 171–178.

Gash, D. M., et al. "Neuronal Transplantation: A Review of Recent Developments and Potential Applications to the Aged Brain." *Neurobiology of Aging,* 6(1985):131–150.

Gignac, M. A. M., and Gottlieb, B. H. "Caregiver's Appraisals of Efficacy in Coping with Dementia." *Psychology and Aging,* 11(1996):214–225.

Goldsmith, M. F. "Attempts to Vanquish Alzheimer's Disease Intensify, Take New Paths." *Journal of the American Medical Association,* 251(1984):1805–1807, 1811–1812.

Gottfries, C. G. "Neurotransmitters in the Brains of Patients with Dementia Disorders." *DMB, Gerontology,* 1(1985):44–47.

Greenwald, B. S., et al. "Neurotransmitter Deficits in Alzheimer's Disease." *Journal of the American Geriatric Society,* 31(1983):310–316.

Gwyther, L. "Letting Go: Separation-Individuation in a Wife of an Alzheimer's Patient." *Gerontologist,* 30(1990):698–702.

Haley, W. E. "The Family Caregiver's Role in Alzheimer's Disease." *Neurology,* 48(May 1997):S25–S29.

Haley, W. E., et al. "Psychological, Social and Health Consequences of Caring for a Relative with Senile Dementia." *Journal of the American Geriatric Society,* 35(1987): 405–411.

Haley, W. E., et al. "Psychological, Social and Health Impact of Caregiving: A Comparison of Black and White Dementia Family Caregivers and Non-Caregivers." *Psychology and Aging,* 10(1995):540–552.

Harris, P. B., and Sterin, G. J., et al. " Insider's Perspective: Defining and Preserving the Self of Dementia." *Journal of Mental Health and Aging,* 5(1999):241–256.

Henderson, V., et al. "Estrogen Replacement Therapy in Older Women." *Archives of Neurology,* 51(1994):896–900.

Henig, R. *The Myth of Senility: Misconceptions About the Brain and Aging.* Doubleday: Anchor Press, 1981.

Henry, J. P. "Relation of Psychosocial Factors to the Senile Dementias." *In The Dementias: Policy and Management,* M. L. Gilhooley et al.,'eds., pp. 38–65. Englewood Cliffs, NJ: Prentice-Hall, 1986.

Hill, P. H., and Henderson, V. "Estrogen Deficiency and Risk of Alzheimer's Disease in Women." *American Journal of Epidemiology,* 140(1994):256–261.

Hirai, Shunsaku. "Alzheimer's Disease: Current Therapy and Future Therapeutic Strategies." *Alzheimer's Disease and Associated Disorders,* 14(2000):S11–S17.

Hyman, B. T., et al. "Alzheimer's Disease: Cell-Specific Pathology Isolates the Hippocampal Formation." *Science,* 225(1984):1168–1170.

Iqbal, K., and Wisniewski, H. "Neurofibrillary Tangles." In *Alzheimer's Disease: The Standard Reference,* B. Reisberg, ed., pp. 48–57. New York: The Free Press, 1983.

Jenike, M. A. *Handbook of Geriatric Psychopharmacology.* Littleton, MA: PSG Publishing Co., Inc., 1985.

Jenike, M. A., et al. "Combination Therapy with Lecithin and Ergoloid Mesylates for Alzheimer's Disease." *Journal of American Psychiatry,* 47(1986):249–251.

Jorm, A. F. "Subtypes of Alzheimer's Dementia: A Conceptual Analysis and Critical View." *Psychological Medicine,* 15(1985):543–553.

Justice, B. *Who Gets Sick: Thinking and Health.* Houston, TX: Peak Press, 1987.

Katzman, R. "The Prevalence and Malignancy of Alzheimer's Disease: A Major Killer." *Archives of Neurology,* 33(1976):217.

Katzman, R. "Current Research on Alzheimer's Disease in a Historical Perspective." In *Alzheimer's Disease: Cause(s), Diagnosis, Treatment and Care,* Z. Khachaturian and T. Radebaugh, eds., pp. 15–29. New York: CRC Press, Inc., 1996.

Kaye, W. H., Sitaram, N., et al. "Modest Facilitation of Memory in Dementia with Combined Lecithin and Anticholinesterase Treatment." *Biological Psychiatry,* 17(1982): 275–280.

Kemper, T. "Neuroanatomical and Neuropathological Changes in Normal Aging and in Dementia." In *Clinical Neurology of Aging,* M. Albert, ed. New York: Oxford University Press, 1984.

Kiecolt-Glaser, J. K., et al. "Spousal Caregivers of Dementia Victims: Longitudinal Changes in Immunity and Health." *Psychosomatic Medicine,* 53(1991): 345–362.

Kitwood, T. "Person and Process in Dementia." *International Journal of Geriatric Psychiatry,* 8(1993):541–545.

Knop, D. S., et al. "In Sickness and in Health: An Exploration of the Perceived Quality of the Marital Relationship, Coping, and Depression in Caregivers of Spouses with Alzheimer's Disease." *Journal of Psychosocial Nursing and Mental Health Services,* 36(1998):16–21.

Kolb, B., and Whishaw, I. *Fundamentals of Human Neuropsychology.* San Francisco: W. H. Freeman and Co., 1980.

Kubler-Ross, E. *On Death and Dying.* New York: Macmillan, 1969.

Lawton, M. P. "Environmental Approaches to Research and Treatment of Alzheimer's Disease." In *Alzheimer's Disease Treatment and Family Stress: Directions for Research,* pp. 340–362. U.S. Department of Health and Human Services, DHHS Publication No. (ADM) 89-1569, 1989.

Leon, J., et al "Alzheimer's Disease Care: Costs and Potential Savings." *Health Affairs,* 17(1998):206–216.

Mace, N. "The Management of Problem Behaviors." In *Dementia Care: Patient, Family, and Community,* N. Mace, ed., pp. 74–112. Baltimore: John Hopkins University Press, 1990.

Mace, N., and Rabins, P. *The 36-Hour Day.* New York: John Hopkin's University Press, 1985.

Mace, N., and Rabins, P. *The 36-Hour Day,* rev. ed. Baltimore: John Hopkins University Press, 1991.

Madrazo, L., et al. "Open Microsurgical Autograft of Adrenal Medulla to the Right Caudate Nucleus in Two Patients with Intractable Parkinson's Disease." *New England Journal of Medicine,* 316(1987):831–834.

Markesbery, W. "Trace Elements in Alzheimer's Disease." In *Alzheimer's Disease: Cause(s), Diagnosis, Treatment and Care,* Z. Khachaturian and T. Radebaugh, eds., pp. 233–236. New York: CRC Press, Inc., 1996.

Mayeux, R. "Putative Risk Factors for Alzheimer's Disease." In *Alzheimer's Disease: Cause(s), Diagnosis, Treatment and Care,* Z. Khachaturian and T. Radebaugh, eds., pp. 39–49. New York: CRC Press, Inc., 1996.

Mayeux, R., et al. "Heterogeneity in Dementia of the Alzheimer's Type: Evidence of Subgroups." *Neurology,* 35(1985):435–461.

McGreer, P., and McGreer, E. "Neuroimmune Mechanisms in the Pathogenesis of Alzheimer's Disease." In *Alzheimer's Disease: Cause(s), Diagnosis, Treatment and Care,* Z. Khachaturian and T. Radebaugh, eds., pp. 217–225. New York: CRC Press, Inc., 1996.

Melton, L. "Neural Transplantation: New Cells of Old Brains." *The Lancet,* 355(June 17, 2000):2142.

Merz, B. "Adrenal-to-Brain Transplants Improve the Prognosis for Parkinson's Disease." *Journal of the American Medical Association,* 257(1987):2691–2692.

Meyer, M. R., et al. "APOE Genotype Predicts When—Not Whether—One Is Predisposed to Develop Alzheimer Disease." *Nature Genetics,* 19(1998):321–322.

Migliorelli, R., et al. "Prevalence and Correlates of Dysthymia and Major Depression Among Patients with Alzheimer's Disease." *American Journal of Psychiatry,* 152(January 1995):37–44.

Miller, J. "Family Support of the Elderly." *Aging and Health Promotion,* Collected works by T. Wells. Rockville, MD: Aspen Publications, 1982.

Mittelman, M., et al. "A Comprehensive Support Program: Effect on Depression in Spouse-Caregivers of AD Patients." *The Gerontologist,* 35(1995):792–802.

Mohs, R. C., et al. "Defining Treatment Efficacy in Patients with Alzheimer's Disease." In *Alzheimer's Disease: A Report of Progress in Research* (Aging, Vol. 19), S. Corkin et al., eds. pp. 351–356. New York: Raven Press, 1982.

Mohs, R. C., Davis, B. M., et al. "Clinical Studies of the Cholinergic Deficit in Alzheimer's Disease." *Journal of the American Geriatric Society,* 33(1985):749–757.

Moore, R. Y. "Parkinson's Disease—A New Therapy?" *New England Journal of Medicine,* 316(1987):872–873.

Nee, L. E., et al. "A Family with Histologically Confirmed Alzheimer's Disease." *Archives of Neurology,* 40(1983):203–208.

O'Connor, J. "Drug Gets Impressive Results in Alzheimer's Patients." *Psychiatric News,* 21(Dec. 5, 1986):1, 7, 25.

Paganini-Hill, A., and Henderson, V. W. "Estrogen Deficiency and Risk of Alzheimer's Disease in Women." *American Journal of Epidemiology,* 140(1994):256–261.

Payne, J. L., et al. "Relationship of Cognitive and Functional Impairment to Depressive Features in Alzheimer's Disease and Other Dementias." *Journal of Neuropsychiatry and Clinical Neurosciences,* 10(Fall 1998):440–447.

Pearlin, L., Turner, H., and Semple, S. "Coping and the Mediation of Caregiver Stress." In *Alzheimer's Disease Treatment and Family Stress: Directions for Research*, pp. 198–217. Washington, DC: U.S. Department of Health and Human Services, 1989.

Pearlin, L., et al. "Caregiving and the Stress Process: An Overview of Concepts and Their Measures." *Gerontologist*, 30(1990):583–594.

Pericak-Vance, et al. "Linkage Studies in Familial Alzheimer's Disease: Evidence for Chromosome 19 Linkage." *American Journal of Human Genetics* 48(1991):1034–1050.

Perry, E. K., and Perry, R. H. "Acetylcholinesterase in Alzheimer's Disease." In *Alzheimer's Disease: The Standard Reference*, B. Reisberg, ed., pp. 93–99. New York: The Free Press, 1983.

Perry, E. K., and Perry, R. H. "A Review of Neuropathological and Neurochemical Correlates of Alzheimer's Disease." *DMG, Gerontology*, 1(1985):27–34.

Peskind, E. "Neurobiology of Alzheimer's Disease." *Journal of Clinical Psychiatry*, 57(Supplement)(1996):5–8.

Peters, B. H., and Levin, H. S. "Chronic Oral Physostigmine and Lecithin Administration in Memory Disorders of Aging." In *Alzheimer's Disease: A Report of Progress in Research* (Aging, Vol. 19), S. Corkin et al., eds., pp. 42–46. New York: Raven Press, 1982.

Prien, R. F. "Psychostimulants in the Treatment of Senile Dementia." In *Alzheimer's Disease: The Standard Reference*, B. Reisberg, ed., pp. 381–386. New York: The Free Press, 1983.

Pruchno, R., and Resch, N. "Husbands and Wives as Caregivers: Antecedents of Depression and Burden." *Gerontologist*, 29(1989):159–165.

Prusiner, S. B. "Some Speculations About Prions, Amyloid, and Alzheimer's Disease." *New England Journal of Medicine*, 310(1984):661–663.

Reisberg, B. *A Guide to Alzheimer's Disease: For Families, Spouses and Friends*. New York: The Free Press, 1981.

Reisberg, B., et al. "Signs, Symptoms and Course of Age-Associated Cognitive Decline." In *Alzheimer's Disease: A Report of Progress in Research* (Aging, Vol. 19), S. Corkin et al., eds., pp. 177–182. New York: Raven Press, 1982.

Reisberg, B., et al. "Effects of Naloxone in Senile Dementia." *New England Journal of Medicine*, 308(1983):721–722.

Reisberg, B., et al. "Memantine in Moderately Severe to Severe Alzheimer's Disease (AD): Results of a Placebo-Controlled 6-Month Trial." Presented at the World Alzheimer's Congress 2000. 7th International Conference on Alzheimer's Disease and Related Disorders, July 13, 2000, Washington, D.C.

Restak, Richard M. *The Brain*. New York: Bantam Books, 1984.

Rogers, J., et al. "Immune-Related Mechanisms of Alzheimer's Disease Pathogenesis." In *Alzheimer's Disease: New Treatment Strategies*, Z. Khachaturian and J. Blass, eds., pp. 147–163. New York: Marcel Dekker, Inc., 1992.

Rosenberg, G. S., et al. "Pharmacologic Treatment of Alzheimer's Disease: An Overview." In *Alzheimer's Disease: The Standard Reference*, B. Reisberg, ed., pp. 329–339. New York: The Free Press, 1983.

Roses, A. "The Metabolism of Apolipoprotein E and the Alzheimer's Diseases." In *Alzheimer's Disease: Cause(s), Diagnosis, Treatment and Care*, Z. Khachaturian and T. Radebaugh, eds., pp. 207–216. New York: CRC Press, Inc., 1996.

Roses, A., et al. "Clinical Application of Apolipoprotein E Genotyping to Alzheimer's Disease." *Lancet*, 343(1994):1564–1565.

St. George-Hyslop, P. H., et al. "The Genetic Defect Causing Familial Alzheimer's Disease Maps on Chromosome 2 L." *Science*, 235(1987):885–889.

Sano, M., et al. "A Controlled Trial of Selegiline, Alpha-Tocoperol, or Both as Treatment for Alzheimer's Disease." *New England Journal of Medicine*, 336(1997):1216–1222.

Schneck, M. K. "Nootropics." In *Alzheimer's Disease: The Standard Reference*, B. Reisberg, ed., pp. 362–368. New York: The Free Press, 1983.

Schulz, R., and Williamson, G. M. "A Two Year Longitudinal Study of Depression Among Alzheimer's Caregivers." *Psychology and Aging*, 6(1991):569–578.

Schulz, R., et al. "Psychiatric and Physical Morbidity Effects of Dementia Caregiving: Prevalence, Correlates, and Causes." *The Gerontologist*, 35(1995):771–791.

Selkoe, D. J., et al. "Conservation of Brain Amyloid Proteins in Aged Mammals and Humans with Alzheimer's Disease." *Science*, 235(1987):873–877.

Selye, Hans. *Stress without Distress.* New York: Dutton, 1974.

Semple, S. "Conflict in Alzheimer's Caregiving Families: Its Dimensions and Consequences." *The Gerontologist*, 32(1992):648–655.

Shihabuddin, L., and Davis, K. "Treatment of Alzheimer's Disease." In *Alzheimer's Disease: Cause(s), Diagnosis, Treatment and Care*, Z. Khachaturian and T. Radebaugh, eds., pp. 257–274. New York: CRC Press, Inc., 1996.

Shomaker, D. "Problematic Behavior and the Alzheimer's Patient: Retrospection as a Method of Understanding and Counseling." *Gerontologist*, 27(1987):370–375.

Shore, P., and Wyatt, R. J. "Aluminum and Alzheimer's Disease." *Journal of Nervous Mental Disease*, 171(1983):353–558.

Shua-Haim, J. R., and Ross, J. S. "Current and the Near Future Medications for Alzheimer's Disease: What can we expect from them?" *American Journal of Alzheimer's Disease*, 14(September/October 1999):294–307.

Siegler, I., and Hyer, L. "Common Crises in the Family Life of Older Persons." In *A Family Approach to Health Care of the Elderly*, D. Blazer and I. Siegler, eds., pp. 33–50. Menlo Park, CA: Addison-Wesley, 1984.

Simpkins, J., et al. "The Potential Role for Estrogen Replacement Therapy in Treatment of the Cognitive Decline and Neurodegeneration Associated with Alzheimer's Disease." *Neurobiology of Aging*, 15(1994):S195–S197.

Sitaram, N., and Weingartner, H. "Cholinergic Mechanisms in Human Memory." In *Alzheimer's Disease: Early Recognition of Potentially Reversible Deficits*, A. I. M. Glen and L. J. Whalley, eds., pp. 159–162. London and New York: Churchill Livingstone, 1979.

Sitaram, N., et al. "Combination Treatment of Alzheimer's Dementia." In *Alzheimer's Disease: The Standard Reference*, B. Reisberg, ed., pp. 355–361. New York: The Free Press, 1983.

Skaff, M., and Pearlin, L. "Caregiving: Role Engulfment and the Loss of Self." *The Gerontologist*, 32(1992):656–664.

Smith, C. M., et al. "Effects of Cholinergic Drugs on Memory in Alzheimer's Disease." In *Alzheimer's Disease: Early Recognition of Potentially Reversible Deficits*, A. I. M. Glen and L. J. Whalley, eds., pp. 148–153. London and New York: Churchill Livingstone, 1979.

Stearn, R., and Davis, K. "Research in Treating Cognitive Impairment in Alzheimer's Disease." In *The Dementias: Diagnosis, Management, and Research*, 2nd ed., M. Weiner, ed., pp. 331–353. Washington, D.C.: American Psychiatric Press, Inc., 1996.

Steffen, A., Futterman, A., and Gallager-Thompson, D. "Depressed Caregivers: Comparative Outcome of Two Interventions." *Clinical Gerontologist*, 19(1998):3–15.

Stephenson, J. "Researchers Find Evidence of a New Gene for Late-Onset Alzheimer's Disease." *Journal of the American Medical Association*, 277(1997):775.

Stewart, W. "Risk of Alzheimer's Disease and Duration of NSAID Use." *Neurology*, 48(1997):626–632.

Strauss, A. L., et al. *Chronic Illness and the Quality of Life.* St. Louis: C. V. Mosby, 1984.

Summers, W. K., Viesselman, J. O., Marsh, G. M., and Candelora, K. "Use of THA in Treatment of Alzheimer-Like Dementia: Pilot Study in 12 Patients." *Biological Psychiatry*, 16(1981):145–153.

Summers, W.K., et al. "Oral Tetrahydroaminoacridine in Long-Term Treatment of Senile Dementia." *New England Journal of Medicine*, 315(1986):1242–1245.

Tagliavini, F, and Pilleri, G. "Neuronal Counts in Basal Nucleus of Meynert in Alzheimer's Disease." *The Lancet* (Feb. 26, 1983):469–470.

Tamminga, N. L., et al. "Alzheimer's Disease: Low Cerebral Somatostatin Levels Correlate with Impaired Cognitive Function and Cortical Metabolism." *Neurology,* 37(1987):161–165.

Tang, M. X., et al. "Effect of Estrogen During Menopause on Risk and Age at Onset in Alzheimer's Disease." *The Lancet,* 348(1996):429–432.

Terri, L. "Behavioral Treatment of Depression in Patients with Dementia." *Alzheimer Disease Association of Disorders,* 8(1994):66–74.

Terri, L., and Gallagher-Thompson, D. "Cognitive-Behavioral Interventions for Treatment of Depression in Alzheimer's Patients." *Gerontologist,* 31(1991):413–416.

Teusink, J. P., and Mahler, S. "Helping Families Cope with Alzheimer's Disease." *Hospital and Community Psychiatry,* 35(1984):152–156.

Thal, L., and Fuld, P. "Memory Enhancement with Oral Physostigmine in Alzheimer's Disease." *New England Journal of Medicine,* 308(1983):720.

Thienhaus, O. J., et al. "Biologic Markers in Alzheimer's Disease." *Journal of the American Geriatric Society,* 33(1985):715–726.

Thompson, E. H., et al. "Social Support and Caregiving Burden in Family Caregivers of Frail Elders." *Journal of Gerontology: Social Sciences,* 48(1993):S245–S254.

Visser, P. J., et al. "Distinction Between Preclinical Alzheimer's Disease and Depression." *Journal of the American Geriatric Society,* 48(May 2000):467–605.

Vitaliano, P., Young, H. M., and Russo, J. "Burden: A Review of Measures Used Among Caregivers of Individuals with Dementia." *The Gerontologist,* 31(1991):67–75.

Volicer, L., et al. "Serotoninergic System in Dementia of the Alzheimer Type." *Archives of Neurology,* 42(Dec. 85):1158–1161.

Weiner, M. "Introduction." In *The Dementias: Diagnosis, Management, and Research,* 2nd ed., M. Weiner, ed., pp. xix–xxiii. Washington, DC: American Psychiatric Press, Inc. 1996.

Weiner, M., and Gray, K. "Differential Diagnosis." In *The Dementias: Diagnosis, Management, and Research,* 2nd ed., M. Weiner, ed., pp. 101–138. Washington, DC: American Psychiatric Press, Inc. 1996.

White, L., et al. "Prevalence of Dementia in Older Japanese-American Men in Hawaii: The Honolulu–Asia Aging Study." *Journal of the American Medical Association,* 276(1996):955–960.

Williamson, G., and Schulz, R. "Coping with Specific Stressors in Alzheimer's Disease Caregiving." *The Gerontologist,* 33(1993):747–755.

Winblad, B., et al. "Biogenic Amines in Brains of Patients with Alzheimer's Disease." In *Alzheimer's Disease: A Report of Progress in Research* (Aging, Vol. 19), S. Corkin et al., eds., pp. 25–34. New York: Raven Press, 1982.

Wisniewski, H. M. "Possible Viral Etiology of Neurofibrillary Tangles, Changes, and Neuritic Plaques." In *Alzheimer's Disease: Senile Dementia and Related Disorders* (Aging, Vol. 7), R. Katzman et al., eds., pp. 555–558. New York: Raven Press, 1978.

Wisniewski, H. M. "Neuritic (Senile) and Amyloid Plaques." In *Alzheimer's Disease: The Standard Reference,* B. Reisberg, ed., pp. 57–61. New York: The Free Press, 1983.

Index

Page references followed by italic *t* indicate material in tables.